CLINICAL
DIABETES

AN ILLUSTRATED TEXT

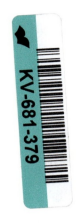

Details are available of a **Slide Atlas of Clinical Diabetes** based on the contents of this book. In the slide atlas format, the material is split into volumes, each of which is presented in a binder together with numbered 35mm slides of each illustration. Each slide atlas volume also contains a list of abbreviated slide captions for easy reference when using the slides. Further information can be obtained from:

Gower Medical Publishing
Middlesex House
34–42 Cleveland Street
London W1P 5FB

Gower Medical Publishing
101 5th Avenue
New York NY 10003
U.S.A.

CLINICAL DIABETES

AN ILLUSTRATED TEXT

Editors:

G Michael Besser MD DSc FRCP
Professor of Endocrinology
Physician in Charge
Department of Endocrinology
St. Bartholomew's Hospital
London, UK

H Jonathan Bodansky MD MRCP
Senior Registrar
The General Infirmary and
    St. James's University Hospital
Leeds, UK

Andrew G Cudworth MD PhD FRCP
Late Professor of Human Metabolism
Consultant Physician
Department of Diabetes and Immunogenetics
St. Bartholomew's Hospital
London, UK

Foreword by:
Arthur H Rubenstein MD
Professor and Chairman
Department of Medicine
The University of Chicago
Chicago
Illinois, USA

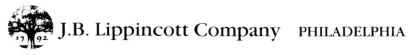 J.B. Lippincott Company PHILADELPHIA

Gower Medical Publishing LONDON • NEW YORK

Distributed in USA and Canada by:
J.B. Lippincott Company
East Washington Square
Philadelphia, PA 19105
USA

Distributed in UK and Continental Europe by:
Harper & Row Ltd
Middlesex House
34–42 Cleveland Street
London W1P 5FB, UK

Distributed in Australia and New Zealand by:
Harper & Row (Australasia) Pty Ltd
PO Box 226
Artarmon, NSW 2064
Australia

Distributed in Southeast Asia, Hong Kong, India and Pakistan by:
Harper & Row Publishers (Asia) Pte Ltd
37 Jalan Pemimpin 02–01
Singapore 2057

Distributed in Japan by:
Igaku Shoin Ltd
Tokyo International
PO Box 5063
Tokyo, Japan

Distributed in Philippines/Guam, Middle East, Latin America and Africa by:
Harper & Row International
10 East 53rd Street
New York, NY 10022
USA

British Library Cataloguing in Publication Data:

Clinical Diabetes.
 1. Man. Diabetes
 I. Besser, G. Michael II. Bodansky,
 H. Jonathan III. Cudworth, Andrew G.
 616.4'62

ISBN 0-397-44565-2 (Lippincott/Gower)

Library of Congress Catalog Card Number: 88-80406

Originated in Hong Kong by Bright Arts (HK) Ltd.
Typeset in London by TNR Productions Ltd.
Text set in Plantin Light; captions set in Helvetica.
Reprinted in Singapore in 1990 by Imago Productions (FE)
Pte Ltd.

Project Editor: David Goodfellow

Design: Ian Spick
Nigel Wright

Illustration: Nigel Wright
Marion Tasker
Michael Rabess
Mark Willey

For Rachel

Foreword

It is always appealing to look at beautiful pictures illustrating aspects of science or medicine. At the same time, one does not usually expect to derive significant information from illustrations, which are often used as an adjunct to a detailed text in scientific publications. In fact, the reason for choosing one particular graph or photomicrograph rather than another to illustrate a particular fact amongst many in a page or two of narrative is not always clear. Often the choice seems to be arbitrary and may depend upon its ready availability to the author, rather than an objective decision carefully designed to enhance the reader's understanding of the subject matter.

Clinical Diabetes: An Illustrated Text differs in several ways from the above description. The illustrations form the central focus of the book and the text is brief and mainly organized to provide a link between the series of pictures in each chapter. Thus the educational impact of the book depends almost entirely upon the subject matter and quality of the illustrations. In this regard the publication is most successful. The graphs and tables are interesting in that they contain a great deal of information; yet they are simple and clear. The photomicrographs have been carefully chosen and those that are reproduced in colour are particularly striking. The schematic illustrations are original and innovative and in many instances provide valuable insights into complicated subjects. The excellence of the book is not surprising because the editors have assembled an outstanding group of contributors. Furthermore, despite the many co-authors, the chapters fit well together and each topic is handled in a uniform manner with minimal overlap. This approach also permits easy reading and adds to the enjoyment of the book.

The publication of a book on diabetes at this time is particularly opportune, because of the recent explosion of knowledge in this field. These new findings are well represented and include up-to-date descriptions of the structure, biosynthesis and action of insulin; the aetiology and pathophysiology of diabetes; and the treatment and complications of this disorder. Thus, although the book will be most valuable for students, house officers and post-graduates in training, it will also appeal to the more sophisticated reader. I would not be surprised if there are many requests from teachers for permission to use selected illustrations in their lectures.

This book is a companion volume to the recently published *Clinical Endocrinology: An Illustrated Text*. The chapter (No. 18) entitled *Hypoglycaemia and Insulinomas* has direct relevance to the material covered in this book on diabetes and readers will benefit from consulting it. I would also guess that they will enjoy this experience so much that they will want to have both texts readily available for their personal use.

AHR

Preface

The understanding of the pathogenesis and metabolic features of diabetes mellitus and its complications has made dramatic advances over the last fifteen years. This understanding has coincided with the advent of new and highly purified insulins and a wider variety of oral hypoglycaemic drugs. As a result, basic and applied research in physiology, biochemistry, virology, immunology, epidemiology and genetics has allowed clinical research workers to bring to the patient and those in the patients' environment, improved management and hope for a better life. While the immediate and acute care has improved, much remains to be done; glimpses of highly significant advances may be caught, even in the areas of the long-term complications which make the existence of many diabetic patients so wretched.

The hope of bringing together the new concepts and developments was behind the planning of this textbook, originally designed with the late Professor Andrew Cudworth, our brilliant colleague and friend, who tragically died so young. He did so much for diabetes, but had many more important contributions to make. The book is highly illustrated using new techniques developed by the publishers. It forms a pair with its sister book, *Clinical Endocrinology*, published in 1987. It is hoped that the two so complement each other that the whole field of endocrinology is integrated and covered by them. The text is aimed widely at the senior student, the postgraduate and the specialist. This book, like its sister, was initially designed as a slide atlas and the principal messages are conveyed in the illustrations, expanded and explained by the text. The starting point of each section is a description of the relevant physiological and biochemical disturbance integrated with the presentation of the altered histopathology, so that clinical features and their management can then be built on to this fundamental knowledge. Causative factors are considered in detail since it is by their study that one might hope to move towards prevention and cure. Dietary factors in management and their interaction with drug therapy have been given an important place. Throughout, a pragmatic and practical, but disciplined approach to the physical and emotional management of the patient's condition has been considered paramount.

Many colleagues have advised and contributed to this work, and our great appreciation and thanks go to them for making it possible, and for their tolerance. Special appreciation is due to David Goodfellow, the publisher's Project Editor, for his invaluable help and expert attention to the book and to Ian Spick, Nigel Wright and Marion Tasker for the design and illustrations which feature so splendidly. The long-suffering staff of Gower Medical Publishing have once again proved talented and delightful colleagues, and we extend our sincere thanks to them.

GMB
JB

Contributors

Jonathan J Benn MA MB BChir MRCP
Lecturer in Medicine, Department of Medicine, St. Thomas's Hospital Medical School, London, UK

Peter H Bennett BSc MB ChB FRCP FFCM
Chief, Epidemiology and Clinical Research Branch, National Institutes of Health, National Institute of Diabetes and Digestive and Kidney Diseases, Phoenix, Arizona, USA

Gian Franco Bottazzo MD MRCP MRCPath
Reader in Clinical Immunology, Department of Immunology, University College and Middlesex School of Medicine, London, UK

Keith D Buchanan MD PhD FRCP
Professor of Metabolic Medicine, Wellcome Research Laboratories, Department of Medicine, The Queen's University of Belfast, Belfast, UK

Eleanor J Dodson BA
Research Fellow, Department of Chemistry, University of York, York, UK

Guy G Dodson BSc MSc PhD
Professor of Biochemistry, Department of Chemistry, University of York, York, UK

M Ivo Drury MD PRCPI FRCOG DSc(Hon) FACP(Hon)
Professor of Therapeutics, University College Dublin; Physician in Charge, Diabetes Unit, Mater Misericordiae Hospital; and Visiting Consultant, National Maternity, Coombe Lying-In and Rotunda Hospitals, Dublin, Eire

Giovanni Federico MD
Department of Paediatrics, University of Pisa, Pisa, Italy

Edwin AM Gale MB FRCP
Senior Lecturer in Medicine, Department of Diabetes and Immunogenetics, St. Bartholomew's Hospital, London, UK

D Robert Gamble MB DipBact FRCPath
Formerly Director, Public Health Laboratory, West Park Hospital, Epsom, UK

Willy Gepts MD PhD
Professor and Head of the Department of Pathology, Free University of Brussels, Brussels, Belgium

Andrew N Gorsuch MA BM BCh MRCP
Senior Registrar, Department of Diabetes and Endocrinology, University College Hospital, London, UK

Anasuya Grenfell MA MRCP
Registrar in Nephrology, St. Phillip's Hospital, London, UK

David R Hadden MD FRCPEd
Consultant Physician, Sir George E Clark Metabolic Unit, Royal Victoria Hospital, Belfast, UK

Simon L Howell DSc
Professor of Endocrine Physiology, Department of Physiology, King's College, London, UK

Rod E Hubbard BA DPhil
Lecturer in Chemistry and Computing, Department of Chemistry, University of York, York, UK

Peter A in't Veld
Research Associate, Department of Pathology, Free University of Brussels, Brussels, Belgium

John T Ireland MD MB ChB FRCPEd
Late Consultant Physician in Medicine and Diabetes, Southern General Hospital, Glasgow, UK

R John Jarrett MD MB BChir FFCM
Professor of Clinical Epidemiology, Division of Community Medicine, United Medical and Dental Schools of Guy's and St. Thomas's Hospitals (Guy's Campus), London, UK

Colin F Johnston PhD
Lecturer in Metabolic Medicine, Wellcome Research Laboratories, Department of Medicine, The Queen's University of Belfast, Belfast, UK

Richard H Jones MA MB BChir FRCP
Senior Lecturer in Medicine, United Medical and Dental Schools of Guy's and St. Thomas's Hospitals (St. Thomas's Campus), London, and Honorary Consultant Endocrinologist, Medway Health Authority, Gillingham, UK

Harry Keen MD FRCP
Professor of Human Metabolism, Unit for Metabolic Medicine, United Medical and Dental Schools of Guy's and St. Thomas's Hospitals (Guy's Campus), London, UK

Eva M Kohner MD FRCP
Consultant Physician and Honorary Senior Lecturer,
Department of Medicine, Royal Postgraduate Medical School,
Hammersmith Hospital, London, UK

Antony B Kurtz PhD FRCP
Thorn Institute of Clinical Sciences, University College and
Middlesex School of Medicine, London, UK

R David G Leslie MD MRCP
Honorary Consultant Physician, Diabetic Department, King's
College Hospital, London, UK

Italo Manocchio DVM
Department of Animal Pathology, University of Perugia,
Perugia, Italy

Dowling D Munro MD FRCP
Consultant Dermatologist, Dermatology Department,
St. Bartholomew's Hospital, London, UK

Mairead MT O'Hare PhD
Research Fellow, Wellcome Research Laboratories,
Department of Medicine, The Queen's University of Belfast,
Belfast, UK

Takashi Onodera PhD
Laboratory of Viral Immunology, National Institute of Animal
Health, Yatabe, Ibaraki, Japan

Donald WM Pearson BSc MB ChB MRCP
Consultant Physician with Special Interest in Diabetes,
Diabetic Clinic, Aberdeen Teaching Hospital, Aberdeen, UK

John C Pickup MA BM BCh DPhil MRCPath
Reader in Chemical Pathology, Division of Chemical
Pathology, United Medical and Dental Schools of Guy's and
St. Thomas's Hospitals (Guy's Campus), London, UK

David A Pyke MD FRCP
Formerly Physician in Charge, Diabetic Department, King's
College Hospital, London, UK

Alan Rees MD MRCP
Lecturer in Medicine, University of Wales, Cardiff, UK

Colin D Reynolds BA PhD MSc
Reader in Biophysics, Department of Physics (Structural
Biophysics Unit), Liverpool Polytechnic, Liverpool, UK

Martin O Savage MA MD FRCP
Consultant Paediatric Endocrinologist, St. Bartholomew's
Hospital, London and Consultant Paediatrician, Queen
Elizabeth Hospital for Children, London, UK

Christopher Shaw PhD
Research Officer, Wellcome Research Laboratories,
Department of Medicine, The Queen's University of Belfast,
Belfast, UK

Kate M Spencer MD MRCP
Senior Registrar, Department of Medicine, Royal Hallamshire
Hospital, Sheffield, UK

John M Stowers MA MB BChir MD FRCP FRCOG
Emeritus Professor of Diabetes and Endocrinology, University
of Aberdeen and Aberdeen Royal Infirmary, Aberdeen, UK

Serge Ng Tang Fui MSc MD MRCP
The Royal Southern Memorial Hospital, Victoria, Australia

Robert B Tattersall MD FRCP
Consultant Physician, Department of Medicine, University
Hospital, Nottingham, UK

Dai JB Thomas MD MRCP
Consultant Physician, Mount Vernon Hospital, Northwood, UK

Antonio Toniolo MD
Institute of Microbiology and Virology, University of Sassari,
Sassari, Italy

John D Ward BSc MD FRCP
Consultant Physician, Royal Hallamshire Hospital,
Sheffield, UK

Acknowledgements

1 Anatomy and Physiology of the Pancreatic Islets
The patients with glucagonoma syndrome (Figs 1.39 and 1.40) were studied in conjunction with Dr Janet M. Marks, Consultant Dermatologist, Royal Victoria Infirmary, Newcastle-upon-Tyne and Dr Fiona M. Stevens, Lecturer in Medicine, The University of Galway.

4 Insulin Molecular Structure and Molecular Behaviour
We are grateful to many for help and discussion in trying to understand the problems of insulin structure. We are particularly grateful to Dorothy Hodgkin and Graham Bentley for their insights.

5 Insulin Action and Metabolism
I am grateful to many colleagues in four continents for their willingness to share ideas, to Bill Deery and Fernando Ribeiro-Neto for guidance on the mechanisms of transmembrane signalling and particularly to Shelley Dearing and Mary-Ann Farabee for their skill and tolerance in the preparation of the manuscript.

6 Diagnostic Criteria, Classification and Presentation of Diabetes
We thank Dr Peter Bennett for Fig. 4.9, Drs R. Cerio and D.M. McDonald for Fig. 4.21, Colin Clements for Fig. 4.23 and Dr John Reidy for Figs 4.25 and 4.26.

9 Aetiology and Pathogenesis of Type I Diabetes: Immunology
We would like to thank the numerous colleagues and friends who contributed tremendously throughout the years to the development of our subject and with whom it was a pleasure to work.

10 Aetiology and Pathogenesis of Type I Diabetes: Viruses
We thank Dr A.L. Notkins for introducing us to this area of research and for his continuous encouragement and support.

We are very obliged to Dr A.B. Jenson for providing histopathology photographs of human cases. We are also grateful to Drs J.W. Yoon, M.J. Dobersen, G.F. Bottazzo, C. Betterle, B. Prabhakar, G. Saggese, G. Federspil, S. Mariotti, A. Corallini, E. Bottone and G. Falcone for illuminating discussions and collaboration. This work has been supported by the Italian Ministry of Education (funds 40% and 60%) and by Novo Farmaceutici Italia through the courtesy of Dr M. Iavicoli.

13 Type II Diabetes: Pathophysiology
We are grateful to many clinical and scientific colleagues for discussions over the years and to Lis Lawrence for her dedication to the word-processor.

19 Diabetes and Surgery
I would like to thank the anaesthetists and surgeons at Basingstoke District Hospital and St. Bartholomew's Hospital, London for allowing me to study their patients.

20 Management of Diabetes in Pregnancy
Thank you to Drs J.M. Stronge and M.E. Foley, National Maternity Hospital, Dublin; Drs N. O'Brien and W. Gorman, Department of Paediatrics, National Maternity Hospital, Dublin; Dr A.T. Greene, Coombe Lying-In Hospital, Dublin; Dr E.W. Lillie, Rotunda Hospital, Dublin; and Dr T. Matthews, Department of Paediatrics, Rotunda Hospital, Dublin.

23 Diabetic Retinopathy
Thank you to Mr John Arnold and Mr Steve Aldington for photographic services.

25 Diabetic Nephropathy
Thank you to Dr G.C. Viberti for making some of his work available and to Dr D.J. Watkins for his advice and criticism.

Contents

1 Anatomy and Physiology of the Pancreatic Islets

Colin F Johnston PhD ● **Christopher Shaw** PhD
Mairead MT O'Hare PhD ● **Keith D Buchanan** MD PhD FRCP

ANATOMY

The pancreas is composed of both exocrine and endocrine elements. The exocrine pancreas consists of numerous lobular acini and ducts. These are held together by connective tissue and are covered by a delicate capsule. The function of the exocrine element is to synthesize, store and secrete digestive enzymes.

Embedded in the sea of exocrine tissues are the islets of Langerhans, originally described in 1869 by Paul Langerhans. These constitute the endocrine element of the pancreas and represent approximately one per cent of the pancreatic mass. The normal adult human pancreas has been estimated to possess 10^5–2×10^6 islets, each containing from a few hundred to several thousand endocrine cells.

Histochemistry

Islets are distinguished from the exocrine parenchyma by their poor affinity for haematoxylin and eosin (H and E) staining (Fig. 1.1). Their cells possess relatively clear cytoplasm. This feature is common to many endocrine cells in other organs and was first described by Feyrter in 1938. The islet is surrounded by a fine capillary network and is encapsulated in collagen.

Several histochemical techniques have superseded haematoxylin and eosin staining by their ability to differentiate between two of the islet cell types. B cells (insulin synthesizing) are demonstrated by Gomori's aldehyde fuchsin technique (Fig. 1.2) and A cells (glucagon synthesizing) by Grimelius' silver technique (Fig. 1.3). B cells constitute the core of the islet and are the most abundant cell type, making up sixty to seventy per cent by volume of the islet. A cells are fewer in number (10–20%) and are distributed either around the islet's periphery or ramify throughout its core.

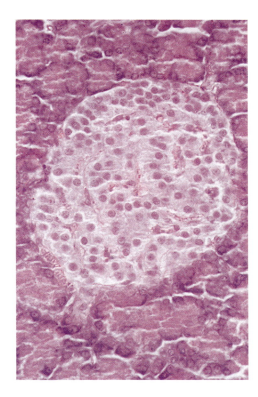

Fig. 1.1 Section of a normal human pancreas showing an islet of Langerhans surrounded by exocrine parenchyma. Islets of Langerhans have a poor affinity for H and E, the stain used here.

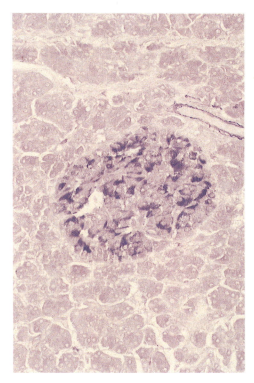

Fig. 1.2 Gomori's aldehyde fuchsin stain of an islet showing differential dark staining of B cells.

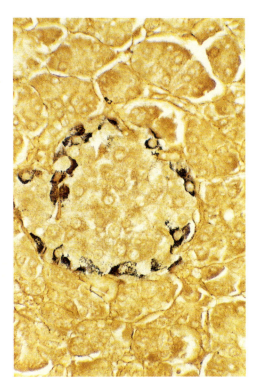

Fig. 1.3 Islet A cells stained darkly with Grimelius' silver.

Immunohistochemistry

Simple histochemistry does not detect a given peptide hormone within an islet cell and fails to detect the presence of cell types other than the A and B cells.

Immunohistochemistry, which utilizes a specific antibody–antigen reaction to localize a given cellular component, is capable of distinguishing the various peptide hormone components contained within different islet cell types. Immunofluorescence, introduced by Coons in 1956, employs a fluorescent second antibody while immunoperoxidase, developed by Sternberger in 1970, uses an enzyme-linked second antibody to localize sites of primary antibody–antigen reactions. The localization of insulin by immunofluorescence is demonstrated in Fig. 1.4.

Glucagon-immunoreactive cells (A cells), somatostatin-immunoreactive cells (D cells) and pancreatic polypeptide-immunoreactive cells (PP cells) can be revealed by the immunoperoxidase technique (Figs 1.5 to 1.7). The glucagon-immunoreactive cells are the commonest non insulin-secreting islet cell type. Somatostatin-immunoreactive cells are much less frequent and make up only five to ten per cent by volume of the islet; they are randomly distributed and their elongated processes appear to touch the other islet cells. This observation suggests that they may have a possible paracrine function. Although PP cells are restricted to a peripheral distribution in the islet, occasional PP-immunoreactive cells occur scattered within the exocrine parenchyma. They make up ten to twenty per cent of the islet.

Electron Microscopy

Prior to secretion from the islet cells, peptide hormones are stored in membrane-bound granules. Under the electron microscope the storage granules of each islet cell type have a distinct appearance (Fig. 1.8). B cell (β) granules have an electron-dense irregular crystalline core with a pronounced electron-lucent halo. A cell (α) granules have a large regular electron-dense core with a small clear halo. D cell (Δ) granules have large, somewhat elliptical, moderately electron-dense, finely granular cores; the granule possesses no halo and the limiting membrane is usually closely applied. PP cells have granules which are smaller than those of B, A or D cells. The granule core is often elliptical and of moderate to high electron density. There is a small clear halo between the core and limiting membrane.

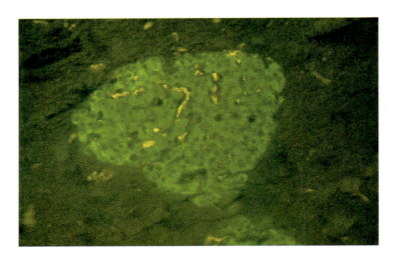

Fig. 1.4 Indirect immunofluorescence localization of insulin in a normal islet. The apple-green fluorescent insulin-immunoreactive cells make up the bulk of the islet.

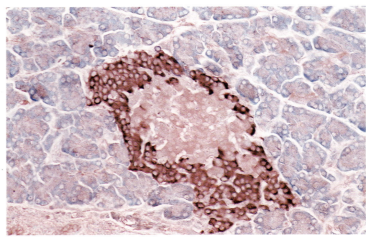

Fig. 1.5 Immunoperoxidase localization of glucagon in a normal islet. The brown reaction product reveals the numerous glucagon-staining A cells lying around the core of unstained B cells.

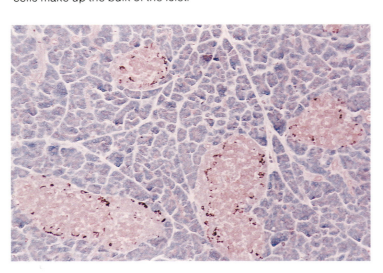

Fig. 1.6 Relatively infrequent somatostatin-immunoreactive cells localized by the immunoperoxidase method in four neighbouring islets from a normal pancreas.

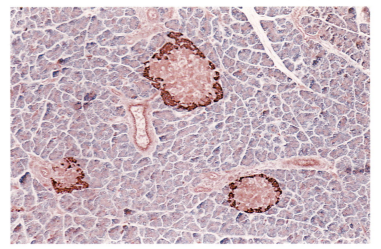

Fig. 1.7 Immunoperoxidase localization of PP- immunoreactive cells which, like those staining for glucagon, occupy a peripheral position within these islets.

DEVELOPMENT

The endocrine component of the pancreas is derived from ductal elements which, in turn, arise from the foregut in the developing embryo. Fig. 1.9 shows the distribution of insulin immuno-reactivity within the pancreas of a twenty-eight-week-old fetus. At this stage of development, B cells occur singly or in small clumps throughout the exocrine parenchyma. There is a great deal of endocrine cell mitotic activity, which is rarely seen in the islets of the adult pancreas. By thirty-two weeks, there are fewer single B cells and more abundant small precursor islets (Fig. 1.10). Exocrine acini are now apparent. Islet size continues to increase and islet cell composition changes towards the pattern seen in the neonatal pancreas. The most striking difference between the pancreas of an early third trimester fetus and that of the neonate is the enormous proliferation of exocrine parenchyma. This is an adaptation which precedes the onset of enteral nutrition.

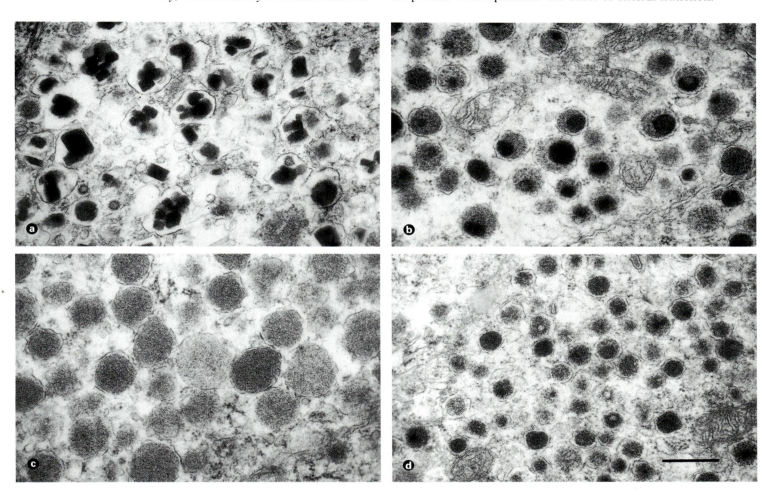

Fig. 1.8 High power electron micrographs of the different islet cell secretory granules:
(a) B cell (β) granules; (b) A cell (α) granules; (c) D cell (Δ) granules;
and (d) PP cell granules. Bar = 0.5μm. By courtesy of Professor W. Gepts.

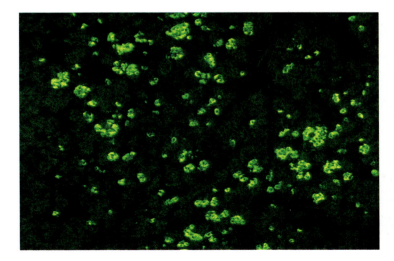

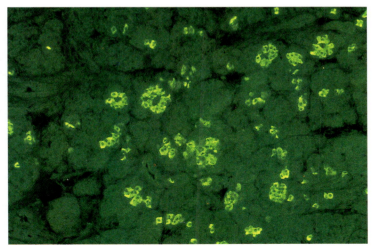

Fig. 1.9 Insulin-immunoreactive cells in the pancreas of a twenty-eight-week-old fetus. B cells occur throughout the exocrine parenchyma.

Fig. 1.10 Insulin-immunoreactive cells in the pancreas of a thirty-two-week-old fetus. There are few single B cells, but small precursor islets are abundant.

1.3

The following account details the chemistry, actions and secretion of glucagon, somatostatin and pancreatic polypeptide. Insulin chemistry and the control of its secretion is discussed in *Chapter 2*.

GLUCAGON
Chemistry
Glucagon is a twenty-nine amino acid polypeptide with a molecular weight of 3485 daltons (Fig. 1.11) which is cleaved from a larger polypeptide precursor molecule called 'proglucagon'. It is synthesized in, and subsequently released from, the A cells of the pancreas. Closely related molecular species of glucagon exist in the gut and are referred to as 'enteroglucagon' or as gut 'glucagon-like immunoreactivity' (GLI). GLI consists of at least three species, however, which include glicentin. This is also produced by the A cells of the islet.

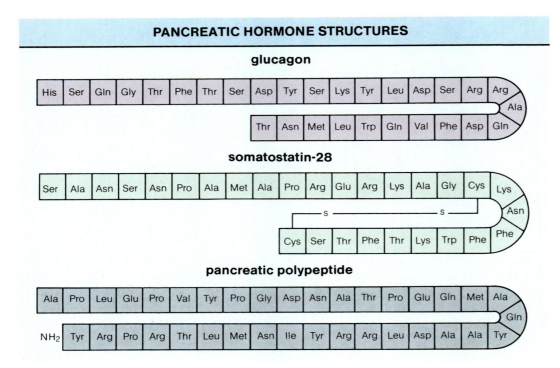

PANCREATIC HORMONE STRUCTURES

Fig. 1.11 Amino acid sequences of human glucagon, somatostatin-28 and pancreatic polypeptide. Somatostatin usually occurs as a cyclic polypeptide, consisting of the carboxyl-terminal fourteen amino acids of somatostatin-28.

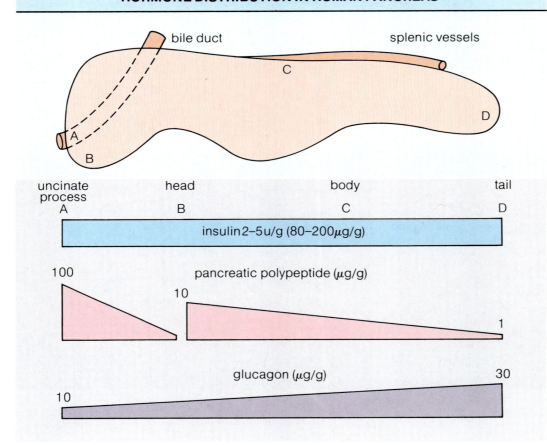

HORMONE DISTRIBUTION IN HUMAN PANCREAS

Fig. 1.12 Distribution of insulin, glucagon and pancreatic polypeptide within the pancreas. The regions A–D indicate sampling points.

Actions

Glucagon and PP are regionally distributed within the pancreas as a whole, unlike insulin and somatostatin. Glucagon is present in highest concentrations in the tail region, whereas PP is predominantly located in the head, in particular in the region corresponding to the uncinate process (Fig. 1.12).

Glucagon's most important actions are glycogenolysis and gluconeogenesis (Fig. 1.13). The hepatic glycogenolytic action is mediated via stimulation of adenylate cyclase activity. Other physiological actions include stimulation of insulin release, lipolysis and ketogenesis. A positive inotropic effect on the heart is seen at pharmacological levels. In the gastrointestinal tract, glucagon inhibits acid secretion and relaxes the gut, although these may also be solely pharmacological effects.

Metabolism

Glucagon has a half-life of a few minutes in the circulation and is rapidly degraded by many tissues, particularly the liver. There are marked differences between portal and peripheral circulating levels.

Regulation of Secretion

A multiplicity of factors control glucagon secretion (Fig. 1.14). Hyperglycaemia inhibits (Fig. 1.15), whereas hypoglycaemia

ACTIONS OF GLUCAGON	
physiological	**pharmacological**
glycogenolysis	positive inotropic effect on the heart
gluconeogenesis	
	reduces gastric acid secretion
lipolysis	
	reduces intestinal motility
ketogenesis	
insulin secretion	

Fig. 1.13 Actions of glucagon.

FACTORS ALTERING GLUCAGON SECRETION	
stimulators	**inhibitors**
amino acids	glucose
gut hormones	somatostatin
hypoglycaemia	insulin
exercise	free fatty acids (FFA)
starvation	α-adrenergic stimulators
stress	
vagal stimulation	
β-adrenergic stimulators	
phosphodiesterase inhibitors	

Fig. 1.14 Factors affecting glucagon secretion.

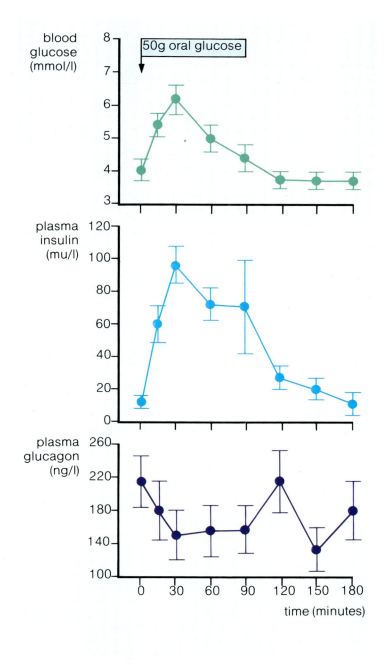

Fig. 1.15 Blood glucose and plasma insulin and glucagon responses to 50g oral glucose in normal human subjects. There is a statistically significant suppression of glucagon at 30 and 60 minutes (mean ± SEM).

stimulates glucagon secretion (Figs 1.16 and 1.17). Amino acids, in particular alanine and arginine (Fig. 1.18), stimulate glucagon release. Indeed, arginine, given as an intravenous infusion, is used as a stimulus to assess glucagon release. An oral protein meal also stimulates glucagon secretion (Fig. 1.19). The vagus nerve exerts a powerful stimulating action. There is an entero–glucagon axis, with cholecystokinin (CCK) in particular stimulating its secretion (Fig. 1.20). Glucagon is released through starvation (Fig. 1.21), exercise and during infections.

SOMATOSTATIN
Chemistry
Somatostatin is a cyclic, fourteen amino acid polypeptide with a molecular weight of 1640 daltons. Larger molecular species, particularly somatostatin-28, have also been characterized and are secreted (see Fig. 1.11). The peptide has been localized throughout the central nervous system, gut and in the D cells.

Actions
All actions of somatostatin are inhibitory (Fig. 1.22). It suppresses the release of many hormones and also exocrine secretions. Insulin, glucagon and pancreatic polypeptide release are sup-

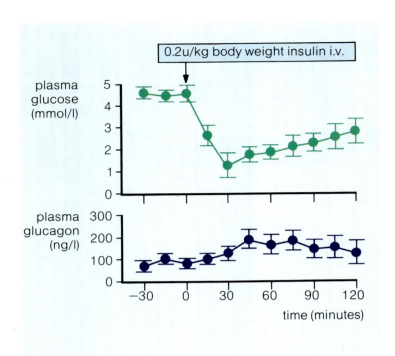

Fig. 1.16 Insulin-induced hypoglycaemia (0.2 units of insulin per kg body weight) in six healthy (mean ± SEM) human subjects causes a prompt glucagon response.

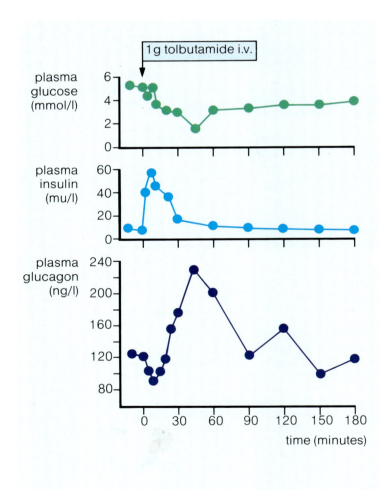

Fig. 1.17 Rapid rise of plasma glucagon demonstrated in a normal human volunteer following 1g tolbutamide intravenously. Plasma insulin rises and glucose falls.

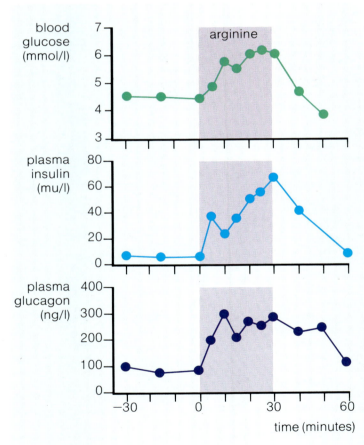

Fig. 1.18 Rapid and sustained glucagon response to intravenous infusion over 30 minutes of 30g L-arginine monochloride. Each point is the mean of seventeen normal human subjects.

pressed. Somatostatin may control pancreatic endocrine function by a paracrine route. It is not known which of these actions are physiologically relevant as many need pharmacological concentrations for their effects.

Release

Somatostatin is released in low concentrations into the circulation following several oral stimuli, particularly the ingestion of fat and protein.

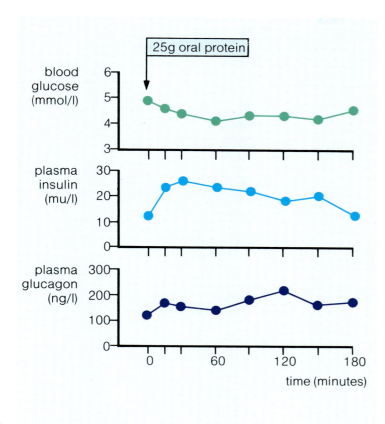

Fig. 1.19 Blood glucose, plasma insulin and glucagon responses to 25g oral protein in twelve normal human subjects. There is a significant increase in pancreatic glucagon at 30, 90, 120, 150 and 180 minutes.

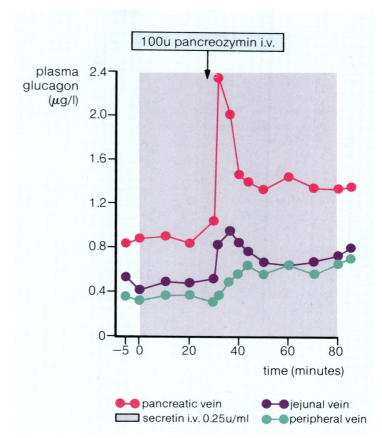

pancreatic vein · jejunal vein
secretin i.v. 0.25u/ml · peripheral vein

Fig. 1.20 Glucagon responses in six dogs to a secretin/ pancreozymin (CCK) challenge. The greater response in the pancreatic vein compared to other sampling sites implies the pancreas is the origin of the stimulated glucagon.

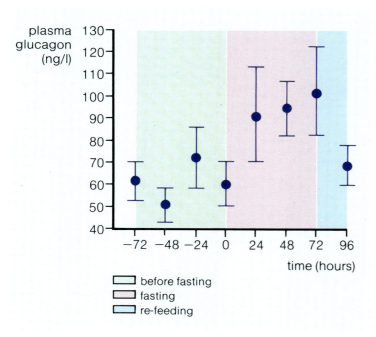

before fasting
fasting
re-feeding

Fig. 1.21 Plasma glucagon elevations during a seventy-two-hour fast in nine healthy human subjects (mean ± SEM).

ACTIONS OF SOMATOSTATIN	
hormonal	**non-hormonal**
inhibition of:	**inhibition of:**
growth hormone	gastric emptying and contraction
thyroid-stimulating hormone (TSH)	pancreatic bicarbonate
insulin	pancreatic enzymes
glucagon	gall bladder contraction
pancreatic poly-peptide (PP)	myoelectric complexes
gastrin	coeliac blood flow
secretin	xylose absorption
gastric inhibitory polypeptide (GIP)	gastric acid secretion
motilin	
enteroglucagon	

Fig. 1.22 Principal actions of somatostatin.

PANCREATIC POLYPEPTIDE
Chemistry
Pancreatic polypeptide (PP) contains thirty-six amino acids and has a molecular weight of 4200 daltons (see Fig. 1.11). It is located in distinct endocrine cells in pancreatic islets and acinar tissue. Two structurally related peptides have recently been isolated; one from the gastrointestinal tract, peptide YY (PYY), and the other from the brain, neuropeptide Y (NPY). With PP, these three peptides constitute the PP family of peptides.

Actions
The physiological role of PP is unknown. Preliminary studies have demonstrated that it can inhibit the stimulation of pancreatic and biliary secretions (Fig. 1.23).

Regulation of Secretion
A variety of factors affect PP release (Fig. 1.24). Fasting, circulating concentrations of PP increase significantly with age (Fig. 1.25). Circulating concentrations show a rapid and dramatic increase following the ingestion of food (Fig. 1.26). Protein is the most potent stimulant for PP release, while fat is slightly less effective (Fig. 1.27). A significant increase in circulating PP is also observed after oral glucose (Fig. 1.28), insulin-induced hypoglycaemia or exercise (Fig. 1.29), while intravenous glucose may suppress levels or have no effect depending upon the duration of the infusion.

An entero-PP axis, with vagal and hormonal components, has been postulated to account for the different effects observed between orally and intravenously administered nutrients. Results concerning this have been conflicting but a CCK-like peptide is the likely candidate for the hormonal component of such an axis.

ACTIONS OF PANCREATIC POLYPEPTIDE

inhibits gall bladder contraction

inhibits pancreatic secretion

Fig. 1.23 Actions of pancreatic polypeptide.

FACTORS ALTERING PANCREATIC POLYPEPTIDE SECRETION

stimulators	inhibitors
protein	somatostatin
fat	intravenous glucose
glucose	
gut hormones	
exercise	
insulin-induced hypo-glycaemia	
stress	

Fig. 1.24 Factors altering plasma PP secretion.

Fig. 1.25 Effect of age on circulating plasma PP concentration in normal subjects (mean ± SEM; n=296).

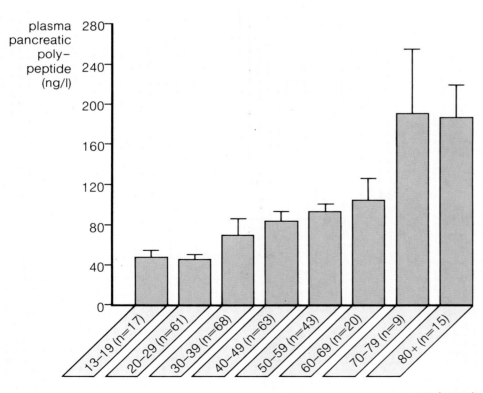

age (years)

PATHOLOGY OF THE PANCREAS

Exocrine Lesions

Lesions of the pancreas can occur in either exocrine or endocrine elements. Primary exocrine lesions often alter the appearance of the endocrine elements. The following two examples of exocrine lesions illustrate both the relative sensitivity of the exocrine tissue and the remarkable resistance of the endocrine tissue to destruction.

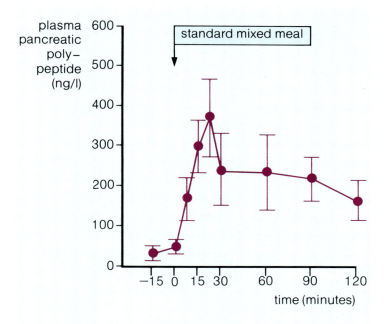

Fig. 1.26 Plasma PP response to a standard mixed meal in twelve subjects (age range 20–68 years). Significant changes in PP concentrations occur at all time intervals following the meal (mean ± SEM).

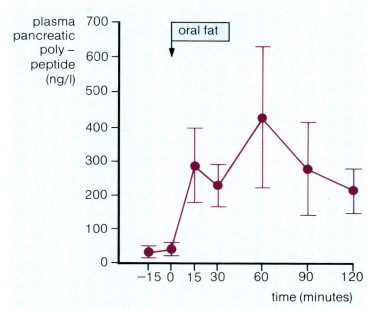

Fig. 1.27 Plasma PP response to oral fat in nine subjects (age range 18–62 years). Significant changes in PP concentrations occur at 15, 30 and 120 minutes (mean ± SEM).

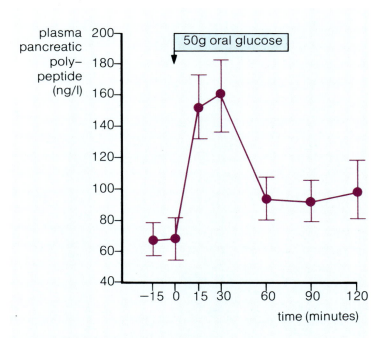

Fig. 1.28 Plasma PP response to 50g oral glucose in sixteen subjects (age range 19–71 years). Significant increases occur at all time intervals following the ingestion of glucose (mean ± SEM).

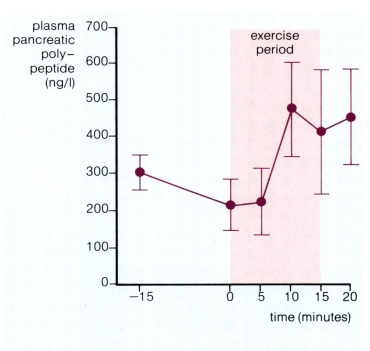

Fig. 1.29 Plasma PP response to a short period of heavy exercise in eight subjects (age range 24–31 years). A significant increase in PP concentration is observed after 10 minutes (mean ± SEM).

Pancreatic ductal occlusion

Occlusion of the pancreatic duct, such as may be caused by the intrusion of a carcinoma, results in generalized acinar atrophy. Fig. 1.30 is a section of the tail of a pancreas from a patient with a large endocrine pancreatic tumour which had caused ductal occlusion.

Cystic fibrosis

Cystic fibrosis, an autosomal dominant disease, with an incidence of one in four thousand live births in the Caucasian population, results in a histological appearance of the pancreas similar to that seen in pancreatic ductal occlusion. In cystic fibrosis, exocrine tissue is progressively replaced by fibrous tissue and fat. The pancreatic islets are largely spared. Fig. 1.31 shows a section of such a pancreas stained to show somatostatin.

Endocrine Lesions

Primary endocrine lesions fall into two broad categories. The first involves islet cell deficiency which is typified by Type I or insulin-dependent diabetes mellitus. The second category involves an excess of islet cells which may be either benign or malignant.

Nesidioblastosis

Nesidioblastosis (Fig. 1.32) is generally associated with hyper-

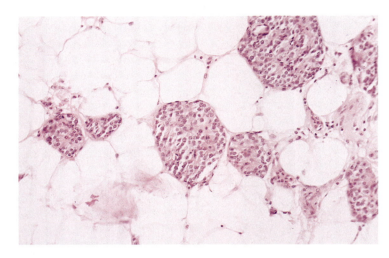

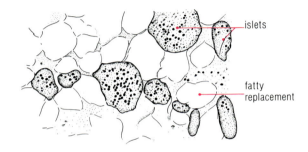

Fig. 1.30 Pancreas from a patient with pancreatic ductal occlusion caused by a large endocrine tumour. The exocrine tissue has atrophied and is replaced with fat. H and E stain.

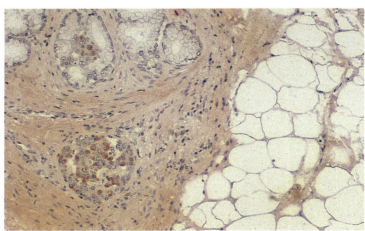

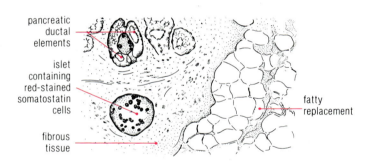

Fig. 1.31 Pancreatic exocrine atrophy in cystic fibrosis. The islet is immunostained for somatostatin. An islet is clearly seen containing a normal quota and pattern of somatostatin-immunoreactive cells. Fibrous tissue and fatty infiltration are evident but there is no normal exocrine tissue.

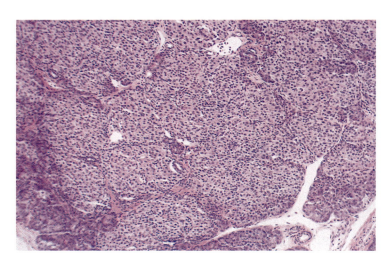

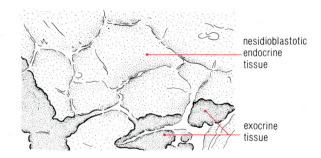

Fig. 1.32 Pancreas from a neonate with nesidioblastosis. There is a massive excess of functional B cells resulting in profound hypoglycaemia. The only effective treatment is either partial pancreatectomy or administration of a long-acting somatostatin analogue. H and E stain.

insulinism resulting from an enormous excess of functional B cells. Islets appear to have been arrested in an early stage of development, are grossly enlarged and are in close association with ductal elements. This condition which occurs in the first few months of life may require eighty to ninety per cent pancreatic resection for cure.

Islet cell hyperplasia

Diffuse islet cell hyperplasia (Fig. 1.33), a similar rare condition to nesidioblastosis, also displays an increase in islet cell mass. However, with this disorder, islets are not arrested in an early stage of development and thus are not associated with ductal elements.

Adenomas

Benign islet cell adenomas are occasionally encountered in adults, particularly in families displaying the multiple endocrine adenomatosis (MEA) Type 1 syndrome. These adenomas may arise from any islet cell type, are frequently multiple and are often concomitant with endocrine tumours of the parathyroid and pituitary glands. Fig. 1.34 shows a small adenoma in a specimen of resected pancreas from such a patient. Fig. 1.35 shows a second microadenoma from the pancreas of the same subject immunostained for insulin.

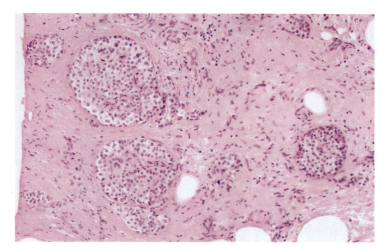

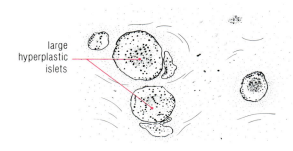

Fig. 1.33 Region of diffuse benign islet cell hyperplasia in a patient with the multiple endocrine neoplasia (MEN) Type 1 syndrome. Additionally, these patients may present with pancreatic tumours which may be either benign or malignant. H and E stain.

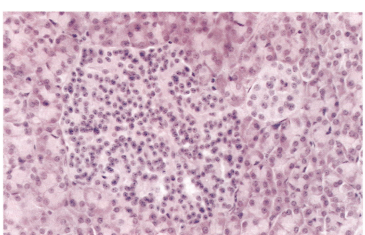

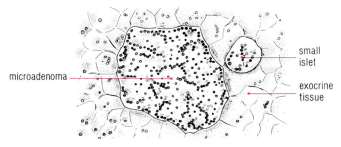

Fig. 1.34 Microadenoma alongside a small normal islet in the pancreas of a patient with the MEA Type 1 syndrome. The microadenoma has retained normal islet physiology but displays an increased density of islet cells. The nuclei of the tumour cells are smaller and more densely staining than those of the normal islets and there is a considerable reduction in cytoplasmic volume. These changes are consistent with neoplastic transformation. H and E stain.

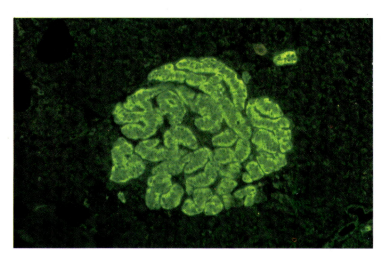

Fig. 1.35 Microadenoma from the pancreas of the same subject as Fig. 1.34 immunostained for insulin. Insulin immunoreactivity is largely located at one pole of each cell. The cells have adopted a ribbon pattern, one of the typical morphological patterns of islet cell tumours.

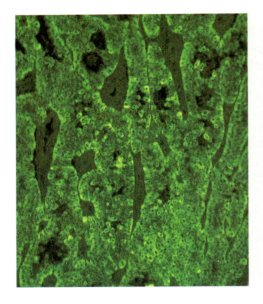

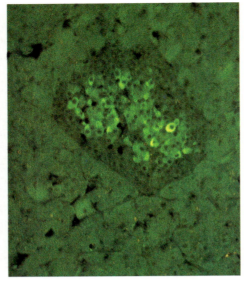

diabetes mellitus

skin rash (necrolytic migratory erythema)

diarrhoea

vulvitis

stomatitis

anaemia

hypoaminoacidaemia

Fig. 1.36 Malignant insulinoma immunostained for insulin. This tumour had metastasized to the liver before the syndrome was diagnosed.

Fig. 1.37 B cells immunostained for insulin from a pancreas containing a malignant insulinoma. The reduction and variability of insulin immunostaining indicates a down-regulation of insulin production.

Fig. 1.38 Clinical features of pancreatic glucagonoma.

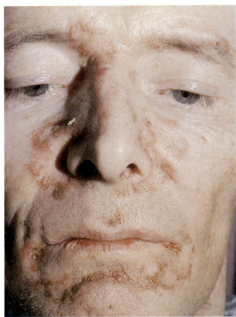

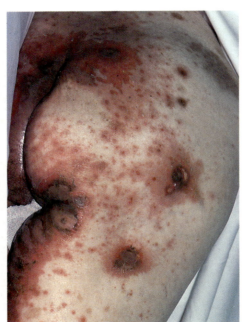

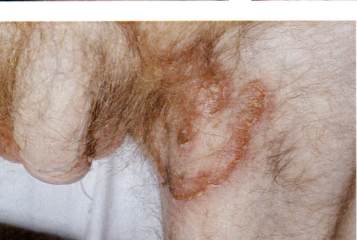

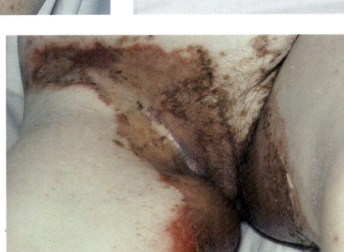

Fig. 1.39 The rash of the glucagonoma syndrome. It is predominantly seen in the dependent areas of the body and the perineal regions.

Malignant islet cell tumours

Islet cell tumours may also be malignant and of a much more aggressive nature. Such tumours have been described containing each of the recognized islet cell types. Fig. 1.36 illustrates a typical staining pattern of an extensive malignant insulinoma. Fig. 1.37 shows an islet, some distance from this tumour, which has been immunostained for insulin. Such islets show a down-regulation of normal B cell insulin production in response to high levels of tumour-derived insulin.

Insulinomas and glucagonomas produce distinctive syndromes, whereas the clinical features produced by somatostatinomas and PP cell tumours are less apparent. The insulinoma syndrome is clinically typified by manifestations of insulin excess; the gluca-gonoma syndrome is equally distinctive (Fig. 1.38). Some islet tumours elaborate hormones which are not associated with the islet cells of the normal adult human pancreas. These hormones include gastrin, vasoactive intestinal polypeptide (VIP), calci-tonin, growth hormone releasing hormone (GHRH), peptide histidine methionine (PHM) and neurotensin. Some of these produce recognized clinical syndromes: gastrinomas give rise to the Zollinger-Ellison syndrome and VIPomas produce the Werner-Morrison syndrome, commonly known as the 'watery diarrhoea hypokalaemic achlorhydria syndrome'.

PANCREATIC HORMONE PATHOLOGY
Pathology of Glucagon

Glucagon has been implicated in the pathogenesis of diabetes mellitus, but current views would suggest that it does not act as a primary aetiological factor, although it may be implicated in certain clinical conditions such as ketoacidosis.

Glucagon deficiency states may be found in diabetes mellitus, where normal glucagon responses to hypoglycaemic stimuli are lost, and in patients with total pancreatectomy. However, clinical problems due to these deficiencies have not been characterized.

Glucagonoma syndrome

This rare syndrome is due to an islet cell tumour secreting glucagon. Most patients have extensive hepatic metastases at the time of diagnosis. The main clinical features are shown in Fig. 1.38. The rash, which is the most dramatic and characteristic feature of the syndrome (Fig. 1.39), can be widespread but is pre-dominantly present in the dependent areas of the body and the perineal regions. It is painful and subject to remissions and re-lapses. Several patients have been described with giant intestinal villi. Fasting hyperglucagonaemia is present and excess glucagon is released following intravenous arginine or tolbutamide (Fig. 1.40).

Fig. 1.40 Massive elevation of glucagon in a patient with the glucagonoma syndrome, with release after intravenous tolbutamide. The control limit for glucagon which is normally up to 300ng/l is not shown in this graph due to the massive difference in scale.

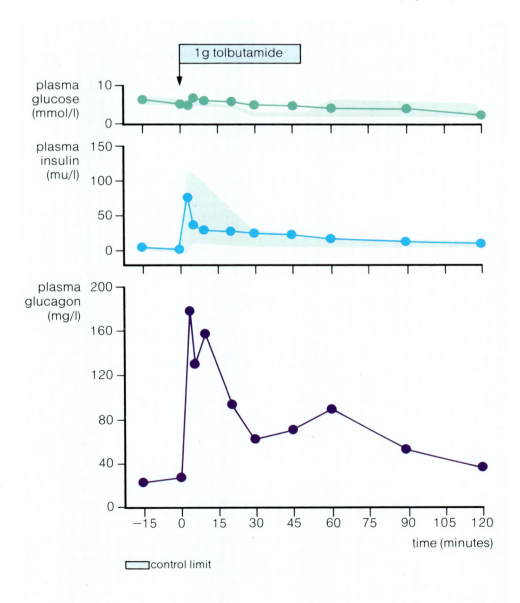

Pathology of Somatostatin

Several patients with a somatostatinoma showing a heterogeneous group of features have been described. As somatostatin cells can be found in other islet cell tumours a clear picture of a pure somatostatinoma syndrome has not been characterized (Fig. 1.41).

Pathology of Pancreatic Polypeptide

Decreased basal PP concentrations and diminished or absent responses to various stimuli have been observed in patients with exocrine pancreatic disease such as chronic pancreatitis and cystic fibrosis, whereas in pancreatic endocrine disease, for example, diabetes mellitus and islet cell tumours, particularly as a feature of MEA Type 1, PP concentrations tend to be elevated.

CLINICAL FEATURES OF SOMATOSTATINOMA

abdominal pains

diarrhoea

diabetes mellitus

steatorrhoea

hypoglycaemia

hypochlorhydria

episodes of headache, flushing and tachycardia

pancreatic islet cell tumour

Fig. 1.41 Principal clinical features associated with somatostatinoma.

CONCLUSION

The anatomy, physiology and some pathological aspects of the pancreatic islets have been reviewed in this chapter. Recent developments in regulatory peptide research include the finding of an extensive peptidergic innervation of both exocrine and endocrine elements. Peptides localized to this system include VIP, gastrin-releasing peptide, calcitonin gene-related peptide and neurotensin, all of which have previously been localized to neural elements in other parts of the body.

The application of techniques of molecular cloning to the genes which encode the precursor molecules of pancreatic peptide hormones has revealed the presence of other putative regulatory peptides encoded by the same genes. For example, differential post-translational processing of the glucagon gene can give rise to the peptides glicentin and oxyntomodulin and, in addition, this gene encodes the amino acid sequences of two glucagon-like peptides, GLP1 and GLP2, the functions of which are at present unknown.

The secretory granules of all cells of the regulatory peptide system, including pancreatic islet cells, appear to contain chromogranin A, a protein with a molecular weight of 70,000 daltons. Although the function of this protein remains unknown, a recently isolated pancreatic regulatory peptide, designated peptide G or pancreastatin, which exhibits a powerful inhibitory action on islet cell hormone release, appears to represent a fragment of chromogranin A.

Our understanding of the anatomy, physiology and biochemistry of the pancreas is continuously increasing and the simplistic concept of separate endocrine and exocrine elements is no longer tenable. The enormous complexity of the peptidergic innervation and the multiplicity of islet cell secretory products requires further extensive research to elucidate possible pathogenic roles in diabetes and other pancreatic and metabolic disorders.

REFERENCES

Cohen S & Soloway RD (1985) *Hormone-producing tumours of the gastrointestinal tract*. Edinburgh: Churchill Livingstone.

Dileepan KN & Wagle SR (1985) Somatostatin: a metabolic regulator. *Life Sciences*, **37**, 2335–2343.

Klöppel G & Heitz Ph eds (1984) *Pancreatic Pathology*. Edinburgh: Churchill Livingstone.

Lefèbvre PJ ed. (1983) *Glucagon*. Berlin: Springer Verlag.

Montague W (1983) *Diabetes and the Endocrine Pancreas: A Biochemical Approach*. London: Croom Helm.

2 Regulation and Mechanism of Insulin Secretion

Simon L Howell DSc

INTRACELLULAR PATHWAY OF INSULIN PRODUCTION

The intracellular pathway involved in the biosynthesis, storage and secretion of insulin by the pancreatic cell is now well understood. The initial biosynthetic product of the pancreatic B cells is the short-lived precursor, pre-proinsulin, which is synthesized on the polyribosomes of the endoplasmic reticulum. Pre-proinsulin is then transported to the cisternae of the endoplasmic reticulum where the 'pre' section is rapidly cleaved off, its half-life being probably only fifteen to thirty seconds. The remaining polypeptide, termed 'proinsulin', then becomes folded in its final conformation to allow correct disulphide bond formation between A and B chains. Once the correct tertiary structure has been adopted, it is transported to the Golgi complex. Here the cleavage of proinsulin to yield insulin and the connecting peptide (C peptide) which links the A and B chains is initiated by proteolytic enzymes with the specificities of trypsin and carboxypeptidase B (Fig. 2.1). After cleavage the insulin and connecting peptide are packaged together in membrane-limited storage granules (β granules), where they are stored until secreted by exocytosis on application of a suitable stimulus. The whole process and the time course of the individual steps are shown

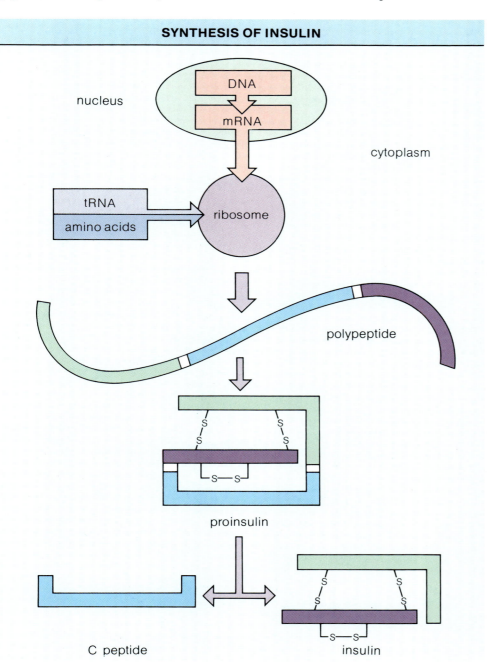

SYNTHESIS OF INSULIN

nucleus

DNA

mRNA

cytoplasm

tRNA

amino acids

ribosome

polypeptide

proinsulin

C peptide

insulin

Fig. 2.1 Biosynthesis of pre-proinsulin and its subsequent conversion to proinsulin and insulin. The conversion to proinsulin is extremely rapid, occurring in less than one minute after its biosynthesis on the ribosome. Proinsulin is already folded in the correct conformation and, when cleaved, yields insulin and C peptide.

in Fig. 2.2, which also indicates the folding of the proinsulin molecules and their storage within the granules as zinc-insulin hexamers.

The mechanism of the secretory process involves exocytosis, that is, the movement of granules towards the plasma membrane where granule membrane and plasma membrane fuse together (Fig. 2.3). This process may be separated into two parts: first, the intracellular movement of granules occurs from the cytoplasmic pool, where they are stored in large numbers of approximately thirteen thousand per cell, to a position close to the plasma membrane and secondly, there is the final fusion process (Fig. 2.4).

REGULATION OF INSULIN SECRETION

The major physiological stimulus for insulin secretion is an increase in serum glucose concentration and this can be elegantly shown during *in vitro* studies with isolated islets of Langerhans. The insulin secretory response of isolated islets to glucose over a range of 0–20mmol/l is shown in Fig. 2.5. It is clear that secretion is initiated at a serum glucose concentration of approximately 5mmol/l, just above the fasting level, and that the overall response is sigmoidal, reaching a plateau at about 20mmol/l. This insulin secretory response to glucose is highly specific; for instance, galactose will not stimulate secretion and the effectiveness of a given

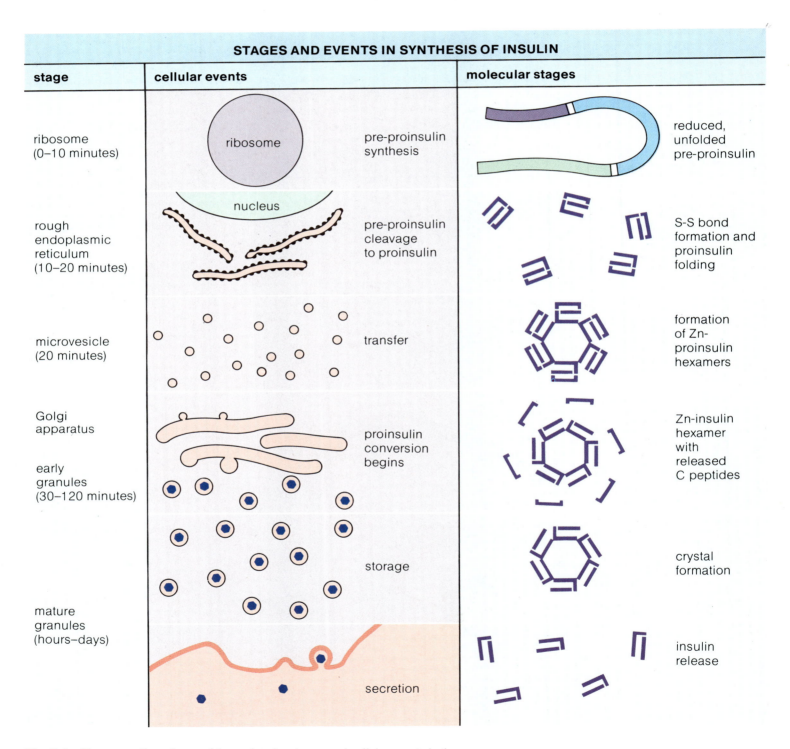

Fig. 2.2 Diagrammatic pathway of the molecular stages and cellular events in the biosynthesis, storage and release of insulin. These events occur within the pancreatic B cells.

carbohydrate stimulus appears to parallel its rate of metabolism by the B cells. This and other evidence has suggested that glucose metabolism and that of other nutrient stimuli are required for the effective stimulation of insulin secretion (the 'substrate site hypothesis').

The time course of the insulin response to glucose has also been studied, both in perfused pancreas preparations and in isolated islets. The response to glucose is initially biphasic with a rapid initial 'spike' followed by a prolonged second phase which continues until the removal of the stimulus (Fig. 2.6). The reason for this biphasic response is not clear. It may reflect either the relative importance of intracellular and extracellular calcium or possibly the physical availability of granules for rapid extrusion. However, not all insulin secretagogues produce a biphasic pattern of release. The hypoglycaemic sulphonylureas, for instance, appear to provoke a single spike of secretion followed by a prolonged period during which release is only slightly greater than the basal levels.

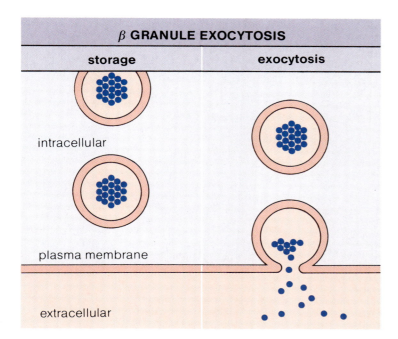

Fig. 2.3 Diagrammatic representation of β granule extrusion by exocytosis. The movement of a β granule close to the plasma (cell) membrane is followed by its fusion with the plasma membrane and release of its contents. This process is called exocytosis.

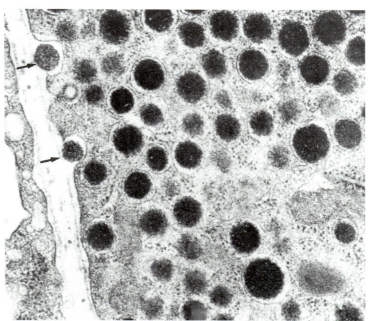

Fig. 2.4 Electron micrograph of a pancreatic islet B cell. The insulin containing β granules are shown, two of which (arrowed) are undergoing exocytosis into the extracellular space.

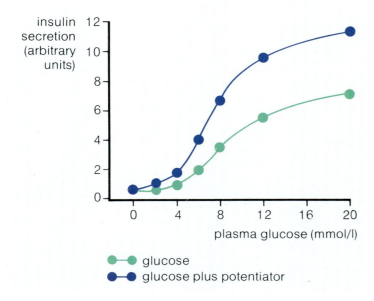

Fig. 2.5 Effect of glucose concentration on insulin secretion. The response to glucose both with and without a secondary stimulus (potentiator) is shown.

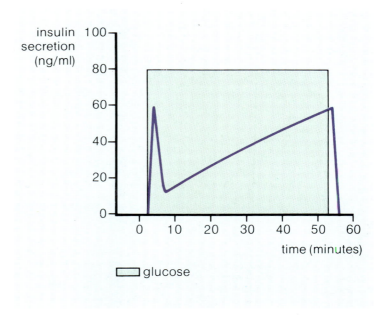

Fig. 2.6 Time course of insulin release from pancreatic islets following stimulation by glucose. The first phase or 'spike' of secretion is followed by a slower rising and more sustained second phase of secretion.

2.3

Many other agents have been shown to influence rates of insulin secretion both *in vivo* and *in vitro*. However, only a small proportion of these are likely to be of physiological, as distinct from pharmacological, importance (Fig. 2.7). Fatty acids, ketone bodies and amino acids may also be considered as physiological stimuli. These are termed primary stimuli in that they do not require the presence of glucose to exert their effects.

The primary stimuli of insulin secretion are believed to exert their effects by altering fluxes of calcium ions across the B cell membrane in order to increase the free intracellular (cytosolic) calcium concentration. By contrast, the secondary stimuli, or potentiators of secretion, may act via alterations in intracellular cyclic adenosine monophosphate (cAMP) concentrations. In this way, the primary stimuli and potentiators act synergistically to promote rates of insulin release (Fig. 2.8 and see Fig. 2.5).

A further way in which calcium may stimulate insulin secretion

FACTORS WHICH INFLUENCE INSULIN SECRETION		
primary stimuli	**potentiators**	**inhibitors**
glucose	secretin	adrenaline
amino acids (arginine and leucine)	pancreozymin	noradrenaline
ketones	GIP (glucose-dependent insulinotropic peptide)	somatostatin
fatty acids	acetylcholine	

Fig. 2.7 Principal factors which influence insulin secretion.

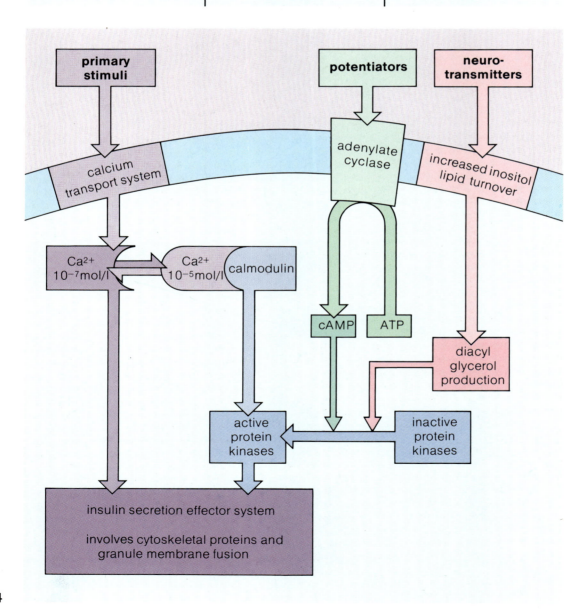

Fig. 2.8 Diagram showing the interactions between primary stimuli (e.g. glucose or amino acids), potentiators (e.g. glucagon or pancreozymin) and neuro-transmitters (e.g. acetylcholine) in the regulation of insulin secretion. Note that cAMP, calcium – calmodulin and diacyl glycerol stimulate separate protein kinases termed a, b and c respectively.

is by the activation of a calcium-phospholipid dependent protein kinase (protein kinase-c). This recently discovered protein kinase may play a role in the regulation of insulin secretion by responding to factors such as acetylcholine. The response is initiated by stimulation of inositol lipid turnover in the membrane which leads to production of diacyl glycerol; this in turn leads to activation of the kinase. It is not yet clear whether protein kinase-c plays a role in the regulation of glucose-induced insulin secretion.

Cyclic AMP and Regulation of Insulin Secretion

It is clear that although cAMP concentrations in the B cells may increase after glucose stimulation, this is not the primary mechanism of action of glucose. The role of cAMP is rather to modulate the effects of glucose stimulation. Therefore, agents which activate B cell adenylate cyclase, such as secretin, pancreozymin and glucagon, will raise cAMP levels in the cells and thus stimulate insulin secretion via activation of cAMP-dependent protein kinase (see Fig. 2.8). This effect may be particularly important in the priming of B cells by gut hormones, including GIP and secretin or both, to the impending arrival of an increased concentration of glucose in the bloodstream. This potentiating effect might explain the greater effect of oral glucose compared to

intravenous glucose in stimulating secretion of insulin. The general role of any gastrointestinal factors in modulating the insulin secretory response is known as the 'entero–insulin axis'.

Role of Calcium in Insulin Secretion

It has long been known that the presence of extracellular calcium is essential for an insulin secretory response to a stimulus. It has also been suggested from radiolabelled calcium ($^{45}Ca^{2+}$) influx and efflux studies that the free intracellular (cytosolic) calcium concentration may be the critically important factor in determining secretory rates. This is indicated by the fact that the higher the cytosolic calcium concentration the greater is the rate of insulin secretion. Glucose is thought to produce this net uptake either by promoting the influx of calcium ions into the cell via specific channels or by reducing its efflux, or both (see Fig. 2.8).

The influx may be increased in part through voltage sensitive calcium channels which are opened following depolarization of the B cell membrane. Conversely, those agents which alter rates of insulin secretion via changes in intracellular cAMP concentration may do so by altering the distribution of calcium, particularly reducing its uptake by mitochondria and by endoplasmic reticular elements, or both (Fig. 2.9). The insulin storage granules

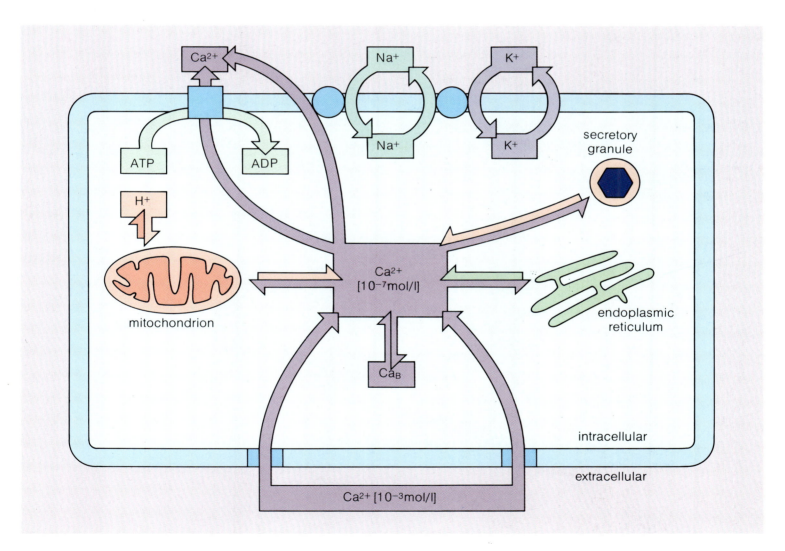

Fig. 2.9 Suggested model for the regulation of intracellular calcium concentration in B-cells. Free intracellular calcium can either be taken up by secretory granules, mitochondria or the endoplasmic reticulum, or it can be bound by specific proteins (Ca_B).

Calmodulin is the most important of these. Intracellular calcium levels can also be influenced by active extrusion by means of various exchange pumps.

also contain calcium, but this does not appear to be in a readily exchangeable pool and may contribute only indirectly to regulation of cytosolic calcium. Several factors which are involved in the maintenance of a cytosolic calcium concentration of $10^{-7}\dot{M}$ in B cells are shown in Fig. 2.9 together with the calcium efflux via Na^+/Ca^{2+} exchange and the Ca^{2+} ATPase (calcium pump).

In addition to calcium uptake by organelles, calcium binding by other proteins (Ca_B) also occurs. The most important of these is probably the ubiquitous calcium-binding protein, calmodulin. Calmodulin, by its interactions with other proteins in the cell, might produce the essential link between the elevation of cytosolic calcium concentrations, elicited by secretagogues, and the activation of the cytoskeleton which leads to intracellular granule movement (Fig. 2.10). This link is likely to be achieved by activation of calcium-calmodulin dependent protein kinase, but may also involve direct activation of the cytoskeleton via calmodulin. Finally, calcium may also influence granule–membrane fusion.

Paracrine Relationships

The location of insulin-secreting B cells in close proximity to the glucagon-secreting A cells and somatostatin-secreting D cells (see *Chapters 1 & 3*) raises the possibility that secretion of each hormone might have local effects on other adjacent cell types. These intra-islet relationships are called paracrine effects; the interactions which have been demonstrated *in vitro* are shown in Fig. 2.11. It is not yet certain whether any or all of the paracrine effects illustrated in Fig. 2.11 are involved in the regulation of insulin secretion *in vivo*.

MECHANISM OF INSULIN SECRETION
Intracellular Transport of Granules

This may involve the microtubule and microfilament elements of the B cell cytoskeleton, since rates of secretion are dramatically altered by treatment of the cells with drugs which interfere with the function of either the microtubules (e.g. colchicine, vinblastine) or the microfilaments (e.g. cytochalasin B, phalloidin).

A schematic model for the possible regulation of microtubules (tubulin), microfilaments (actin) and of myosin during the insulin secretory process is shown in Fig. 2.12. It is suggested that microtubules provide the static directional system, while microfilaments, perhaps with actomyosin as the functional contractile unit, provide the motile forces for granule movement.

Granule to Membrane Fusion

Granules will ultimately reach a position close to the plasma membrane which may be determined by van der Waal's forces and electrostatic repulsion. The final fusion may be regulated either by local alterations in the membranes, perhaps by phosphorylation of membrane proteins, or by neutralization of the negative charges following a local influx of calcium ions across the plasma membrane on stimulation of secretion. The latter possibility is illustrated schematically in Fig. 2.13.

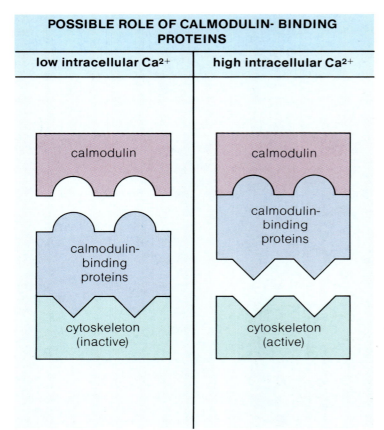

Fig. 2.10 Possible mechanism of the regulation of cytoskeletal function by calcium. The binding of calmodulin, calmodulin-binding proteins and the cytoskeleton is changed in the presence of free calcium ions.

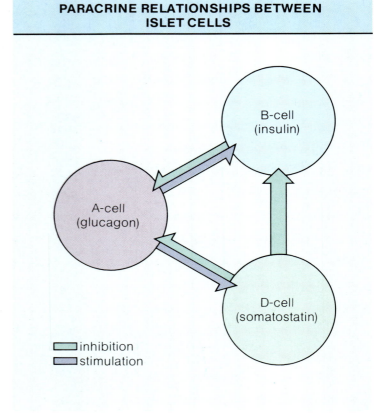

Fig. 2.11 Some of the paracrine relationships which have been suggested between the A, B and D cells of the islets of Langerhans.

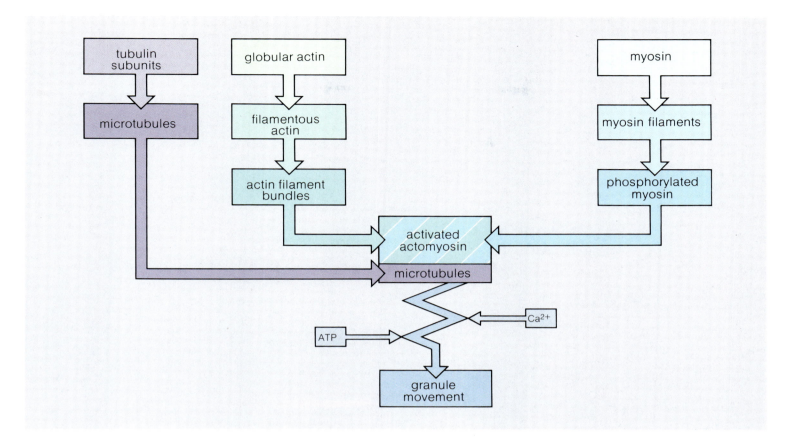

Fig. 2.12 Possible mechanism of granule movement within the B cell. There is thought to be an interaction between microtubules and microfilaments, with actomyosin as the functional contractile unit.

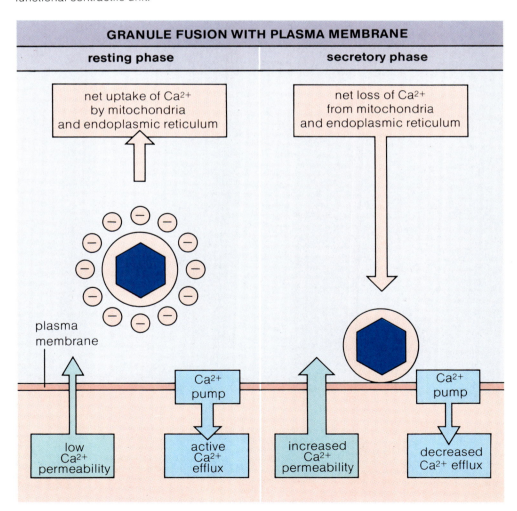

GRANULE FUSION WITH PLASMA MEMBRANE

resting phase	secretory phase

net uptake of Ca^{2+} by mitochondria and endoplasmic reticulum

net loss of Ca^{2+} from mitochondria and endoplasmic reticulum

plasma membrane

low Ca^{2+} permeability

Ca^{2+} pump

active Ca^{2+} efflux

increased Ca^{2+} permeability

Ca^{2+} pump

decreased Ca^{2+} efflux

Fig. 2.13 Possible effect of a rise in intracellular calcium on the fusion of β granules with the B cell plasma membrane. The increase in intracellular calcium causes a reduction in the net negative charge on the granule membrane. This, in turn, increases the probability of fusion of the granule membrane with the plasma membrane, with consequent exocytosis of the granule content.

2.7

REFERENCES

Hedeskov CJ (1980) Mechanism of glucose-induced insulin secretion. *Physiological Reviews*, **60**, 442–509.

Howell SL (1984) The mechanism of insulin secretion. *Diabetologia*, **26**, 319–327.

Montague W (1983) *Diabetes and the Endocrine Pancreas: A Biochemical Approach*. London: Croom Helm.

Wallis M, Howell SL & Taylor KW (1985) *The Biochemistry of Polypeptide Hormones*. Chichester: John Wiley.

Wollheim CB & Sharp GW (1981) Regulation of insulin release by calcium. *Physiological Reviews*, **61**, 914–973.

3 Morphology of the Normal and Diabetic Endocrine Pancreas

Willy Gepts MD PhD ● **Peter A in't Veld**

MORPHOLOGY OF THE ENDOCRINE PANCREAS

The human endocrine pancreas is composed of $10^5-2 \times 10^6$ islets of Langerhans scattered throughout the pancreatic parenchyma. These micro-organs typically contain several hundred endocrine cells arranged around a capillary network. Most islets have a diameter of 100–200μm and account for 1–2% of the total gland volume.

Islet Cell Type Distribution

At least four different islet cell types have been identified on the basis of the ultrastructure of their secretory granules and their immunohistochemical staining characteristics (see *Chapter 1*).

The distribution of these cell types within the islet and throughout the pancreas as a whole is not random, but has a precise topography. The posterior duodenal part of the gland, derived from the ventral primordium and supplied by the superior mesenteric artery, contains islets mainly composed of pancreatic polypeptide or PP cells (Fig. 3.1), while the islets in the tail, body and head regions, derived from the dorsal primordium and supplied by the coeliac artery, contain mainly B cells (Fig. 3.2). The dorsally derived lobe contains few PP cells but most of the A cells, in contrast to the ventrally derived lobe which contains few A cells but most of the PP cells.

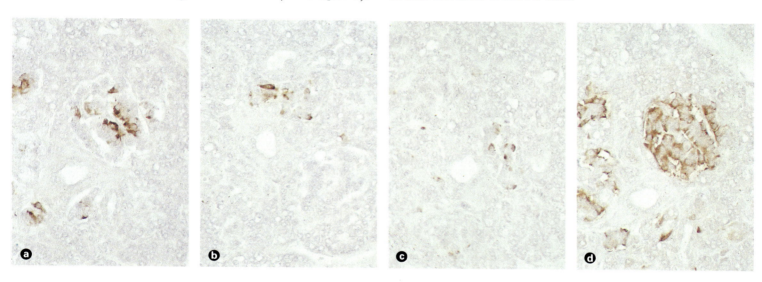

Fig. 3.1   Human islet of Langerhans from the ventrally derived head region. Four consecutive paraffin sections are shown, stained with the peroxidase-antiperoxidase technique of Sternberger for insulin (a), glucagon (b), somatostatin (c) and pancreatic polypeptide or PP (d) and demonstrate the relative abundance of PP cells.

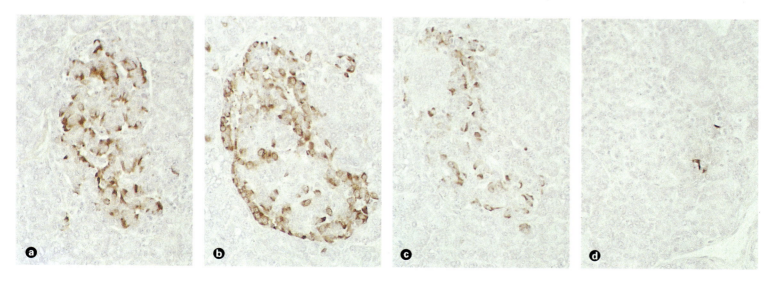

Fig. 3.2   Human islet of Langerhans from the dorsally derived body region. The relative abundance of B and A-cells is demonstrated. Staining as in Fig. 3.1.

Intra-Islet Communication

Though islet cell function is mainly determined by the plasma concentrations of glucose and other metabolites, there is increasing evidence for the existence of a number of pathways modifying the effect of these primary stimuli.

In many mammalian species, islets are composed of a central core of B cells surrounded by a peripheral layer of A cells. D cells are generally in contact with both islet cell types. Such an arrangement suggests intra-islet interactions between the various types of islet cells. Indeed, several islet hormones have been shown to affect each other's secretion levels. It has been proposed that the localization of the various cell types within the islet is determined by the blood flow pattern, the afferent artery initially perfusing the B cell compartment and subsequently the non-B cell compartment. It should be stressed, however, that the blood perfusion pattern for human islets is poorly understood and that the available data on rodent material is equivocal. Moreover, zones of separate islet cell types are not always evident in human material.

An intra-islet endocrine pathway may not be the only communication link between islet cells; hormones released within the islet may also affect the function of neighbouring endocrine cells through a paracrine route. This is supported by the occasional presence of long, cell processes protruding from D and PP cells. Like the processes of gastric D cells, these protrusions may end in synapse-like terminals on endocrine target cells.

A third type of pathway affecting islet cell function is formed by

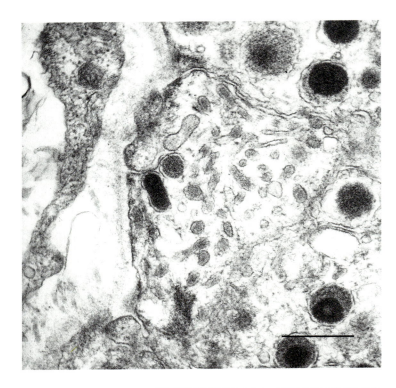

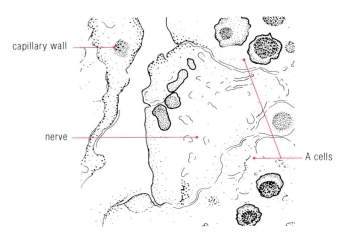

Fig. 3.3 Islet cell innervation. A nerve fibre, resembling a cholinergic nerve terminal, is shown adjoining two A cells and a capillary wall. TEM; bar=0.5μm.

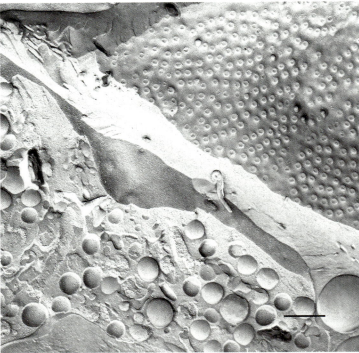

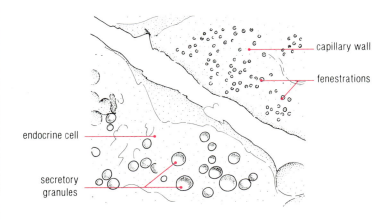

Fig. 3.4 Freeze-fracture replica of an islet capillary showing the fenestrated capillary wall and part of an endocrine cell with cytoplasmic secretory granules. TEM; bar=0.5μm.

the autonomic nervous system. Nerve fibres penetrate the islets alongside the blood vessels (Fig. 3.3). Both adrenergic and cholinergic fibres have been identified, while some peptidergic fibres have been shown to contain somatostatin-like and vasoactive intestinal polypeptide-like immunoreactivity.

Islets contain many capillaries that surround the endocrine cells in such a way that most cells are bordered by at least one capillary. The endothelial cells lining these vessels contain small pores closed by a diaphragm (Fig. 3.4). Such fenestrated capillaries are characteristic of many glands and may be responsible for the fast transfer of chemical messengers between the blood and the intercellular space. Blood flow through the islets accounts for approximately ten per cent of the total pancreatic blood flow and is under the control of both glucose and adrenaline.

Apart from blood-borne or locally-acting substances, islet cell function may also be modulated through direct cell-to-cell interactions via gap junctions (Fig. 3.5). These membrane specializations contain channels, 15–20 Å wide, that bridge the membranes of apposed cells. They have been shown to exist both between homologous and heterologous islet cells and may mediate electrical and metabolic coupling, through the diffusion of substances with a molecular weight of less than 1200 daltons.

The regulation of B cell insulin-secreting islets is a complex process that is dependent upon the structural organization of the endocrine pancreas. The study of islet morphology may therefore greatly contribute to a better understanding of islet function and its disorders.

PANCREATIC PATHOLOGY IN HUMAN DIABETES
Despite increasing evidence in recent years for the heterogeneity of diabetes, its pancreatic pathology is still mainly represented by two distinct entities: (i) insulin-dependent (IDDM) or Type I diabetes and (ii) non-insulin dependent (NIDDM) or Type II diabetes.

Pancreatic Pathology in Type I Diabetes
Type I or insulin-dependent diabetes is usually characterized by a sudden clinical onset in a lean person, a tendency to ketosis, low plasma insulin and low extractable insulin in the pancreas.

The pancreas of Type I diabetic patients is often small and reduced in weight. This change does not result from a congenital hypoplasia, but is the consequence of a progressive atrophy developing in the course of the disease (Fig. 3.6). The atrophy mainly affects the areas with few PP cells and spares the PP cell rich areas.

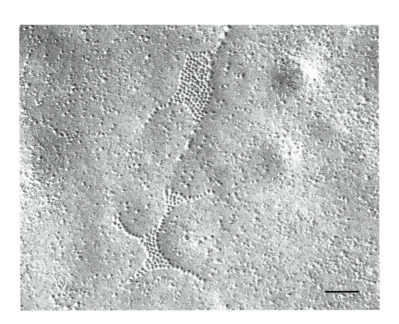

Fig. 3.5 Freeze-fracture replica showing part of the membrane P-face, that backing onto the protoplasm, of an endocrine cell from the central part of a human islet. The aggregates of 9nm particles correspond to gap junctions. TEM; bar=0.1 μm.

Fig. 3.6 Weight of the pancreas in fifteen acute cases (death occurring < 6 months after diagnosis) and sixteen chronic cases (death occurring from 1–37 years after diagnosis) of Type I diabetes (Gepts, 1965).

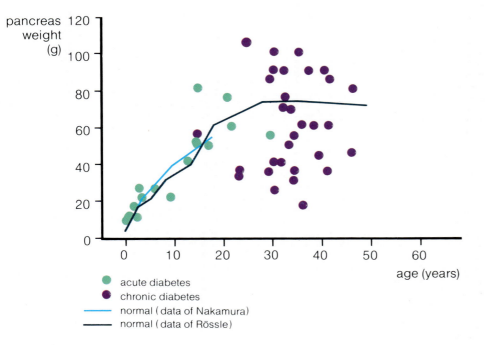

In Type I diabetes the islets show pathognomonic changes. By the time of the clinical onset of the disease, most islets are composed of thin cords of small cells arranged in a variable amount of fibrous stroma (Fig. 3.7). Historically, such islets have been considered to be atrophic, but recent evidence suggests they are composed of about two-thirds glucagon cells and one-third somatostatin cells (Fig. 3.8). Pseudo-atrophic islets do not contain B cells. B cell-containing islets are rare in the pancreas of Type I diabetic patients even at the clinical onset of the disease (Fig. 3.9).

Insulitis is the most characteristic lesion of the islets in Type I

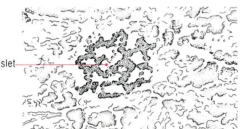

Fig. 3.7 Pseudo-atrophic islet in the pancreas of a Type I diabetic patient. The islet is composed of narrow cords of small cells, which can be shown by immunocytochemical staining to contain glucagon or somatostatin (see Fig. 3.8). Gomori's chromium haematoxylin-phloxine stain.

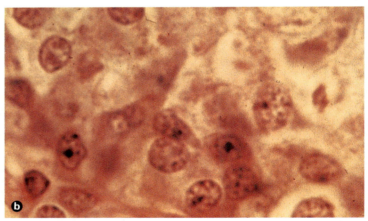

Fig. 3.8 Pseudo-atrophic islet in the pancreas of a Type I diabetic patient. The islet has been stained for glucagon (blue cells) and for somatostatin (brown cells) with the peroxidase-antiperoxidase technique of Sternberger, using specific antibodies to glucagon and to somatostatin.

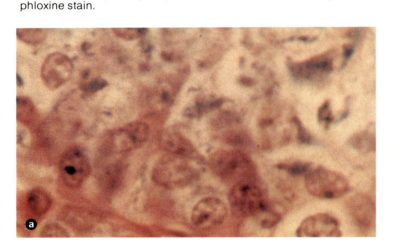

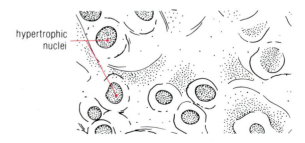

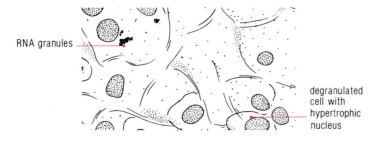

Fig. 3.9 Islet of a recently diagnosed Type I diabetic patient showing B cells with cytological features of functional hyperactivity. There is nuclear hypertrophy, degranulation and an increased RNA content of the cytoplasm. (a) Dominici-erythrosine-orange stain. (b) after incubation of the section with ribonuclease the RNA granules are removed.

diabetes. In most cases it is represented by an infiltration of lymphocytes either in or around the islets or both (Fig. 3.10), but in rare cases polymorphonuclear cells are also present (Fig. 3.11).

Insulitis has been found in those diabetic patients who have died shortly after clinical onset. It is more common in very young diabetic patients (Fig. 3.12). Insulitis is an elusive lesion; it is

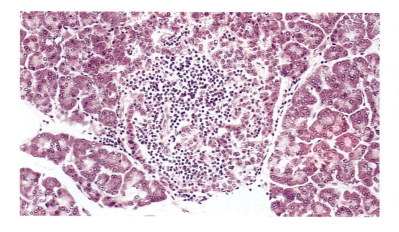

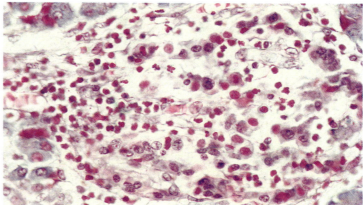

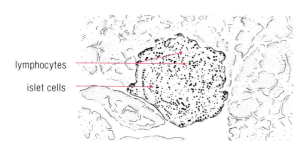

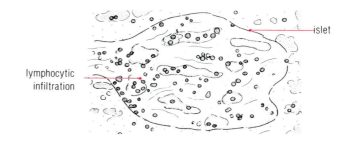

Fig. 3.10 Islet of a recently diagnosed Type I diabetic patient showing a diffuse lymphocytic infiltration (insulitis) with onset of atrophy of the islet cell cords. H and E stain.

Fig. 3.11 Islet of a recently diagnosed Type I diabetic patient showing a diffuse inflammatory infiltrate composed of lymphocytes and many polymorphonuclear cells. Gomori's chromium haematoxylin-phloxine stain.

Fig. 3.12 Insulitis and age at onset of diabetes. Insulitis is more common in young patients.

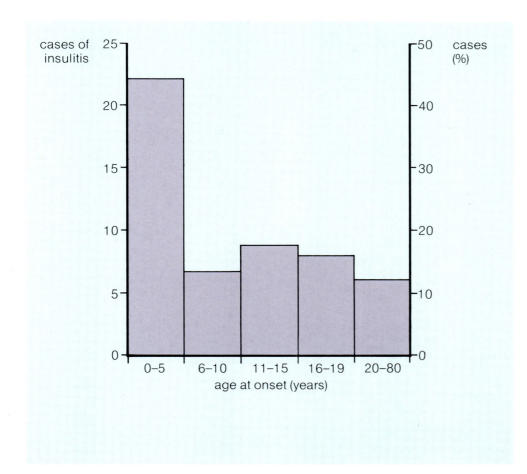

rarely detectable after a clinical duration of more than six months to one year. It usually affects only a few islets and almost exclusively those that still contain B cells (Fig. 3.13).

A profound numerical reduction of the B cells in Type I diabetes has been demonstrated previously with crude quantitative methods. Recently, this has been confirmed by studies performed with sensitive immunocytochemical techniques and more refined morphometric methods (Fig. 3.14). No quantitative changes in the other three types of islet cells (A, D and PP) have been demonstrated (Fig. 3.14).

B cells remain present, albeit in low numbers, in fifty per cent of the insulin-dependent subjects who have had the disease for less than ten years and in ten per cent of those with disease of longer duration. These morphological findings are consistent with clinical studies which have demonstrated the preservation of some B cell function for many years after the clinical onset of Type I diabetes. Both clinical and morphological studies indicate that the later in life Type I diabetes appears, the better the chances of B cell survival.

With a prolonged duration of Type I diabetes, a progressive distortion of the islet architecture develops. This distortion results not only from the disappearance of the B cells but also from an increasing tendency of the A and D cells to leave the confines of the individual islets and to spread as single cells into the exocrine parenchyma (Fig. 3.15).

Evidence of B cell regeneration is scarce in the pancreas of Type I diabetic patients. It can only be detected in subjects who died shortly after the diagnosis of diabetes. In some cases, it is represented by a proliferation of centroacinar cells; in others by an endocrine differentiation of ductal cells called 'nesidioblastosis' (Fig. 3.16).

Pathogenic Considerations in Type I Diabetes

Type I diabetes is mainly characterized by a severe insulin deficiency resulting from a profound numerical reduction of the B cells. The bulk of evidence suggests that in the usual cases of Type I diabetes the B cells are destroyed by an autoimmune process triggered, in genetically susceptible individuals, by various and still poorly defined environmental factors, which may include viruses and chemical agents (see *Chapter 10*). Contrary to the classical opinion, Type I diabetes is not an acute disease. At the time of clinical onset, the pancreatic pathology represents the end result of a long struggle between the regenerative capacity of the B cells and the putative destructive factors.

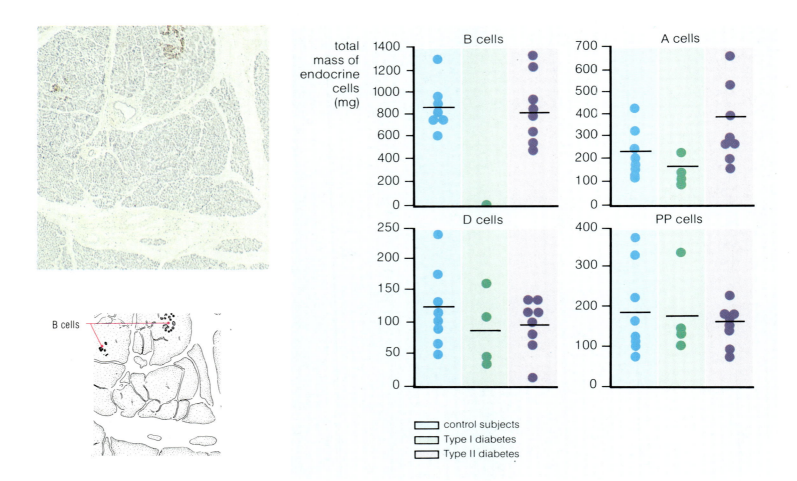

control subjects
Type I diabetes
Type II diabetes

Fig. 3.13 Low power magnification of pancreatic tissue from a recently diagnosed Type I diabetic patient. There are several pseudo-atrophic islets without insulitis. Only two islets which still contain B cells (stained brown) are affected by insulitis. Indirect immunoperoxidase staining method with an antibody to insulin.

Fig. 3.14 Estimated total mass of each endocrine cell type in the pancreas of control and diabetic subjects. Mean values are indicated (Rahier *et al.*, 1983).

Pancreatic Pathology in Type II Diabetes

Type II or non-insulin dependent diabetes is a heterogeneous disorder in which some subjects have deficient insulin secretion, while others, particularly the obese, are hyperinsulinaemic and insulin-resistant.

Except in cases where deposits of amyloid are abundant, there are no distinct differences between the general appearance of the islets in Type II diabetic patients and elderly non-diabetic subjects. Therefore, a diagnosis of Type II diabetes usually cannot be made from the histology of the islets alone.

Amyloidosis (Fig. 3.17), formerly called 'islet hyalinosis', is the most typical, though not most specific, change of the islets in

PERCENTAGES OF ENDOCRINE CELLS OUTSIDE ISLETS						
	insulin cells (%)		glucagon cells (%)		somatostatin cells (%)	
	isolated	small clusters	isolated	small clusters	isolated	small clusters
control subjects	4.1 (1.7–7.0)	12.6 (7.0–15.7)	3.8 (0.5–5.5)	3.5 (1.1–6.0)	4.3 (0.6–7.2)	5.9 (0.0–10.0)
Type I diabetes	100	0	5.1 (1.2–8.0)	6.9 (5.3–9.1)	15.5 (12.6–19.4)	10.9 (7.2–15.6)
Type II diabetes	3.7 (1.6–6.2)	9.5 (4.4–16.4)	2.9 (0.6–6.1)	1.1 (0.0–2.2)	2.7 (1.1–4.8)	3.1 (0.8–9.6)

Fig. 3.15 Percentages of the different endocrine cells present outside the islets in non-diabetic and diabetic subjects. The mean and range are shown for each case (Rahier *et al.*, 1983).

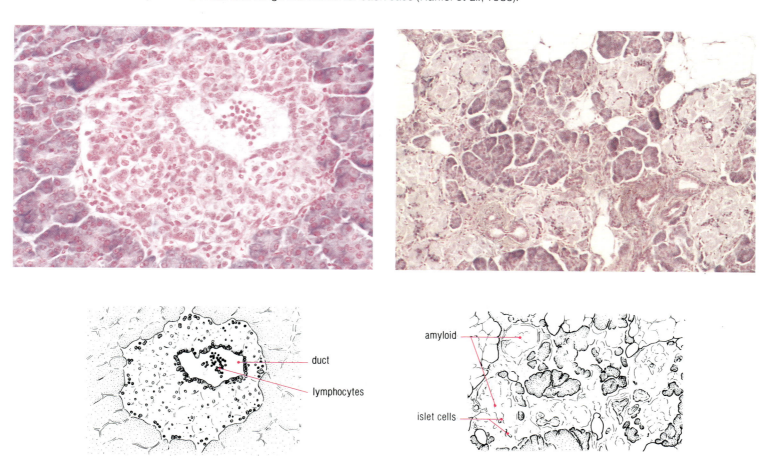

Fig. 3.16 Regenerative islet in the pancreas of a recently diagnosed Type I diabetic patient. Newly formed islet cells are derived from the epithelium of a duct. Lymphocytes are present in the lumen of the duct and in some places at the periphery of the islet (insulitis). H and E stain.

Fig. 3.17 Severe amyloidosis (islet hyalinosis) in the islets of a Type II diabetic patient. Gomori's chromium haematoxylin-phloxine stain.

Type II diabetes. Its incidence is clearly related to age: it is rarely found in diabetic patients under forty years of age, but fifty per cent of those over the age of seventy have amyloid in at least some of their islets. Islet amyloidosis is also observed, although with a much lower frequency and severity, in elderly non-diabetic subjects. Recent studies have revealed that islet amyloid contains insulin B chains. The pathogenic significance of islet amyloidosis remains undetermined.

Crude estimates of the total number of B cells in Type II diabetic patients have indicated an average reduction of 50–60%. However, a wide range of values and considerable overlap are evident, which may reflect heterogeneity in both the diabetic and non-diabetic populations.

Pathogenic Considerations in Type II Diabetes

Taken together, the morphological changes of the endocrine pancreas in Type II diabetes provide no satisfactory explanation for the disease. The lack of consistent cytological features of hyperfunction of the B cell, in the presence of long-lasting hyperglycaemia, suggests either an inherited or an acquired functional defect. However, it is likely that in the majority of cases a complex interplay between hyperglycaemic hyperinsulinaemia with insulin resistance and an absolute or relative functional B cell defect is involved.

REFERENCES

Gepts W (1965) Pathologic anatomy of the pancreas in juvenile diabetes mellitus. *Diabetes*, **14**, 619–633.

Gepts W & De Mey J (1978) Islet cell survival determined by morphology. An immunocytochemical study of the islets of Langerhans in juvenile diabetes mellitus. *Diabetes*, **27** (suppl. 1), 251–261.

Gepts W & LeCompte PM (1981) The pancreatic islets in diabetes. *American Journal of Medicine*, **70**, 105–115.

Klöppel G (1984) Islet histopathology in diabetes mellitus. In *Pancreatic Pathology*. Edited by Klöppel G & Heitz Ph. pp.154–192. Edinburgh: Churchill Livingstone.

Orci L (1982) Macro- and micro-domains in the endocrine pancreas. *Diabetes*, **31**, 538–565.

Pipeleers D (1984) Islet interactions with pancreatic B cells. *Experientia*, **40**, 1114–1126.

Rahier J, Goebbels RM & Henquin JC (1983) Cellular composition of the human diabetic pancreas. *Diabetologia*, **24**, 366–371.

Westermark P & Wilander E (1983) Islet amyloid in Type 2 (non-insulin-dependent) diabetes is related to insulin. *Diabetologia*, **24**, 342–346.

4 Insulin Molecular Structure and Molecular Behaviour

Eleanor J Dodson BA ● **Guy G Dodson** BSc MSc PhD
Rod E Hubbard BA DPhil ● **Colin D Reynolds** BA PhD MSc

The chemical structure of insulin was established by Sanger and his co-workers in Cambridge in the 1950's (Fig. 4.1). The three-dimensional structure of insulin in the crystalline two-Zn form was first determined in 1969 by Dorothy Hodgkin and her co-workers in Oxford. The crystal structure explains much of the hormone's physical and chemical behaviour and is the basis for the arguments concerning its mechanism of action at the receptor.

In the two-Zn insulin crystal, six insulin molecules are organized as a hexamer whose construction is illustrated in

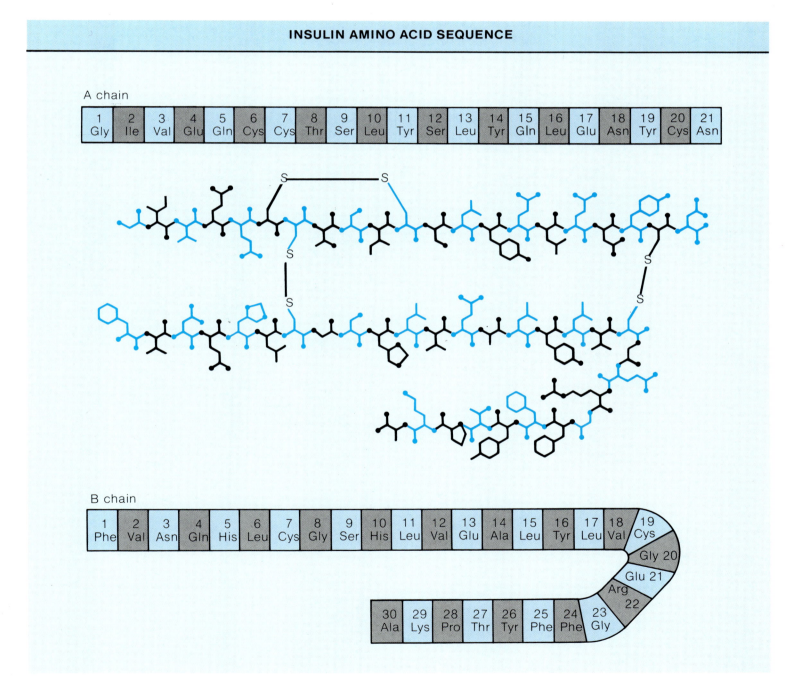

INSULIN AMINO ACID SEQUENCE

A chain

1	2	3	4	5	6	7	8	9	10	11	12	13	14	15	16	17	18	19	20	21
Gly	Ile	Val	Glu	Gln	Cys	Cys	Thr	Ser	Leu	Tyr	Ser	Leu	Tyr	Gln	Leu	Glu	Asn	Tyr	Cys	Asn

B chain

1	2	3	4	5	6	7	8	9	10	11	12	13	14	15	16	17	18	19
Phe	Val	Asn	Gln	His	Leu	Cys	Gly	Ser	His	Leu	Val	Glu	Ala	Leu	Tyr	Leu	Val	Cys

Gly 20
Glu 21
Arg 22

30	29	28	27	26	25	24	23
Ala	Lys	Pro	Thr	Tyr	Phe	Phe	Gly

Fig. 4.1 Amino acid sequence of pig insulin.

4.1

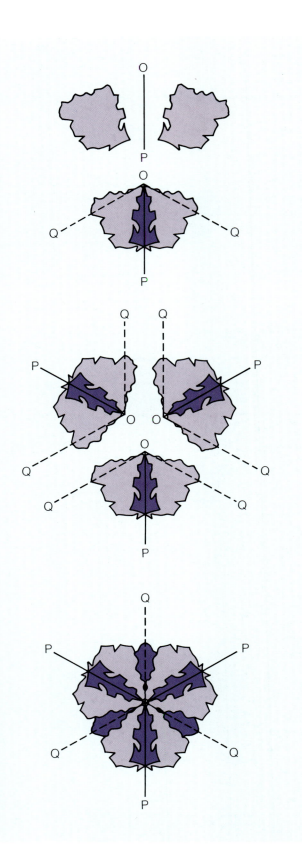

Fig. 4.2. It is made up of three identical dimers related by a threefold axis of rotation. The two insulin molecules in the dimers have very similar, but not identical, three-dimensional structures. These differences in structure, produced by packing within the crystal, only affect some side-chains on the dimer surface. Thus, the dimer structure contains an approximate twofold axis which lies perpendicularly to the threefold exact crystal axis passing through the hexamer centre. In solution, the hexameric structure is free of crystal contacts and contains symmetrical dimers.

The atomic parameters of the insulin molecule in two-Zn insulin have been defined crystallographically using X-ray

INSULIN MOLECULAR CHAIN

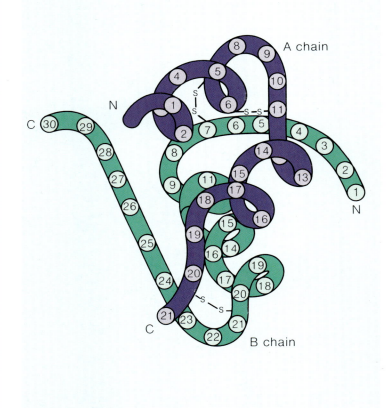

Fig. 4.2 Schematic representation of insulin's pattern of aggregation to the hexameric state from the monomer, via the dimer. O–P is the twofold axis of symmetry relating to the two insulin molecules within the natural dimer which occurs in solution in the absence of zinc ions. In the presence of zinc ions, the insulin dimers assemble to a hexamer through the coordination of the B_{10} histidines (tenth amino acid in the B chain) with the metal ions. The two-Zn hexamer has threefold rotational symmetry and the dimers are also related by a twofold symmetry axis along the line O–Q. This property of assembly is exploited by proinsulin in nature. In the B cell, which is rich in zinc, proinsulin forms zinc-containing hexamers. The proinsulin hexamer has great stability and solubility.

Fig. 4.3 Folding of the polypeptide backbone (main-chain) in the insulin molecule. The amino termini are represented by 'N' and the carboxyl termini by 'C'. The direction of view is along the local twofold axis (O–P in Fig. 4.2). The three disulphide bonds are shown.

diffraction data which extend to 1.5A spacing. This has defined their positions accurately to within 0.2Å. Research into the structure of other insulin crystals continues in the U.K., China and Japan (Dodson *et al.*, 1981).

PIG INSULIN
Main-Chain Structure
The folding of the two-Zn insulin A and B chains is illustrated in Fig. 4.3. The A chain contains two roughly anti-parallel helical structures, which consist of amino acids A_1–A_{10} and A_{14}–A_{20}. They are connected by an extended stretch of peptide between A_{11}

and A_{13}. The B chain has a central well-defined length of α-helix between B_9 and B_{20}. At each end of this, the chain turns sharply into extended structure (B_1–B_7 and B_{22}–B_{30}).

Side-Chain Structure
Internal
All globular proteins have non-polar interiors and polar exteriors. Consequently the interior of the insulin monomer is non-polar. The side-chains which are buried, or which are in contact with the non-polar core, are shown within the skeleton of the main-chain structure in Fig. 4.4.

INSULIN SIDE-CHAIN STRUCTURE

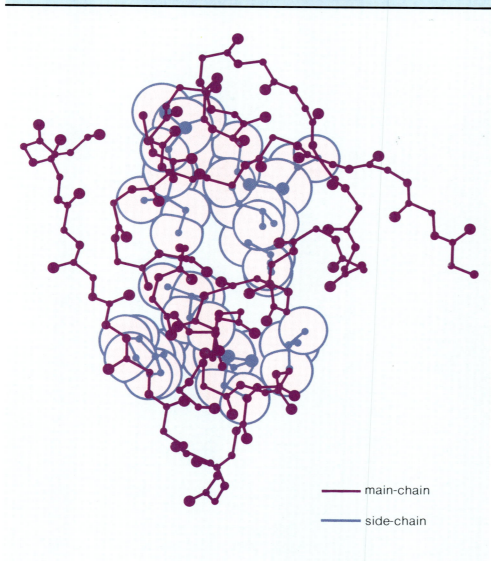

—— main-chain

—— side-chain

Fig. 4.4 Internal side-chain structure in the pig insulin molecule. The buried side-chain groups are shown with their van der Waals radii represented as spheres. The side-chains are all non-polar.

The surface of the insulin monomer contains two distinct non-polar surfaces involved in dimer and in hexamer formation. The view perpendicular to the dimer-forming surface is shown in Fig. 4.5. It is possible to see how the non-polar side-chains and extended main-chain atoms are organized together to form the framework for a well-defined surface which is buried by the formation of the dimer. The more polar regions form the surface of the hexamer.

The non-polar surfaces which are buried by the formation of the two-Zn insulin hexamer (see Fig. 4.2) are shown in Fig. 4.6. The A chain polar surface residues and the B chain residues, B_5, B_7, B_{21}, B_{22} and B_{27}–B_{30}, are not involved in aggregation to the hexamer and are on the surface. There is no secondary structure developed on hexamer formation, which is in contrast to the β-sheet formed on dimer formation, and only weak H-bonds are present. The complete atomic structure of the insulin monomer viewed in the direction of the local twofold axis is shown in Fig. 4.7.

Monomer Structure

The two molecules in the dimer (the asymmetric unit of the crystal in two-Zn insulin) show small but distinct differences. These are most marked at the A chain N terminus and the B chain C terminus (Fig. 4.8).

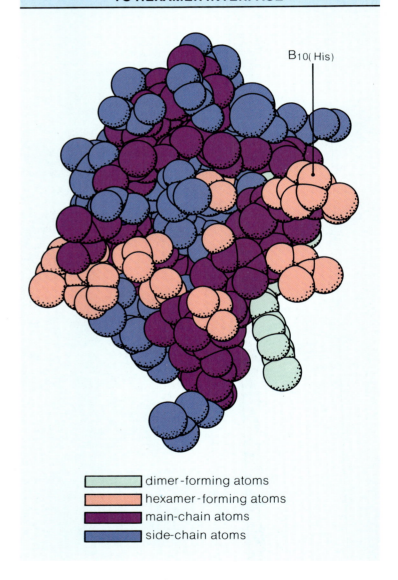

INSULIN STRUCTURE VIEWED PERPENDICULARLY TO DIMER INTERFACE	**INSULIN STRUCTURE VIEWED PERPENDICULARLY TO HEXAMER INTERFACE**

B_{10}(His)

dimer-forming atoms
hexamer-forming atoms
main-chain atoms
side-chain atoms

dimer-forming atoms
hexamer-forming atoms
main-chain atoms
side-chain atoms

Fig. 4.5 Insulin molecule viewed perpendicularly to the dimer-forming surface. Each atom is drawn as a sphere representing its van der Waals radius (the non-bonded contact distance). The surface of the molecule is shown with its proper shape and structure. When formed, the dimer is stabilized by anti-parallel, β-sheet, H-bonding contacts.

Fig. 4.6 Insulin molecule viewed perpendicularly to the hexamer-forming surface (perpendicular to O–Q in Fig. 4.2). Each atom is drawn as a sphere representing its van der Waals radius. There are both hydrophilic and hydrophobic residues involved in hexamer formation. The zinc coordination is via the hydrophilic B_{10} histidine and water molecules.

INSULIN STRUCTURE

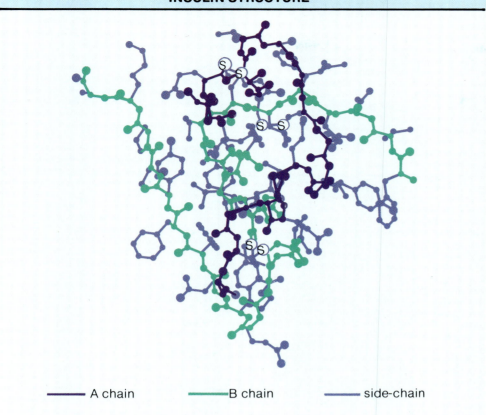

Fig. 4.7 Complete structure of the insulin molecule showing all atomic positions.

— A chain   — B chain   — side-chain

TWO-Zn INSULIN DIMER STRUCTURE

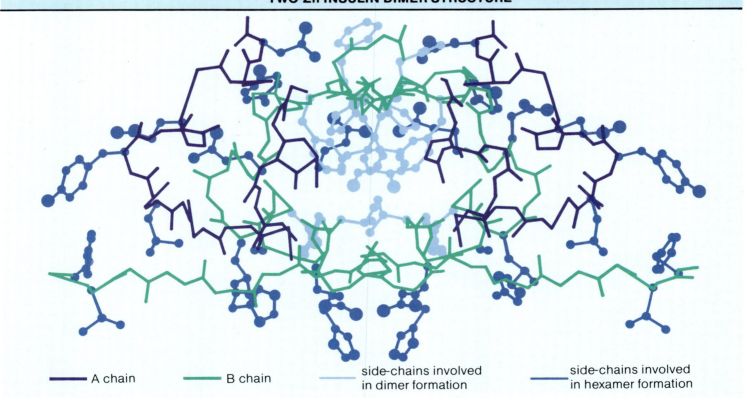

— A chain   — B chain   — side-chains involved in dimer formation   — side-chains involved in hexamer formation

Fig. 4.8 Insulin dimer from the two-Zn insulin hexamer viewed down the direction of the threefold crystal axis. There are minor but significant differences in the structure of the two molecules at A_1–A_5, B_{29} and B_{30}. Only the residues buried by dimer and hexamer formation are shown.

The structural changes in the A chain N terminus bring about some different internal interactions. The folding of the main chain structure in both of the two-Zn molecules is shown in Fig. 4.9a. In addition to the changes in the A chain N terminal helix, B_{25} phenylalanine and residues B_{28}–B_{30} take different conformations. Much larger structural changes are present in the closely related four-Zn insulin crystal (Fig. 4.9b).

The variations found in the structure of insulin in the different crystals raise questions about the molecule's structure when free in solution as a monomer. It has been possible, however, to determine the crystal structure of the monomer. One particular conformation (molecule 1 in Fig. 4.9) found in all the insulin crystal forms studied so far, is strikingly similar to that of the insulin monomer in the crystal.

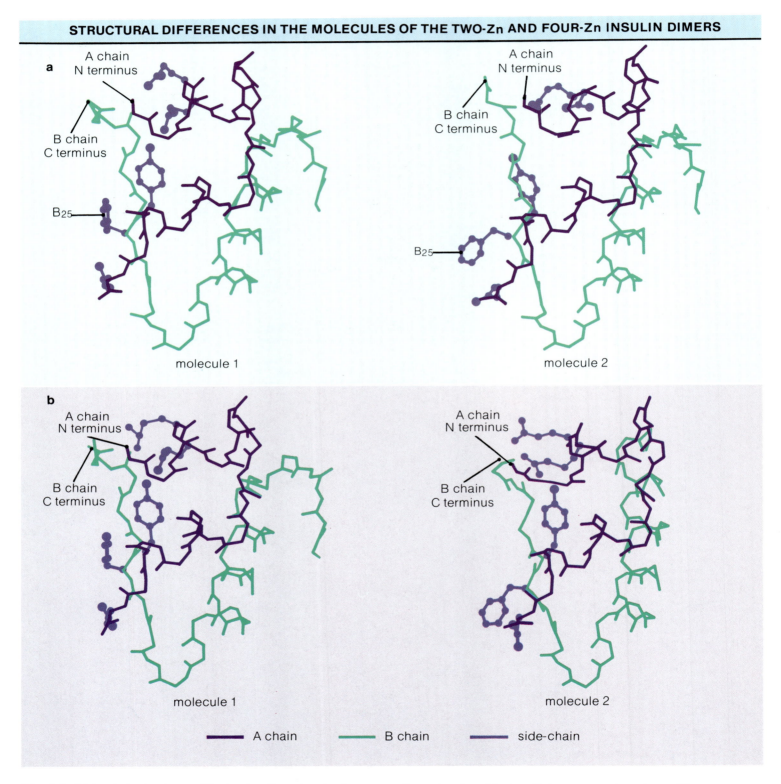

STRUCTURAL DIFFERENCES IN THE MOLECULES OF THE TWO-Zn AND FOUR-Zn INSULIN DIMERS

a

A chain N terminus

B chain C terminus

B_{25}

molecule 1

A chain N terminus

B chain C terminus

B_{25}

molecule 2

b

A chain N terminus

B chain C terminus

molecule 1

A chain N terminus

B chain C terminus

molecule 2

—— A chain   —— B chain   —— side-chain

Fig. 4.9 Main-chain structures of the two insulin molecules from the dimers of (a) the two-Zn insulin hexamer and (b) the four-Zn insulin hexamer. There are small but significant differences between the molecules of the two-Zn hexamer and very large differences between the molecules of the four-Zn hexamer.

HUMAN INSULIN

Human insulin has an amino acid sequence slightly different to that of pig insulin which has been widely used in the treatment of diabetes (see Fig. 4.1). In human insulin, the B chain C terminal residue, B_{30}, is threonine; in pig and beef insulin it is alanine. There are also two additional amino acid differences between beef insulin and human (and also pig) insulin in the A chain. The structure of human insulin, however, has been analysed carefully, because of its lower antigenicity.

A comparison of the accurately refined human and pig two-Zn insulin crystal structures reveals that the two species are essentially identical. This can be seen in Fig. 4.10 which compares the two complete dimer structures. There are significant differences of more than 0.3A only at B_{30}, where the amino acid

HUMAN AND PIG INSULIN STRUCTURES

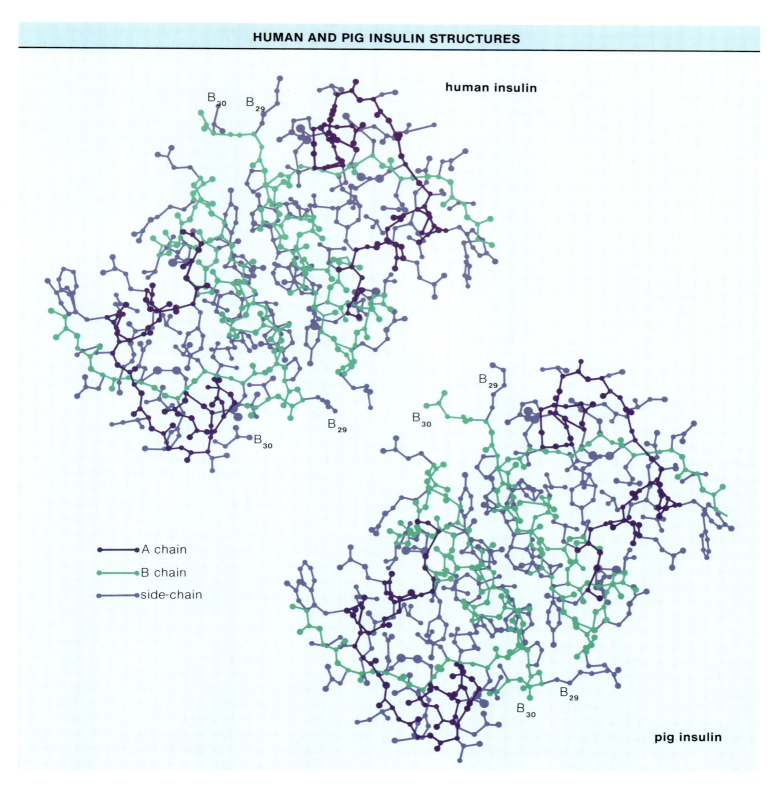

A chain
B chain
side-chain

Fig. 4.10 Structure of the dimers from human and pig two-Zn insulin hexamers viewed in the direction of the local twofold axis. The very close similarity in structure is clear.

change occurs, and in the adjacent lysine at B_{29}. The extra bulk and the H-bonding capacity of the threonyl hydroxyl group in human insulin results in restructuring of the water molecules surrounding the B_{30} side-chain. These structural changes are not significant in terms of the hormone's biological activity. However, they may affect the molecule's packing in the crystal which involves contacts at B_{29} and B_{30}. The small, but distinct, differences in the behaviour of human and pig two-Zn insulin crystals probably stem from these different interactions between the hexamer structures in the crystal lattice.

STRUCTURE AND BIOLOGICAL ACTIVITY OF INSULIN

A survey of the forty or so known insulin sequences in various species reveals that there is a group of residues common to them all. Those invariant residues which are on the hormone surface (Fig. 4.11), and which actually form a distinct region, are possibly involved in interactions between insulin and its receptor. Both A and B chain residues are involved and some of these are also present on the dimer-forming surface.

The indications from sequence variation concerning the binding region in insulin have been supported, to some extent, by chemical studies. For example, many modifications of the surface invariant residues reduce insulin's potency but they also disturb its three-dimensional structure. However, no simple chemical modification of a side-chain has yet been produced in which the action of insulin is abolished without any significant disturbance of its structure. Such a modification would of course lead to the identification of the side-chains critically involved in the expression of activity.

One modification that does apparently remove activity without altering the molecule's three-dimensional structure is a short cross-link between the α-amino group of A_1, and the B chain C terminus. Thus it seems that the interaction between the insulin molecule and its receptor is a complex one, possibly requiring structural changes in the hormone. The ability to undergo these changes properly may be necessary for high potency. This would explain the effects of chemical modification which only reduce potency but which do not abolish activity altogether. Finally, it may be that the flexibility exhibited by the insulin molecule in the crystal is a reflection of the structural changes it undergoes in binding to its receptor.

Recently, a des-B_{30} insulin, cross-linked at A_1–B_{29} through its main-chain, has been shown to be without biological activity. This single chain insulin crystallizes and has a three-dimensional structure very similar to the native hormone. Its inactivity suggests the residues at the B chain C terminus must move away before, or during, binding to the receptor.

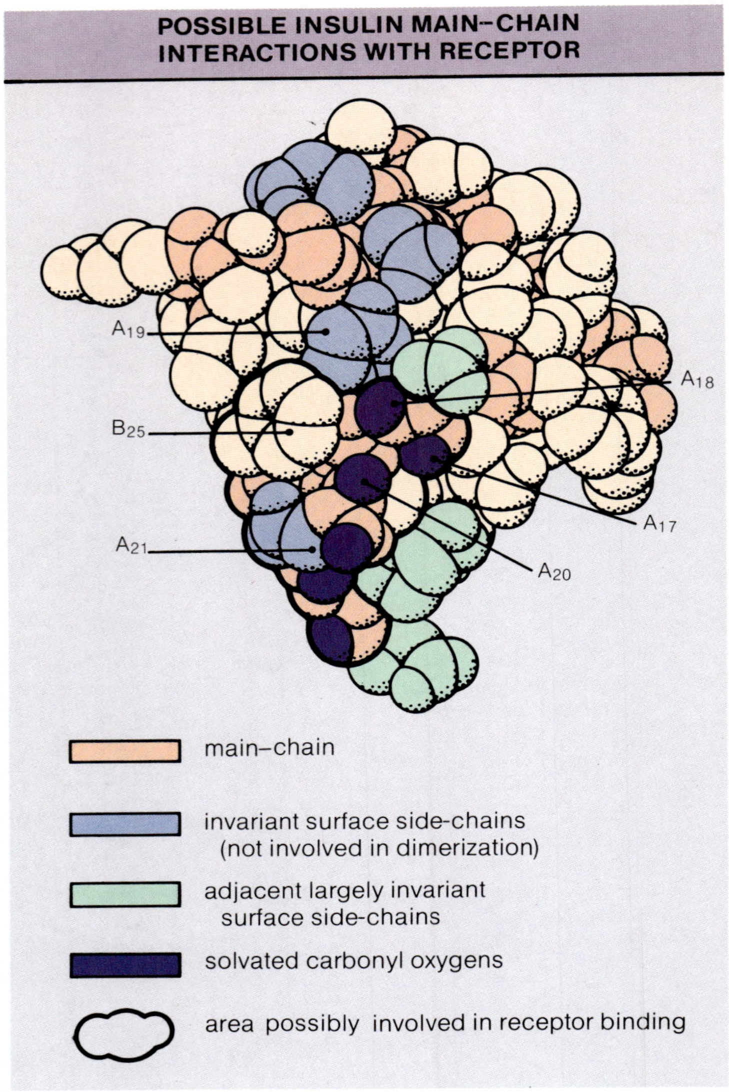

POSSIBLE INSULIN MAIN–CHAIN INTERACTIONS WITH RECEPTOR

main–chain

invariant surface side-chains (not involved in dimerization)

adjacent largely invariant surface side-chains

solvated carbonyl oxygens

area possibly involved in receptor binding

Fig. 4.11 Insulin molecule receptor site. The molecule is shown here viewed in the direction of the dimer local axis with the dimer-forming surface on the left. Atoms are represented by their van der Waals radii. The invariant residues on the surface are indicated. There is evidence that the region about and including the carbonyl oxygens of A_{17}, A_{18} and A_{20} is involved in receptor binding and the subsequent biological activity of the molecule.

REFERENCES

Baker EN, Blundell TL, Cutfield JF, Cutfield SM, Dodson EJ, Dodson GG, Hodgkin DC, Hubbard RE, Isaacs NW, Reynolds CD, Sakabe K, Sakabe N & Vijayan M (in press). The structure of 2 Zn pig insulin crystals at 1.5Å resolution. *Philosophical Transactions of the Royal Society of London*.

Blundell TL, Dodson GG, Hodgkin DC & Mercola DA (1972) Insulin: the structure in the crystal and its reflection in chemistry and biology. *Advances in Protein Chemistry*, **26**, 279–402.

Chothia C, Lesk A, Dodson G & Hodgkin D (1983) Transmission of conformational change in insulin. *Nature*, **302**, 500–505.

Dodson GG, Glusker J & Sayre D eds (1981) Section V. Insulin: biology, chemistry and structure. In *Structural Studies on Molecules of Biological Interest*, pp.407–590. Oxford: Oxford University Press.

5 Insulin Action and Metabolism

Richard H Jones MA MB BChir FRCP

GENERAL CONSIDERATIONS

In a normal individual, insulin is continuously present in physiologically active concentrations. Complete insulin withdrawal, for example, by pancreatectomy, results in a profound metabolic disturbance within hours. It can be calculated that a subject of normal weight secretes approximately 50u (2mg or 340nmol) of insulin per day, giving a lifetime requirement of about 9mmol (50g). Throughout life the modulation of secretion rate and of pathways of deactivation maintains the metabolic balance between hypoglycaemia and excessive circulating and tissue concentrations of many energy substrates.

The overall fuel economy of the body depends upon an immensely complex interaction of neurological and humoral pathways which are far from completely understood, but the dominant position of insulin in this system is undisputed. It is clear that the increase in insulin secretion upon the ingestion of food both reduces the production and release of metabolic substrates from tissue stores and ensures appropriate uptake and disposal of the nutrients absorbed by the gut.

A summary of the major influences of insulin on substrate balance is given in Figs 5.1 and 5.2. Hepatic glucose production, from both glycogen and gluconeogenic substrates (alanine and lactate), is markedly inhibited. Glucose uptake and oxidation is stimulated in many tissues. In muscle, synthesis of glycogen is increased and in fat cells increased production of α-glycerophosphate leads to the incorporation of glucose carbon in triglyceride (TG) stores. Glucose uptake by the liver is largely independent of the insulin concentration and may increase or fall depending on the portal vein glucose concentration. In man, the major stimulation of non-esterified fatty acid (NEFA) synthesis occurs in the liver with subsequent transfer as TG in very low density lipoprotein (VLDL) to adipose tissue. In the fat cell, activation of lipoprotein lipase increases the availability of NEFA from the circulating lipoprotein for synthesis of intracellular TG, while the lipolytic pathways are strongly inhibited.

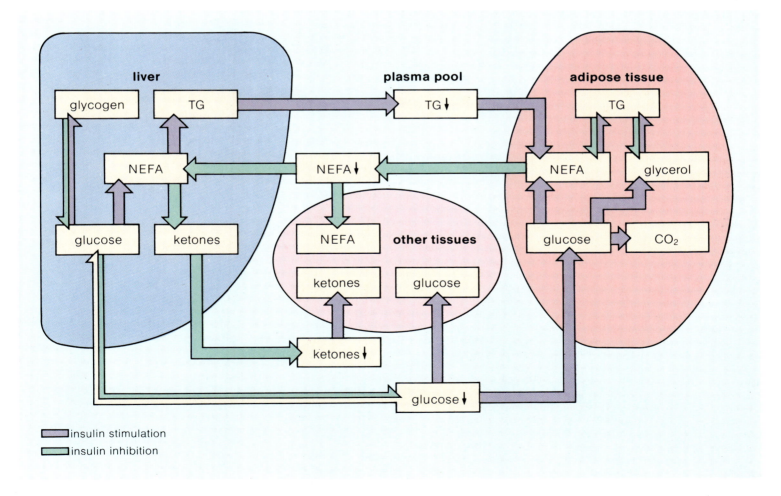

Fig. 5.1 Major effects of insulin on glucose and lipid metabolism. The effect on the plasma concentration of metabolites is indicated.

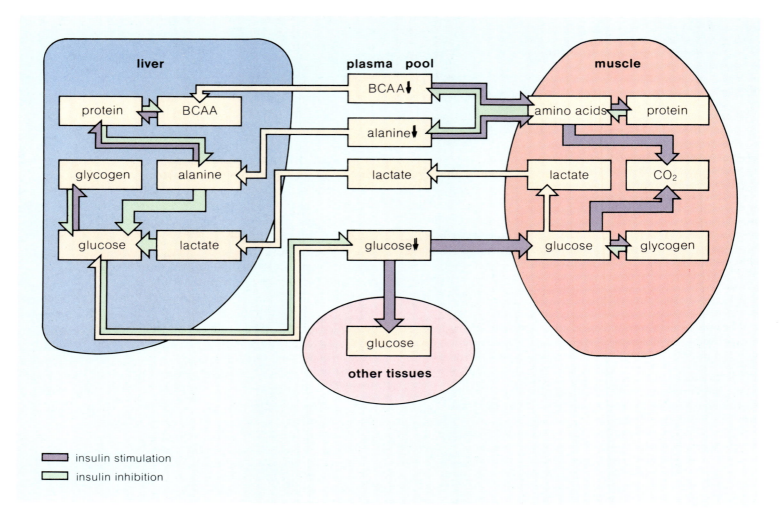

Fig. 5.2 Major effects of insulin on glucose and amino acid metabolism. Not all the pathways shown are influenced by insulin.

The effect on the plasma concentration of metabolites is indicated.

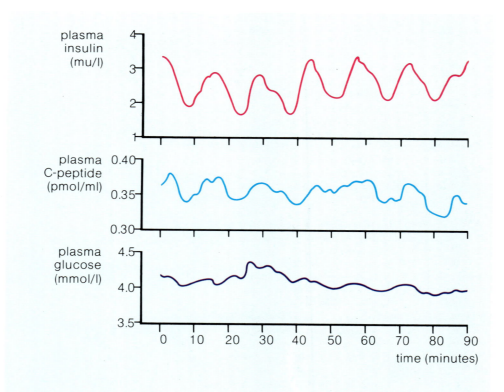

Fig. 5.3 Pulsatility of basal insulin secretion. The most marked fluctuations are apparent in portal vein insulin concentrations. In many subjects, regular oscillations in insulin concentration are detectable in peripheral blood despite the damping effect exerted by the liver. The figure shows observations made in one individual. From Lang *et al.* (1979), by courtesy of the New England Journal of Medicine.

Insulin also exerts considerable influence on protein metabolism (see Fig. 5.2). Uptake of amino acids and synthesis of protein are increased and proteolysis is inhibited. In muscle, insulin also increases oxidation of branched-chain amino acids (BCAA).

Of the many energy substrates, glucose appears to be subject to the tightest homoeostatic control. The glucose turnover rate, largely under the influence of insulin, can be increased at least sixfold after a meal, ensuring that arterial glucose concentrations remain within a very narrow range. Glucagon, growth hormone, cortisol and catecholamines all include among their many effects the ability to increase blood glucose concentration. Except in the unphysiological circumstances of hypoglycaemic stress, their patterns of secretion are not primarily determined by glucose concentration, indicating a less than dominant role for these hormones in glucose homoeostasis.

In the basal state, a careful analysis of plasma insulin concentrations, by methods which eliminate noise from the data, indicates a rhythmic periodicity in the rate of secretion, which is probably caused by a degree of pulsatility; pulses occur with a cycle time of approximately thirteen minutes in normal man (Fig. 5.3). The observation of a tendency to glucose fluctuations, with the same frequency but approximately two minutes in advance of the insulin cycle, may indicate that such pulsatility is merely a property of the servo mechanism which relates insulin secretion to glucose concentration. Alternatively it may represent the existence of an endogenous pancreatic pacemaker for insulin secretion, independent of any external stimulus. After ingestion of food a number of stimuli to the pancreatic B cells, described in detail in *Chapter 2*, combine to induce a rapid increase in insulin secretion. The concentration rises rapidly to a peak between thirty and sixty minutes, returning steadily to basal values when intestinal absorption is complete (see *Chapter 1*).

The volume of distribution and the pathways of metabolism have a major influence on the concentration of insulin reaching the target tissues. A worked example is shown in Fig. 5.4. If it is assumed that in one minute the pancreas secretes a pulse of 60mu of insulin into a portal flow of 1500ml of blood, the concentration reaching the liver will be 40mu/l above the concentration in the splanchnic veins. At least forty per cent of the insulin is removed in its first pass through the liver, resulting in a delivery of an additional 36mu/min into the systemic circulation. This can only result in a rise of insulin concentration at peripheral sites of 6mu/l above the basal arterial level.

Fig. 5.5 shows the insulin concentrations in the portal vein and hepatic vein and artery following a glucose load in normal dogs. It is clear that the liver is exposed to a considerably greater concentration of insulin than any other tissue. This illustration, although crudely adequate, involves a number of over-simplifications. First, the final concentration of insulin reaching, for example, a muscle or fat cell, will be determined not only by blood flow rate, that is cardiac output, but also by other elements of the distribution space (or plasma volume), the permeability of capillary membranes to insulin and by its further dilution in the extravascular extracellular space. In addition, the important role of metabolism, or the destruction of the hormone, in influencing final concentrations at the cellular level has been ignored. Removal by glomerular filtration, for example, will reduce the quantity of the hormone effectively delivered and local degradation by the tissues themselves could potentially exert a powerful influence on the amount reaching the receptors.

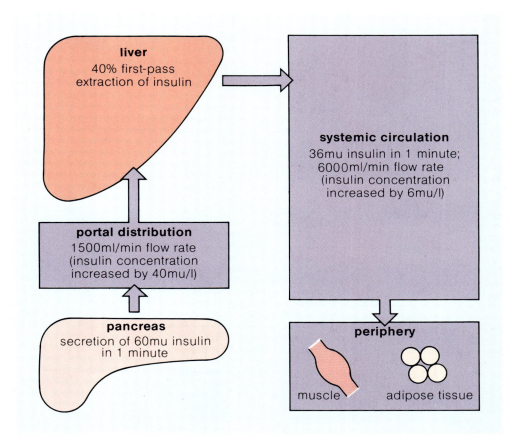

Fig. 5.4 Influence of insulin distribution on tissue exposure to endogenous insulin. The combined effects of portal delivery and first-pass hepatic extraction lead to an increase in the peripheral insulin concentration which is considerably less than the increment to which the liver is exposed.

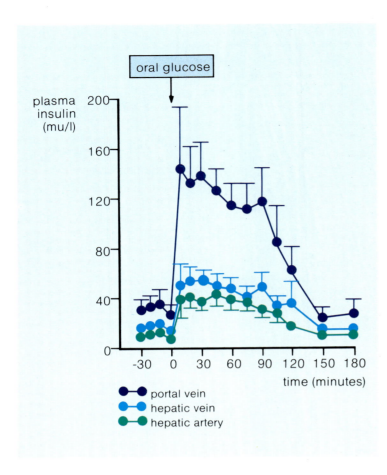

Fig. 5.5 Plasma insulin concentrations before and after oral glucose (1 g/kg body weight) in nine normal conscious dogs. The portal vein levels are approximately three times higher than the arterial levels both in the basal state and after oral glucose. The magnitude of hepatic extraction is apparent in the difference between the portal and hepatic venous plasma concentrations (mean ±SEM). From Chap et al. (1986), by courtesy of Rockefeller University Press.

Fig. 5.6 illustrates one aspect of these mechanisms. The combination of insulin degradation in the tissue itself and a relative barrier to insulin passage across the capillary endothelium results in a lower concentration of insulin in the immediate environment of the target cell. In most tissues, the mode of transport is probably simple diffusion, but endothelial cells have been shown to translocate insulin from their intraluminal to extravascular surfaces in vesicles. This activity could further influence tissue exposure, particularly in the central nervous system or other tissues where tight junctions exist between endothelial cells.

INSULIN AT THE CELLULAR LEVEL

The use of insulin labelled with radioactive iodine led rapidly to the demonstration of specific binding sites for the hormone on the outer plasma membranes of isolated cells. The relevance of these sites to insulin action was initially unclear as they could be found in a wide variety of cell types including many not regarded as targets for insulin. Furthermore, early studies with fat cells suggested quite different dose response relationships for insulin binding and insulin action (Fig. 5.7), such that the maximum biological effect was achieved when only a small proportion of the detectable binding sites was occupied.

It is now established that such insulin binding is indeed related to biological action. The most convincing evidence comes from many studies involving insulins either from different animal species or which have been chemically modified. Reduction or abolition of binding potency has in every case been associated with an equivalently reduced insulin effectiveness. Particularly convincing is the case of turkey insulin, which both possesses an increased ability to displace radiolabelled mammalian insulins from cells or membranes and is in addition more biologically potent than other insulins *in vitro*.

Fig. 5.6 Influence of endothelial permeability and local degradation of insulin on the concentration of insulin at the surface of the target cell.

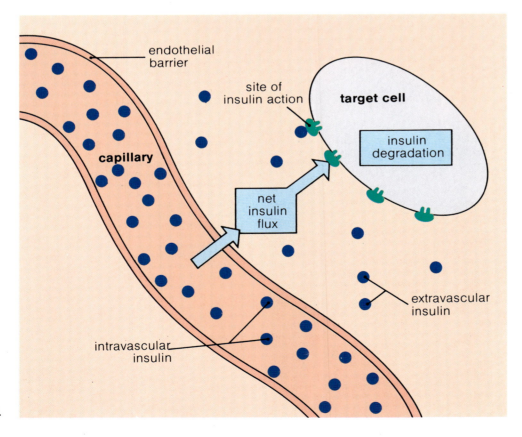

Why then are the dose response relationships of binding and action so different? Several possible explanations have emerged. First, as previously indicated, the liver and peripheral tissues are exposed, under normal circumstances, to widely different concentrations of insulin. The effects of insulin on hepatic metabolism, although of major importance, have been more difficult to study *in vitro* than the influence of the hormone on adipocyte metabolism.

However, recent evidence suggests that in the liver the range of concentrations which affects, for example, amino acid uptake, is more closely related to the number of occupied receptors than is the case in peripheral tissues. The implication, as illustrated in Fig. 5.8, is that modulation of hepatic response and of peripheral response to insulin is tuned to the range of concentrations to which these tissues are exposed under physiological conditions.

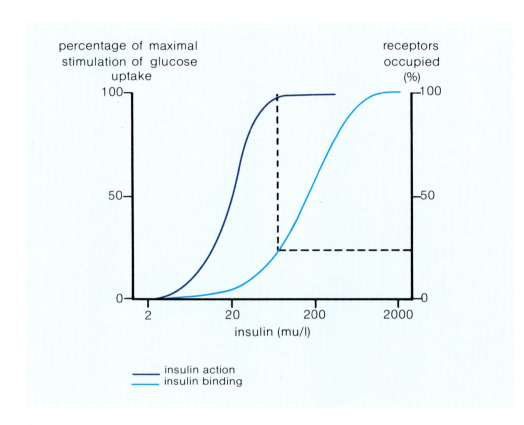

Fig. 5.7 Dose response curves for insulin action on adipocytes. Full activity is achieved with twenty-five per cent of the receptor number occupied. The degree to which receptor number exceeds that required to stimulate fully the metabolic responses of the cell varies in different tissues. In peripheral target cells, the binding of insulin is not the rate-limiting step.

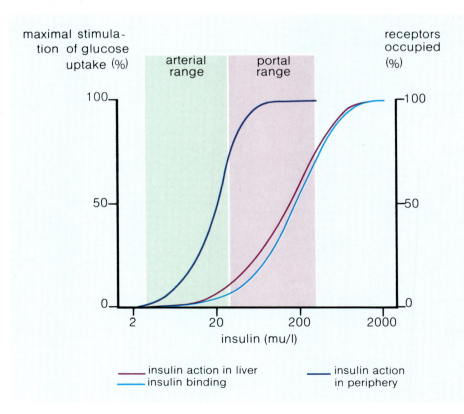

Fig. 5.8 Dose response curves for insulin action in the liver. Hepatic response to insulin is more closely related to the dose response curve for binding than the response in the periphery. In both cases, the sensitivity of the tissue is appropriate for the range of insulin concentrations to which it is exposed.

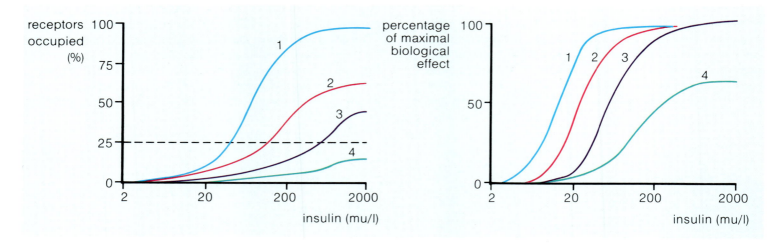

Fig. 5.9 Theoretical curves to illustrate one of the implications of 'spare' insulin receptors. The initial relationship between binding and action is defined such that a maximal effect is achieved with twenty-five per cent of the receptors occupied by insulin (curve 1). This represents the condition illustrated in Fig. 5.7, that is full activity at twenty-five per cent receptor occupancy. Curves 2–4 demonstrate the effects on binding and biological action of progressive decrements in receptor number. In curves 2 and 3, the total number of receptors exceeds twenty-five per cent of the original total so that a sufficient number can still be occupied to achieve a full effect; there is no loss of responsiveness. The response curves for action are, however, shifted to the right indicating a loss of tissue sensitivity to insulin. Only if the total receptor number falls below twenty-five per cent of the original (curve 4) is there a loss of maximal activity (responsiveness) as well as sensitivity.

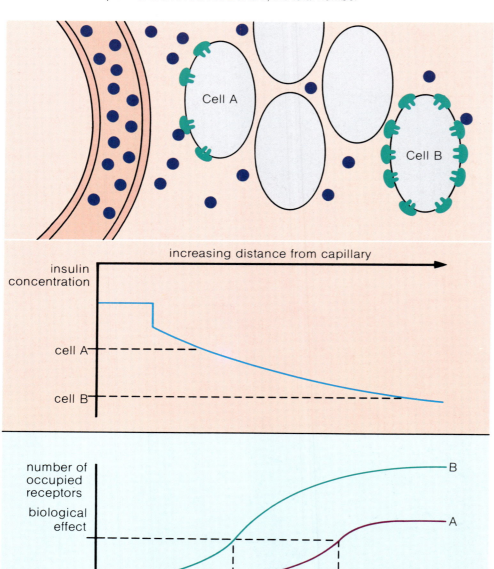

Fig. 5.10 Effect of insulin concentration on cell surface receptor number. The upper diagram and graph show the gradient of insulin concentration that exists with increasing distance from the capillary. The lower graph illustrates how, by modulating the number of receptors in the plasma membrane, each cell can manifest a similar biological effect. The development of an inverse relationship between ambient hormone concentration and cell surface receptor number is termed 'down-regulation'.

Secondly, it is clear that there are important actions of insulin other than the rapid metabolic effects with which it is primarily associated. It also has important actions on cell growth and development which are relatively slow in onset and which may be more closely related to receptor occupancy over a greater range than, for example, the increase in glucose transport.

Thirdly, the condition illustrated in Fig. 5.7 allows a change in the number of receptors on the cell surface to occur without loss of the maximal responsiveness to insulin. The effect of such a change is illustrated diagrammatically in Fig. 5.9.

A number of factors may influence cell receptor number and may be involved in some types of pathological insulin resistance. One factor is insulin itself. High ambient insulin concentrations induce a reduction in the number of insulin receptors, a phenomenon known as down-regulation. A possible physiological role for this effect is illustrated in Fig. 5.10. It can be seen that cells adjacent to a capillary will be exposed to relatively higher concentrations of insulin than those deeper in the tissue. By down-regulation, the response of each cell in the tissue to a given circulating insulin concentration could be similar in spite of this tissue gradient.

Finally, it is now understood that insulin degradation is initiated by receptor binding and that this process is proportional to receptor occupancy. The number of insulin receptors required by an organism may be influenced by factors related to the termination of the insulin signal as well as factors which give an appropriate magnitude of metabolic response to the hormone. Whatever the reasons, it would appear that, at least in adipose tissue, the sequence of biochemical steps which leads from insulin's interaction with the receptor to the final measured metabolic response, the initial binding event, is not the rate-limiting step.

The Insulin Receptor

Recognition that the experimentally observed specific sites for insulin are indeed linked to insulin action justifies their designation as insulin receptors and has led to intense exploration of their structure and properties. The intact receptor (Fig. 5.11) is a glycoprotein with an approximate molecular weight of 400,000 daltons consisting of four glycosylated polypeptide chains covalently linked by disulphide bonds. The molecule is a dimer consisting of two α-subunits (MW approximately 120,000 daltons), which include binding sites for insulin, and two β-subunits (MW approximately 80,000 daltons), which are involved in initiating at least some of the actions of insulin. In some tissues, one or more functions of the receptor may require association of the complex with other polypeptides, possibly by hydrophobic rather than covalent bonding. Recently, such association has been reported with class I antigens of the major histocompatibility complex and other possible candidates will be considered below.

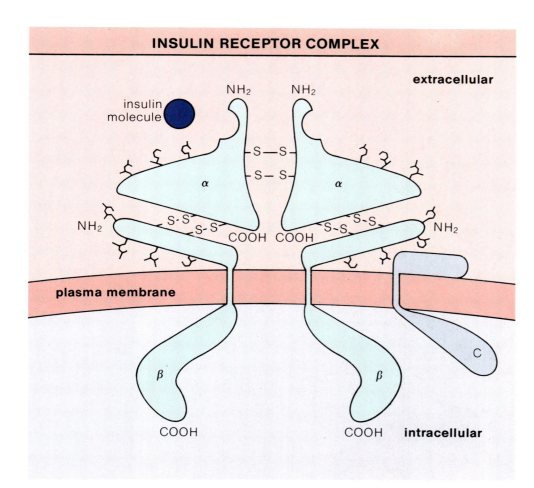

INSULIN RECEPTOR COMPLEX

Fig. 5.11 Insulin receptor complex. The α-subunits are entirely extracellular but the β-subunits have an intracellular and an extracellular domain. The α- and β-subunits are linked by disulphide bonds as are the two halves of the heterodimeric complex. The α-subunit is approximately twenty times the size of its ligand, insulin. The possibility of important interactions with other membrane proteins by non-covalent bonding is represented by the structure 'C'. The shapes of the subunits, spatial relationships between them, positions of the insulin-binding and glycosylation sites and number and positions of the disulphide bonds are imaginary.

Recently two separate groups have successfully isolated and sequenced the human cDNA which codes for the insulin receptor precursor. There appears to be only one copy of this sequence in the human genome located on the short arm of chromosome 19 (Fig. 5.12). The gene codes for a linear sequence of 1382 amino acids comprising a signal peptide of twenty-seven residues, the α-subunit (735 residues), which ends with a cleavage site of four basic amino acids (Arg-Lys-Arg-Arg) and the β-subunit (620 residues). Examination of the sequence has revealed a number of important functional domains. Only the β-subunit contains a run of hydrophobic residues capable of spanning the plasma membrane implying that after insertion the α-subunit is entirely extracellular. It has long been known that the α-subunit includes the site responsible for the binding of insulin, but until more is known of the folding and cross-linking of the peptide no such site can be identified. One particular region of the α-subunit, residues 155–312, is particularly rich in cysteine units suggesting that the tertiary structure may depend considerably on disulphide bonds. The α-subunit includes thirteen potential asparagine-linked glycosylation sites and the β-subunit, four such sites on the N-terminal, or extracellular, side of the transmembrane sequence. The intracellular segment of the β-subunit has been shown to include an ATP binding site, residues known to be associated with phosphokinase activity in other proteins and regions with considerable homology with a group of oncogene products. Both the α- and β-chains reveal a number of similarities with the receptor for epidermal growth factor (EGF).

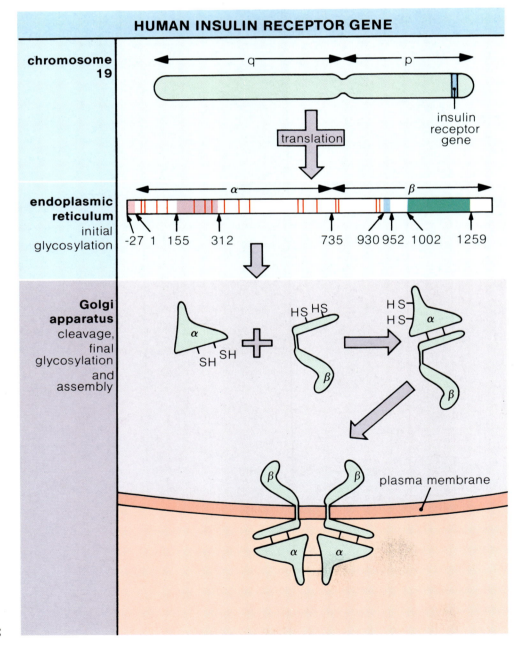

HUMAN INSULIN RECEPTOR GENE

Fig. 5.12 Human insulin receptor gene. It is located between positions 13.2 and 13.3 on the short arm of chromosome 19. After translation of a single chain receptor precursor, initial glycosylation occurs in the endoplasmic reticulum. Cleavage into the α- and β-chains, their combination into monomers and their glycosylation are completed in the Golgi apparatus. The precursor protein has an initial amino acid signal peptide (−27 to −1) and there is a cysteine-rich region in the α-subunit (155–312). In the β-subunit, the hydrophobic transmembrane sequence runs from 930–952 and tyrosine kinase activity occurs at 1002–1259. The single red vertical lines represent positions of potential asparagine-linked glycosylation. Some or all of the final association into heterodimers may require insertion into the plasma membrane.

The peptide molecular weights of the initial α and β sequences, 84,214 and 69,703 daltons respectively, are both considerably less than those of the processed subunits, indicating a major degree of glycosylation before final insertion into the plasma membrane. At least some of this glycosylation appears to occur in the endoplasmic reticulum during translation and before transfer to the Golgi apparatus, where the peptide is cleaved into the α- and β-chains and where final glycosylation occurs. Either before or during insertion into the plasma membrane, many but perhaps not all of the disulphide linked α-β units are combined in pairs to form complete α_2-β_2 heterodimeric complexes.

Insulin Action

The association of insulin with its receptor results in transmission of a signal or signals to the cell interior and can lead to the destruction of the hormone. The mechanisms of these processes and the relationships between them are still largely unknown despite the fact that an understanding of them has been and remains a major goal of cell biology. There is a strong possibility that the established kinase activity of the receptor β-subunit is integrally concerned with at least some aspects of signal transmission. Binding of insulin to the α-subunit leads specifically to activation of the kinase and phosphorylation of one or more tyrosine residues also in the β-subunit (autophosphorylation). This process is associated with phosphorylation of one or more substrates within the cell, predominantly phosphorylation of serine residues. It is not clear whether this serine kinase activity is intrinsic to the β-subunit or involves the activation of a separate but associated serine kinase (Fig. 5.13).

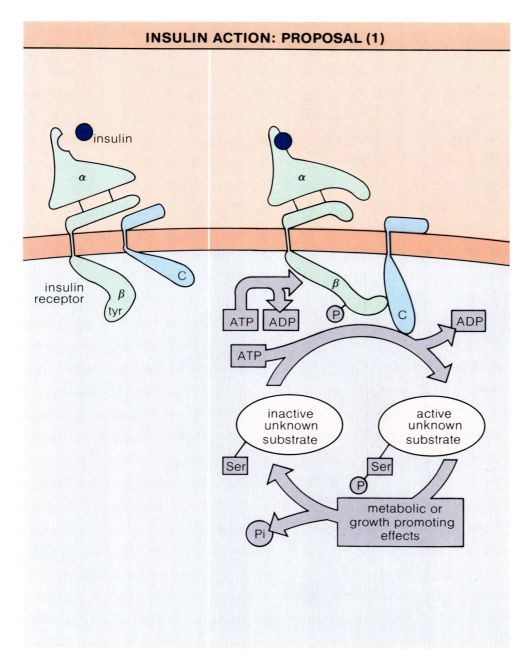

INSULIN ACTION: PROPOSAL (1)

Fig. 5.13 Insulin action: proposal (1). Representation of the insulin receptor as a tyrosine kinase. Association of insulin with its receptor causes a conformational change which allows the tyrosine kinase of the β-subunit to autophosphorylate one or more of its own tyrosine residues. The activated receptor as represented here stimulates a separate serine kinase (C) in the membrane to phosphorylate a serine residue of an unknown cytoplasmic substrate. This change either activates or disinhibits intracellular pathways sensitive to the action of insulin.

Many of the insulin-induced changes in intracellular enzyme activity are associated with changes in their degree of phosphorylation. It is an attractive concept that this newly but clearly established function of the insulin receptor may initiate a cascade of phosphorylation steps leading to the metabolic effects of insulin. However, evidence that this may be too simple an idea is beginning to emerge. It has been reported that some anti-insulin receptor antibodies are capable of exerting insulin-like effects but do not activate the receptor kinase. It may be that the kinase activity, in common with similar activity of EGF receptors, is related to the growth promoting activities of insulin rather than the metabolic effects.

A number of proposals for mechanisms of insulin action have involved the generation of relatively small molecular weight materials which could act as 'second messengers' for the hormonal signal within the cell.

It has been suggested that receptor occupancy could result, by proteolysis, in the generation of one or more active peptides either from the receptor itself or from an unknown substrate (Fig. 5.14). Attempts to substantiate this proposal by isolation and full characterization of such peptides have not yet succeeded, in spite of intense effort, casting increasing doubt upon their existence.

Many hormone and neurotransmitter receptors, when activated by their ligands, interact with proteins which can bind the nucleotide, guanosine triphosphate (GTP). The best characterized of these 'G' proteins either stimulate or inhibit the enzyme, adenylate cyclase, with consequent changes in cyclic AMP levels.

Although insulin induces a fall in tissue cyclic AMP, it is clear that insulin action is not adequately explained by this effect alone. There is increasing evidence that other 'G' proteins exist with the potential for targets other than adenylate cyclase. The possibility that a subunit of such a protein could constitute a second messenger for insulin is illustrated in Fig. 5.15.

Many hormones and neurotransmitters whose effects are mediated by an increase in cytosolic calcium have been shown to activate phospholipase C. This enzyme catalyses the hydrolysis of the membrane phospholipid, phosphatidylinositol, 4,5-bisphosphate to yield inositol trisphosphate (IP_3) and diacylglycerol (DAG), both of which may act as second messengers within the cell. Insulin has been shown to increase the phospholipid substrate for this hydrolysis and to increase levels of diacylglycerol. However, with insulin the increases in IP_3 are either very transient or do not occur. It has recently been proposed that insulin acts through an analogous stimulation of a different membrane phospholipase specific for glycolipid in which the phosphoinositol moiety is linked to carbohydrate. The products of this hydrolysis are diacylglycerol and a complex carbohydrate–phosphate material containing inositol and glucosamine, potentially capable of mediating some of the actions of insulin (Fig. 5.16). This suggestion awaits confirmation but is attractive in that its novelty explains the difficulties previously experienced in understanding insulin action and because of its analogies with other examples of biological message transmission.

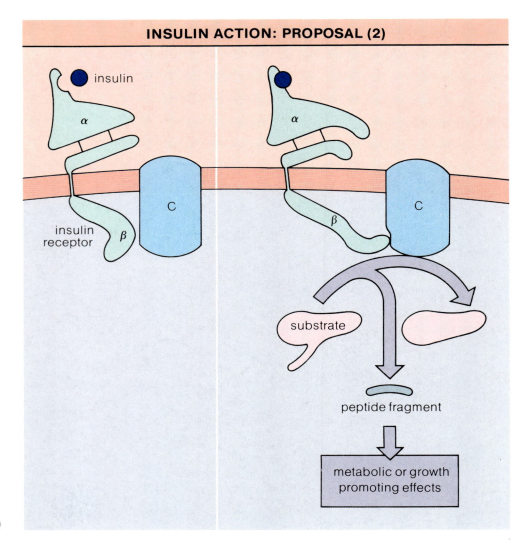

INSULIN ACTION: PROPOSAL (2)

insulin

α

α

insulin receptor

β

β

C

C

substrate

peptide fragment

metabolic or growth promoting effects

Fig. 5.14 Insulin action: proposal (2). The receptor-associated protein is represented as a protease (C) which generates a peptide second messenger after activation by the occupied receptor.

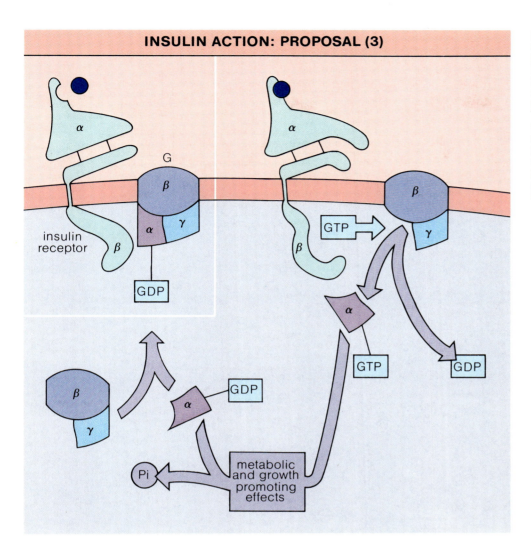

INSULIN ACTION: PROPOSAL (3)

Fig. 5.15 Insulin action: proposal (3). The activated receptor interacts with GTP-binding protein (G) and facilitates the binding of GTP and release of GDP from the nucleotide-binding site. In the GTP state, the dissociation of the G protein α-subunit from the βγ-complex results in signal generation. The α-subunit is represented here as the mobile second messenger. In exerting its action, the GTP-α subunit loses inorganic phosphate. The GDP state favours reassociation with the βγ-complex and the G protein is reconstituted. An alternative possibility is that the βγ-complex may constitute an active moiety.

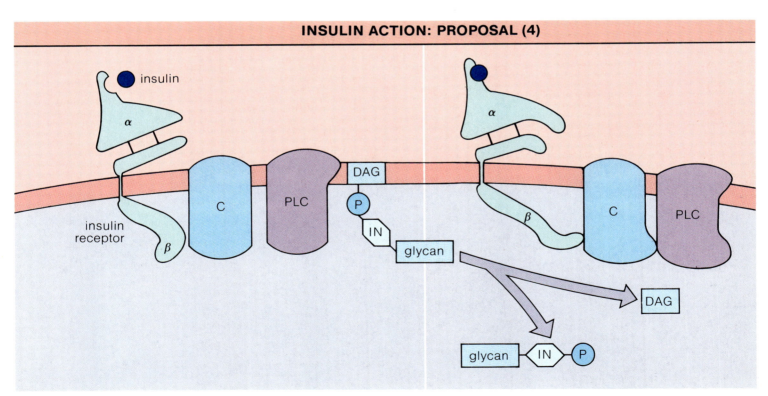

INSULIN ACTION: PROPOSAL (4)

Fig. 5.16 Insulin action: proposal (4). Activation of the insulin receptor leads to activation of a specific membrane phospholipase C (PLC), via a postulated coupling protein (C), which could itself be a G protein. The substrate of PLC, a glycolipid which contains inositol-phosphate (PIN), is hydrolysed to release diacylglycerol (DAG), itself a second messenger, and an inositol-phosphate glycan which could serve to mediate actions of insulin at intracellular sites (Saltiel et al., 1986).

The mechanisms of insulin action so far considered involve the concept that the hormonal signal could be transferred to either intracellular enzymes or organelles while the insulin receptor complex remains at the cell surface. In addition to these possibilities, it is now clearly established that the complex can be ingested by endocytosis as the first step in what has been termed the 'insulin receptor itinerary'.

Processing of the Insulin–Receptor Complex

Binding to its receptor may have one of three consequences for the insulin molecule: it may either dissociate intact from the receptor, undergo a structural change to a less active form before release or enter a pathway which results in its degradation to either small peptides or individual amino acids. Similarly the receptor component may be induced to enter a cycle which includes early structural modification and then either complete destruction or reprocessing and reinsertion at the cell surface.

The microanatomy of these processes has been established but the controlling events are not understood. Shortly after insulin binding, complexes which are initially separated cluster together in pits in the cell membrane lined on the inside surface by the protein, clathrin. Invagination of this section of the cell membrane and pinching off from the surface leads to the formation of intracellular coated vesicles in which the previously extracellular face of the receptor along with the bound insulin is contained within the lumen (Fig. 5.17). During this process and before internalization is complete some of the insulin is structurally modified and may be released from the cell; a larger proportion of the insulin remains within the cell. The partially degraded insulin

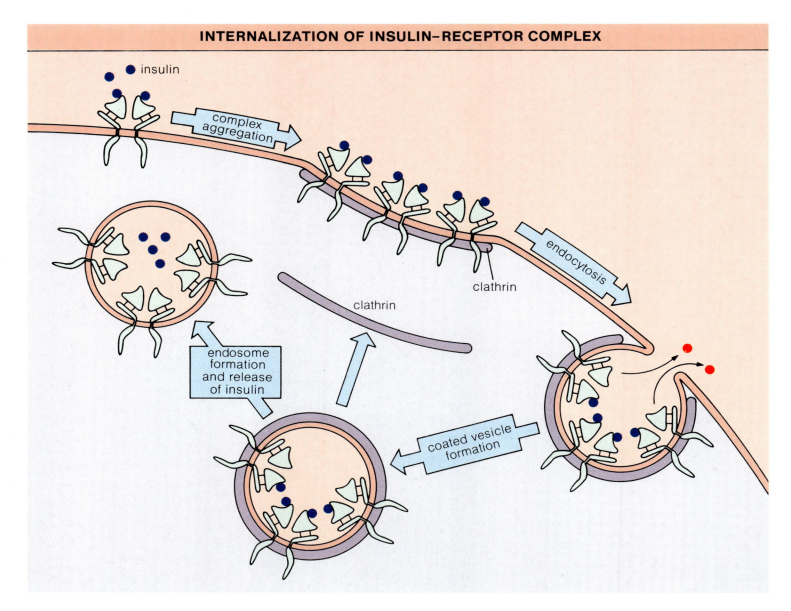

INTERNALIZATION OF INSULIN–RECEPTOR COMPLEX

insulin

complex aggregation

endocytosis

clathrin

clathrin

endosome formation and release of insulin

coated vesicle formation

Fig. 5.17 Internalization of the insulin–receptor complex. After clustering in clathrin-coated pits, invagination leads to the formation of intracellular coated vesicles. There is the possibility of partial processing and release of some of the bound insulin at this stage.

Removal of the clathrin produces a low-density uncoated vesicle, the endosome. A proton pump in this organelle lowers the pH of the lumen, inducing dissociation of the insulin–receptor complex.

retains a similar molecular weight to the hormone itself but has altered electrophoretic mobility, reduced immunoreactivity and impaired biological activity. The site or sites of cleavage have not been firmly identified but may lie near the C terminus of the insulin **B** chain. The coated vesicle loses its clathrin which is thought to return to the cell surface. The vesicle itself is now recognized as a specific intracellular organelle, the endosome, inside of which the generation of an acidic pH results in dissociation of the ligand from the receptor.

From this point the routes followed by the receptors and the now uncoupled insulin appear to diverge, with transfer of insulin to lysosomes, where its complete proteolysis subvenes, and restoration of the receptors to the cell surface, possibly after reprocessing in the Golgi apparatus. The method by which this separation occurs is not understood but its efficiency is considerable with endocytotic internalization resulting in degradation of up to two-hundred times more insulin on a molar basis than of insulin receptors (Fig. 5.18). Clearly the majority of internalized receptors are successfully recycled to the cell surface, but the degree to which receptor degradation is also increased by insulin-stimulated endocytosis may in part explain the phenomenon of down-regulation (see Fig. 5.10).

Very little if any of the internalized insulin reappears at the surface of the cell. Several intracellular enzymes have been described that are capable of actively degrading insulin, but in intact cells or tissues access to these systems is almost entirely via initial binding to the plasma membrane binding sites. As a result of this, the kinetics and specificity of insulin degradation closely reflect the kinetics and specificity of receptor binding rather than those of the intracellular enzymes ultimately responsible for the degradation process.

The insulin receptor itinerary offers further possibilities for mechanisms of insulin action. For example, there have been suggestions that some intracellular binding sites may be targets for internalized insulin, or it is possible that the endosomes with activated β-subunits on their outer surfaces could influence intracellular processes. There is little doubt that rapid metabolic responses to insulin can be initiated from the cell surface. Internalization of the insulin–receptor complex may have as its only major function the termination of the insulin signal, but it remains possible that other events of physiological importance, perhaps concerning the control of cell growth, could depend upon this process. It is still not known how insulin acts nor with any precision how the degradation process occurs. It is now clearly recognized that both action and degradation are sequelae of binding to the same population of specific recognition sites. This dual role for the receptors has important implications at the level of the whole animal or human subject.

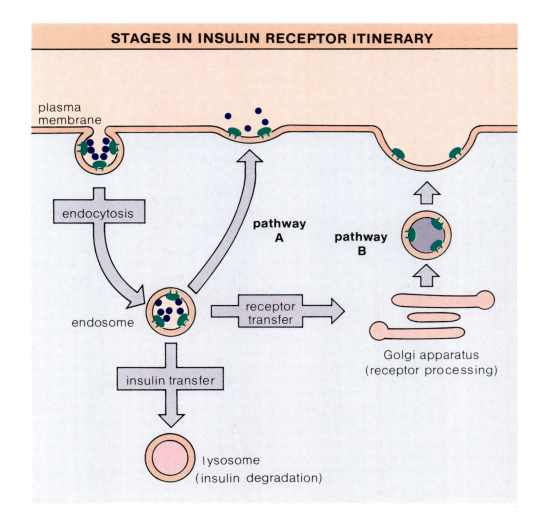

STAGES IN INSULIN RECEPTOR ITINERARY

plasma membrane

endocytosis

endosome

insulin transfer

pathway A

pathway B

receptor transfer

Golgi apparatus (receptor processing)

lysosome (insulin degradation)

Fig. 5.18 Further stages in the insulin receptor itinerary. Most of the insulin and a few of the receptors are transferred to lysosomes where they are proteolytically reduced to small peptide fragments and individual amino acids. Most of the receptors are processed in the Golgi apparatus from where, along with those that have been newly synthesized, they are returned to the plasma membrane (pathway B). A 'short loop' may exist (pathway A) which could allow a more rapid recycling and offer a further possible route for the release of partially processed insulin.

PHYSIOLOGY OF INSULIN RECEPTOR FUNCTION

There is a paradox which can be simply stated: for a given input of insulin into an intact subject, the biological effect will be a direct function of the number and affinity of binding sites, and of the concentration of insulin achieved; the concentration achieved will itself be negatively correlated with the number and affinity of binding sites. As has been shown, the time course of insulin concentration in plasma after, for example, a bolus intravenous injection, is determined by multiple factors of distribution and metabolism. An increase in receptor number will appear on analysis of time course data as both an increased distribution space, to allow for increased receptor bound insulin, and an increased clearance rate, because of the greater rate of insulin internalization. To quantify the behaviour of these interactions requires mathematical modelling techniques which are only now

beginning to reach the required level of sophistication. An example of a relatively simple model designed to incorporate these ideas is illustrated in Fig. 5.19.

It is possible even without advanced computation to appreciate the importance of this phenomenon by making relatively simple physiological observations. Figs 5.20 and 5.21 illustrate one example of this. Chemically modified insulins with widely varying affinities were infused into dogs at equimolar rates and the clearance rates and hypoglycaemic effects monitored. Fig. 5.20 shows the relationship of the rate of clearance from the plasma and previously determined *in vitro* potency. Fig. 5.21 demonstrates the effect this phenomenon has on hypoglycaemic activity. The most dramatic observation is that as the potency of an insulin is progressively reduced from one hundred per cent (native insulin) the reduced clearance permits higher concentrations sufficient to

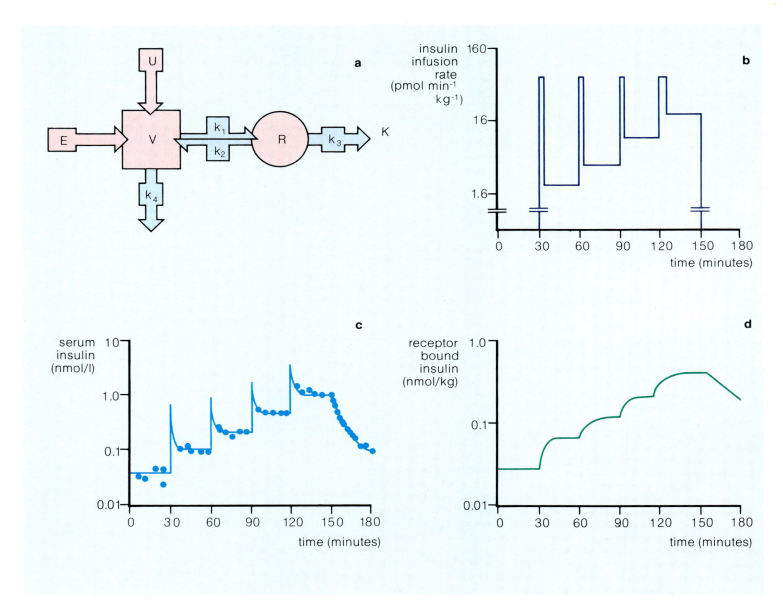

Fig. 5.19 Simple computer model of insulin distribution and metabolism. (a) endogenous insulin (E) or infused insulin (U) enters an initial, rapidly mixing compartment (V) which will include the plasma volume and a proportion of the extracellular space. The rate constants k_1 and k_2 control the rates of association (k_1) and dissociation (k_2) of insulin from a population of tissue receptors (R). Insulin may leave the system from the receptors (k_3). Pathways of removal which are not receptor dependent, for example, glomerular filtration, are accommodated in k_4. The graphs illustrate how this model can be fitted to a set of data from one normal subject infused intravenously with insulin. (b) shows the infusion rates used and the circles in (c) the measured serum concentrations. The curve in (c) is the concentration profile predicted by the model after computer optimization of the values for V, R and the rate constants. Quantification of receptor-bound insulin *in vivo* as plotted in (d) is not accessible except by modelling techniques such as these. From Jones *et al.* (1984), by courtesy of Springer Verlag.

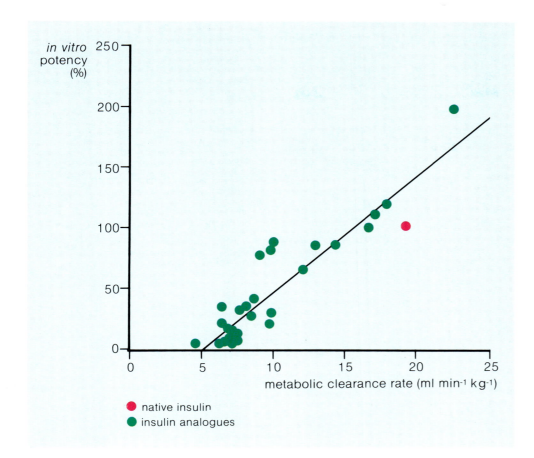

in vitro potency (%)

metabolic clearance rate (ml min⁻¹ kg⁻¹)

● native insulin
● insulin analogues

Fig. 5.20 Metabolic clearance rates of insulin and its analogues. Clearance rates were determined by infusion into dogs at a plasma concentration of 5nmol/l. Values have been plotted against the respective *in vitro* potencies of the analogues, with native insulin defined as 100% potent; the correlation is clear (r = 0.94; p<0.001). The data suggest that a clearance rate of approximately 5ml min⁻¹ kg⁻¹ is attributable to non receptor-mediated systems, but that at a plasma concentration of 0.5nmol/l (approximately 75mu/l) 80% of insulin metabolism is receptor initiated. The data point at the top right of the graph is turkey insulin which has a higher receptor affinity than mammalian insulins *in vitro* and is metabolized more quickly *in vivo* than native insulin.

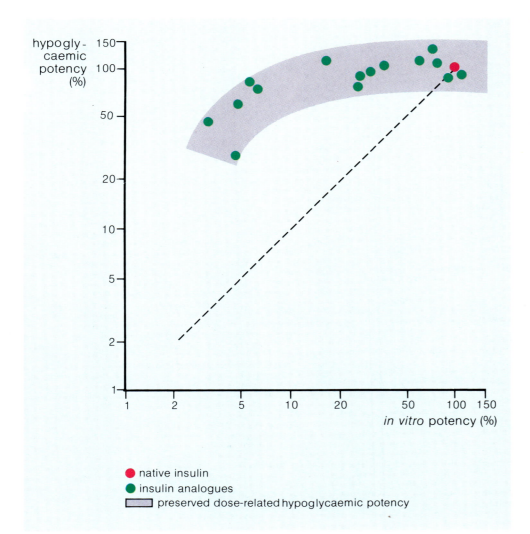

hypogly- caemic potency (%)

in vitro potency (%)

● native insulin
● insulin analogues
▨ preserved dose-related hypoglycaemic potency

Fig. 5.21 Hypoglycaemic potency of insulin and its analogues. Analogues with a variety of receptor affinities have been examined for their *in vitro* biological potencies (lipogenesis in isolated adipocytes) and on a dose-related basis for their hypoglycaemic potencies *in vivo*. The reciprocal relationship between affinity and clearance rate (see Fig. 5.20) results in the preservation of dose-related hypo-glycaemic potency over a wide range of affinities with native insulin defined as 100% potent. If hypoglycaemic potency is expressed in terms of plasma concentration rather than dose, the data points are scattered around the line of identity (broken line).

maintain a similar hypoglycaemic effect. This relationship only breaks down to a major extent when affinity has been reduced by ninety per cent.

The major influence of receptor number and affinity is not on the overall hypoglycaemic activity of a given input of insulin but rather on its time course. With a large number of high affinity receptors a pulse of insulin will produce a brisk response which is quickly terminated. Conversely, with a small number of low affinity receptors, a similar pulse will produce a slower more prolonged effect. It may be that in evolutionary terms the optimal structure of the insulin molecule and that of its receptor are not those that achieve the highest binding affinity between the two, but rather those that produce a time course of response to insulin appropriate to the feeding and exercise habits of the animal.

An additional twist to the story concerns the influence of hepatic extraction on intraportally secreted insulin. It is clear that the number of hepatic insulin receptors and the affinity of insulin for them will exert a powerful influence on the ratio of insulin concentrations between the liver and periphery. For example, a large number of very high affinity hepatic receptors may leave the periphery seriously insulin deficient. This effect has been demonstrated in reverse by studies in which a low affinity diacetyl analogue of insulin with a binding potency relative to native insulin of approximately twenty-five per cent was infused intraportally into dogs. This functional alteration resulted in a considerably reduced hepatic extraction of the analogue with a relative redistribution of both the material itself and its biological effectiveness to peripheral tissues. These arguments impinge powerfully on interpretations of pathological states such as insulin resistance with or without diabetes and the cause of diabetes in subjects with mutant insulins. Some of the major implications in pathophysiology will be reviewed in *Chapter 13*.

REFERENCES

Chap Z, Ishida T, Chou J, Hartley CJ, Entman ML, Brandenburg D, Jones RH & Field JB (1987) First-pass hepatic extraction and metabolic effects of insulin and insulin analogues. *American Journal of Physiology*, **252**, 209–217.

Chap Z, Jones RH, Chou J, Hartley CJ, Entman ML & Field JB (1986) Effect of dexamethasone on hepatic glucose and insulin metabolism after oral glucose on conscious dogs. *Journal of Clinical Investigation*, **78**, 1355–1361.

Cockram CS, Jones RH & Sönksen PH (1985) The biological properties of insulins with tyrosine replaced by phenylalanine at positions 14 and 19 of the A chain. *Diabetic Medicine*, **2**, 241–244.

Ebina Y, Ellis L, Jarnagin K, Edery M, Graf L, Clauser E, Ou J, Masiarz F, Kan YW, Goldfine ID, Roth RA & Rutter WJ (1985) The human insulin receptor cDNA: the structural basis for hormone-activated transmembrane signalling. *Cell*, **40**, 747–758.

Gammeltoft S & Van Obberghen E (1986) Protein kinase activity of the insulin receptor. *Biochemical Journal*, **235**, 1–11.

Jones RH, Sönksen PH, Boroujerdi MA & Carson ER (1984) Number and affinity of insulin receptors in intact human subjects. *Diabetologia*, **27**, 207–211.

Lang DA, Matthews DR, Peto J & Turner RC (1979) Cyclic oscillations of basal plasma glucose and insulin concentrations in human beings. *New England Journal of Medicine*, **301**, 1023–1027.

Saltiel AR, Fox JA, Sherline P & Cuatrecasas P (1986) Insulin-stimulated hydrolysis of a novel glycolipid generates modulators of cAMP phosphodiesterase. *Science*, **233**, 967–972.

Taylor R (1984) Insulin receptor assays – clinical application and limitations. *Diabetic Medicine*, **1**, 181–188.

Ullrich A, Bell JR, Chen EY, Herrera R, Petruzzelli LM, Dull TJ, Gray A, Coussens L, Liao Y-C, Tsubokawa M, Mason A, Seeburg PH, Grunfeld C, Rosen OM & Ramachandran J (1985) Human insulin receptor and its relationship to the tyrosine kinase family of oncogenes. *Nature*, **313**, 756–761.

Diagnostic Criteria, Classification and Presentation of Diabetes

Serge Ng Tang Fui MSc MD MRCP   ● **Harry Keen** MD FRCP

Diabetes mellitus (DM) is a disorder of multiple aetiology, characterized by hyperglycaemia, glycosuria and a wide spectrum of clinical and pathological manifestations. Diagnosis of the metabolic disorder is straightforward when patients present with typical symptoms, such as thirst, polyuria and weight loss. Glycosuria is invariably heavy, often associated with ketonuria, and blood glucose concentration is so grossly and unequivocally elevated that a single measurement confirms the diagnosis.

Problems in diagnosis arise when routine testing of either asymptomatic subjects or patients with unrelated or non-specific symptoms reveals lesser degrees of glycosuria and random blood glucose levels which are not grossly elevated. Diagnosis then depends on the level of blood glucose, measured under specific conditions and related to diagnostic criteria which mark the cutoff point between normal and abnormal. In most populations,

however, blood glucose concentrations, like blood pressure and other biological variables, show no natural demarcation between normal and abnormal (Fig. 6.1) making the diagnostic cutoff point arbitrary.

Over the past two decades, the glycaemic criteria defining diabetes have been revised and reset at considerably higher levels than those in the past, and a category of 'impaired glucose tolerance' (IGT) has been interposed between normal and diabetic levels (Fig. 6.2). The recommendations proposed by the Expert Committee of the World Health Organisation (WHO, 1980), with a view to international standardization, embody this trend and have been widely accepted. A revised version of these recommendations has been published in a more recent report (WHO, 1985).

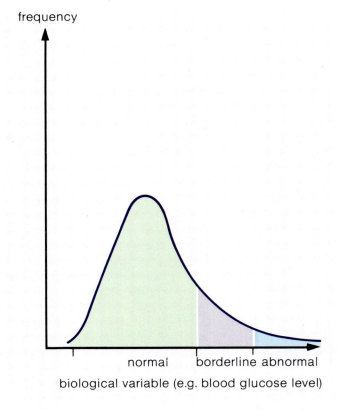

Fig. 6.1 The arbitrary definition of biological abnormality. Many biological variables, including blood glucose concentration and blood pressure, are distributed in the 'positively skewed continuous distribution' of frequency as shown here. Cutoff levels are arbitrary, although they represent a form of probability distinction; the top few per cent being 'abnormal', the next ten or so per cent being 'borderline' and the rest considered 'normal'.

Fig. 6.2 Revised oral glucose tolerance test (OGTT) criteria for diabetes mellitus. The revised criteria (WHO, 1980 and 1985) are compared to those previously recommended by WHO (1965). Values between the two curves are now defined as 'impaired glucose tolerance' (IGT). Note that in 1965, only the two-hour value was recommended for diagnosis and that intermediate values are not diagnostic.

EVOLUTION OF THE DIAGNOSTIC CRITERIA FOR DIABETES

A brief account of the evolution of the modern diagnostic concept of diabetes helps to understand the problems in diagnosis and the basis of the new criteria. Four main stages can be recognized in this evolution. In the earliest or *descriptive period* (Fig. 6.3), diabetes was recognized by its distinctive and dramatic clinical features. Polyuria was noted in ancient Egyptian script hieroglyphs. The term 'diabetes' is usually attributed to Arateus who, in the first century A.D., described it as an uncommon disorder characterized by intractable thirst, polyuria, weight loss, dehydration and early death. Sweetness of the urine was also recorded in ancient Hindu and Chinese writings, but not until the eighteenth and nineteenth centuries was this identified in Europe to be due to glucose and subsequently to excessive glucose in the blood.

Glycosuria, ketonuria and hyperglycaemia distinguished diabetes mellitus from other polyuric syndromes and set a milestone for the *chemical* or *diagnostic period* (Fig. 6.4). Nevertheless, clinical features distinguished what is now recognized as insulin-dependent diabetes mellitus (IDDM). Soon, it became apparent that similar chemical abnormalities could be detected in older and usually obese patients with milder and more insidious symptoms. The concept of diabetes expanded considerably to include this less acute, more numerous, non-lethal clinical variant, now termed non insulin-dependent diabetes mellitus (NIDDM).

The discovery of insulin and its life-saving property by Banting and Best in 1921, marked the start of the *therapeutic period* (Fig. 6.5). It confirmed the concept of a deficiency of insulin action as the basic abnormality in diabetes and gave rise to the differentiation between IDDM and NIDDM. The prolonged survival of young diabetic patients following the introduction of insulin revealed the delayed complications of the disease, affecting the small vessels of the retina and renal glomeruli, damaging

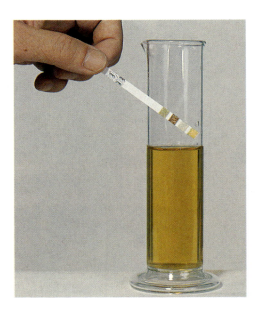

Fig. 6.3 Evolution of the diagnostic concept of diabetes: (1) the ancient descriptive period. Along with this early Egyptian record (The Ebers Papyrus, 1550 B.C.), there were early Chinese and Indian descriptions of the various clinical features of diabetes. Arateus in the first century A.D. gave the first comprehensive clinical description.

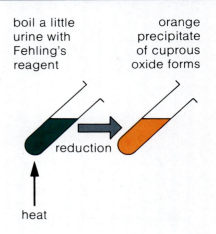

original chemical identification of glucose in urine – Fehling's test

boil a little urine with Fehling's reagent

orange precipitate of cuprous oxide forms

reduction

heat

Fig. 6.4 Evolution of the diagnostic concept of diabetes: (2) the chemical or diagnostic period. Chemical identification of glucose levels in urine and later in blood, usually by reduction of copper salts, removed reliance upon the sense of taste; for example, in Fehling's test (1848), copper sulphate solution changes from blue to orange when boiled with solutions containing glucose or other reducing sugars.

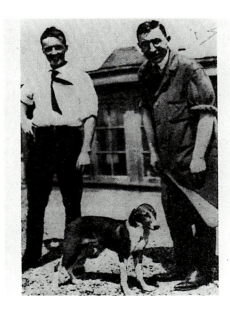

Fig. 6.5 Evolution of the diagnostic concept of diabetes: (3) the therapeutic period. The discovery of insulin by Banting and Best (1921) was followed by its rapid exploitation for world supply. Oral hypoglycaemic agents appeared in the 1940's and 1950's. Banting (right) and Best are shown here with the first dog to receive insulin.

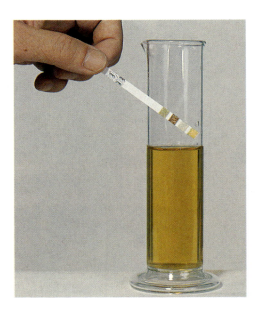

Fig. 6.6 Evolution of the diagnostic concept of diabetes: (4) the modern or screening period. Enzyme-based glucose detection in urine gave rise to simple and sensitive routine screening tests, which were later extended to blood glucose.

the peripheral nerves and accelerating atherosclerotic change in the larger arteries supplying the heart, brain and lower limbs.

Simple and sensitive biochemical tests have made urine analysis for glucose, ketones and protein a routine investigation. This constitutes the *screening period* (Fig. 6.6). Increasingly, glycosuria and hyperglycaemia were detected in patients with few or none of the classical symptoms, and often even in apparently healthy subjects undergoing routine medical examination for insurance or employment purposes. As diagnosis became more chemical and less clinical, the original concept of diabetes as an uncommon and lethal clinical syndrome greatly expanded to make it one of the commonest disorders, ranging from the acute, polysymptomatic IDDM to the clinically silent forms of NIDDM. Sustained hyperglycaemia, in the untreated state, with or without symptoms, and with a propensity to a set of complications, of which retinopathy and nephropathy are the most specific clinically, has come to underlie the modern concept of diabetes.

The Oral Glucose Tolerance Test (OGTT)

In over eighty per cent of patients presenting clinically, the diagnosis of diabetes is established by a single blood glucose estimation at presentation; the level is unequivocally raised, with random venous plasma values well above 11.1 mmol/l (200 mg/dl) or fasting values well above 7.8 mmol/l (140 mg/dl). However, the drive towards early chemical diagnosis, in the hope of preventing long-term complications, stimulated the search for more sensitive methods of detecting hyperglycaemia even in the absence of symptoms and signs. The oral glucose tolerance test (Fig. 6.7) was developed to assess the ability to maintain blood glucose homeostasis following a standard oral glucose challenge. The use of an intravenous glucose challenge (IVGTT) has been largely restricted to research studies. The blood glucose level, two hours after the oral glucose load, was shown to be most reliable in detecting defective glucose utilization and plays an important part in the interpretation of blood glucose responses.

In the past, there has been considerable variation in the application and interpretation of the OGTT, with respect to the size of the glucose load (50g, 75g, 100g or per kg body weight), the timing and the type of blood samples (venous or capillary, plasma or whole blood), the analytical methods employed and the question of age correction of the result. The lowest two-hour blood glucose level considered diagnostic of diabetes in middle-aged subjects ranged between 5.6 and 11.1 mmol/l (100–200 mg/dl) and overlapped the highest value accepted as normal, ranging between 5.6 and 10.0 mmol/l (100–180 mg/dl). The same test result could therefore be interpreted as diabetic or normal depending upon the set of criteria used. Thus population prevalence rates would vary more than tenfold. This situation was clearly unsatisfactory both for the individual at diagnosis and for epidemiological estimates of the prevalence of diabetes.

Population and Long Term Follow-up Studies

The earlier criteria that were used made the assumption that blood glucose values exceeding an arbitrary normal range, which was derived from small samples of young healthy subjects, were diagnostic of diabetes. In the absence of specific symptoms or signs, or some independent, non-glycaemic marker of the diabetic state, there was no means of validating these diagnostic criteria. Thus there remained much doubt, especially for the large number of older people with blood glucose values that were only slightly above the normal range.

Population studies in the 1960's, such as that conducted in Bedford, U.K. (Fig. 6.8), showed that glucose tolerance, estimated

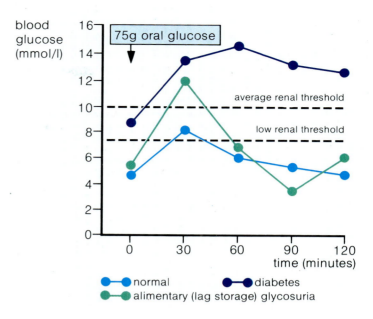

Fig. 6.7 The oral glucose tolerance test (OGTT). WHO recommendations (1980 and 1985) for the performance and interpretation of OGTT are now widely accepted (see Fig. 6.11). After an overnight fast, blood is taken before and up to two hours after a 75g glucose load. Typical curves are illustrated for normal and diabetic responses. In normal subjects, the blood glucose concentration returns to near fasting level by two hours. In diabetic patients, it is often raised under fasting conditions, remains raised at two hours and returns to fasting values only after some considerable delay.

The average renal threshold for glucose is about 10mmol/l (180mg/dl). If it is exceeded, the glucose concentration in the urine rises steeply. If the renal threshold is low, as in young people, or if it falls, as sometimes happens in pregnancy, glycosuria will occur with normal rises of blood glucose. If glucose is rapidly absorbed from the small bowel, the accelerated glycaemic rise may exceed the renal threshold with resulting glycosuria (alimentary or lag storage glycosuria); this is often followed by a fall in blood glucose to below fasting values. This type of curve is, however, not pathological. Fasting, one-hour and two-hour samples are usually taken for OGTT. In practice, capillary blood obtained by either finger of ear-lobe prick is more conveniently obtained than venous blood. Non-fasting capillary blood values are usually higher than venous values (see Fig. 6.12).

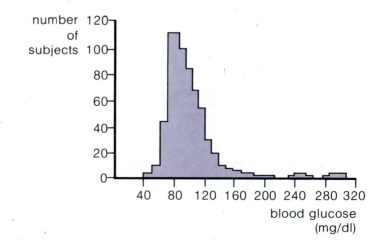

Fig. 6.8 Capillary blood glucose concentrations two hours after 50g oral glucose in a population sample from Bedford, U.K. The values form a unimodal frequency distribution which is positively skewed to the right. The pattern is characteristic of the majority of reported populations and quite distinct from the bimodal distribution in the Pima Indians and the Micronesians of Nauru (see Fig. 6.9).

in this case from capillary blood glucose values two hours after 50g of oral glucose, formed a continuous distribution, skewed toward the higher values. There was no natural demarcation apparent between 'normal' and 'diabetic' values (see also Fig. 6.2). There was no evidence in the distribution of these data to support the diagnostic values then prevailing, nor any other for that matter. The Bedford study met this problem by interposing between clearly normal and diabetic responses a stratum of intermediate responses which was termed 'borderline diabetes'. This was defined as a two-hour capillary blood glucose level between 6.7 and 11.1 mmol/l (120–200 mg/dl). This zone of diagnostic uncertainty has acquired a variety of names such as subclinical, latent, early and chemical diabetes. People with responses falling within it were nevertheless classed as diabetic, carrying many of the clinical, economic and psychosocial implications of the diagnosis.

Subsequent evidence suggested that this was unjustified for three reasons. First, prospective follow-up studies over ten years showed that only one to two per cent per year of subjects with 'borderline diabetes' deteriorated to frankly diabetic levels (two-hour blood glucose levels ≥ 11.1 mmol/l or ≥ 200 mg/dl). One

third reverted to normal tolerance. Secondly, clinically significant, specific microvascular complications were not seen in the borderline group during the ten years of follow-up. Lastly, in two populations, the Pima Indians of Arizona and the Micronesians of Nauru, with an exceptionally high prevalence of diabetes of approximately fifty per cent, the distribution of two-hour blood glucose levels was bimodal, with the division between normal and diabetic components lying at about 11.1 mmol/l (Fig. 6.9). Retinal and renal complications were found almost exclusively in subjects in the upper glycaemic group.

These data strongly suggested that the diagnostic cutoff point for diabetes should lie at or about a two-hour blood glucose level of 11.1 mmol/l rather than at the previously accepted lower level of about 7.8 mmol/l (140 mg/dl), which included subjects with 'borderline diabetes'. However, in subjects with intermediate two-hour values, the chance of worsening to diabetes, although comparatively low, was still higher than in those with clearly normal OGTT responses. The risk of atherosclerotic arterial disease was also twice as high in the borderline group as in normal subjects and there was some evidence that it carried increased risks in pregnancy. These were the main considerations leading to

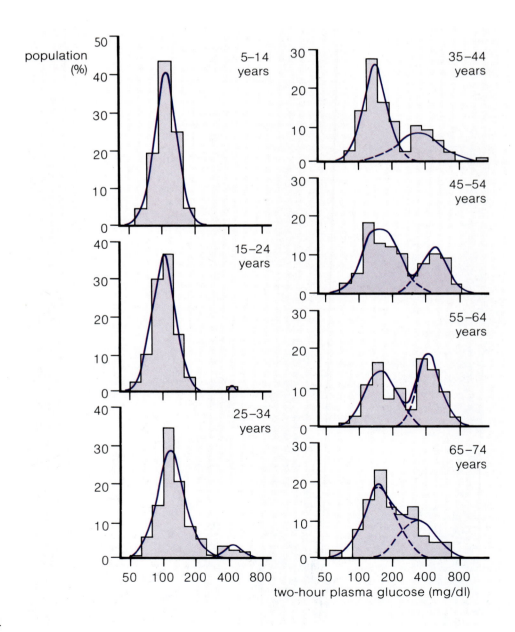

Fig. 6.9 Bimodal distribution of two-hour plasma glucose in the Pima Indians of Arizona. The transition point occurs at a plasma glucose level of approximately 11.1 mmol/l (200mg/dl), the value now accepted to be diagnostic of diabetes mellitus. A similar bimodal distribution occurs in the Micronesians of the Pacific Island of Nauru. Both populations are relatively isolated, very obese, comparatively inbred and with a very high prevalence of diabetes (about 50% at age fifty years). Data for females are shown and each graph represents a different age group.

the recent revision of criteria for diagnosing diabetes and the creation of the new subdiabetic category of 'impaired glucose tolerance' (IGT).

New Diagnostic Criteria for Diabetes Mellitus (DM)

By the late 1970's, three authoritative bodies, the European Association for the Study of Diabetes (EASD, 1979), the National Diabetes Data Group (NDDG, 1979) of the U.S. National Institute of Health and the World Health Organisation (WHO, 1980) had appointed expert committees to review diagnostic criteria and methodology, with the objective of rationalizing, standardizing and, if possible, achieving international agreement. Their recommendations, although differing in detail, shared many fundamental features. There was common agreement that the lesser degrees of glucose intolerance should no longer be classified as DM (borderline or otherwise) but as the newly defined category of IGT. Diagnostic values for diabetic OGTT were therefore raised above previous values as shown in Fig. 6.10.

All three groups agreed that the OGTT is often unnecessary to establish the diagnosis of diabetes. In patients with characteristic symptoms such as thirst and polyuria, diagnosis can usually be confirmed by a single unequivocally raised plasma glucose level; for example, a random value greater than 11.1 mmol/l or a fasting value greater than 7.8 mmol/l. When symptoms are not present, blood glucose raised above these limits, either in a casual blood sample or in the OGTT, should be demonstrated on more than one occasion to confirm the diagnosis. There were small differences between the three bodies in the number and timing of OGTT samples required to fulfil the criteria, but the simpler recommendations of WHO (1980) and their more recently revised recommendations (WHO, 1985) are now widely accepted.

A two-hour venous plasma glucose level between 7.8 and 11.1 mmol/l in the absence of fasting hyperglycaemia (<7.8 mmol/l), should be classed as IGT. A value between the fasting and the two-hour points exceeding 11.1 mmol/l is also required by NDDG to qualify for IGT.

All three groups recommended that OGTT be performed under standard conditions as detailed in Fig. 6.11, as significant variation may occur under different test conditions.

DIAGNOSTIC CRITERIA FOR DIABETES USING VENOUS PLASMA GLUCOSE VALUES

Fig. 6.10 Diagnostic criteria for DM and IGT: (1) venous plasma. Illustrated is the interpretation of venous plasma glucose values derived from a random (non-fasting) sample and from standardized samples taken during an OGTT following 75g of oral glucose. If typical symptoms are present, a single random venous plasma glucose concentration of 11.1 mmol/l (200mg/dl) or more or a single fasting value of 7.8mmol/l (140mg/dl) or more confirms the diagnosis of DM; an OGTT is unnecessary. If typical symptoms are absent, the finding of these values strongly supports the diagnosis but requires confirmation with a further abnormal value. An OGTT is only indicated if random or fasting values are not clearly elevated.

PROCEDURE FOR OGTT

glucose load: adults: 75g in 250–300ml of chilled water*
children: 1.75g/kg body weight
drink within 5 minutes

preceding diet and activity: unrestricted carbohydrate (>150g daily) and physical activity for at least 3 days before test

fasting period: 10–16h on the night before test
pure water allowed
test in the morning

timing of samples: before and 2h after oral glucose (also at 30, 60 and 90 minutes if required)*
remain seated and no smoking through test

types of samples: venous or capillary; whole blood or plasma
note type for interpretation

precautions: note any drugs (e.g. thiazide diuretics, corticosteroids) which may influence OGTT responses
note departures from desirable OGTT conditions

*NDDG recommends 100g glucose load plus additional 3h sample in pregnancy

Fig. 6.11 Standard procedure for an oral glucose tolerance test.

The above blood glucose values refer to venous plasma, but venous or capillary whole blood or capillary plasma may also be used with appropriate adjustments to the values as shown in Fig. 6.12.

Diagnosis of Diabetes in Pregnancy (Gestational DM)
Diabetic women, usually with insulin-dependent diabetes (IDDM), who become pregnant require special care (see *Chapter 20*). However, glucose intolerance may first be detected during pregnancy, often in the last trimester, and this may require attention as more severe degrees of intolerance are associated with increased fetal and perinatal mortality and morbidity. A previous history of obstetric problems, such as stillbirth, large babies and either respiratory difficulties or hypoglycaemia in the newborn should also alert the physician.

Glycosuria may be detected during pregnancy and is of particular significance if it occurs in the fasting state, for instance, in an early morning test; later in the day, it may be due to the low renal threshold of pregnancy. The further investigation of glycosuria represents one of the indications for OGTT. The WHO criteria for diagnosing gestational diabetes and IGT are shown in Fig. 6.13, along with the O'Sullivan and Mahan criteria which are still widely used. Following delivery, glucose tolerance should be reassessed. It may remain abnormal, although it usually reverts to normal. In the latter case, the risk of NIDDM or IGT later in life is considerably increased.

DIAGNOSTIC CRITERIA FOR DIABETES WHEN NOT USING VENOUS PLASMA

	random sample (mmol/l)			standardized OGTT (mmol/l)		
	diabetes likely	diabetes uncertain	diabetes unlikely		diabetes	IGT
venous blood	≥10.0	4.4 – <10.0	<4.4	fasting	≥6.7	<6.7
				2h	≥10.0	6.7 – 10.0
capillary blood	≥11.1	4.4 – <11.1	<4.4	fasting	≥6.7	<6.7
				2h	≥11.1	7.8 – 11.1
capillary plasma	≥12.2	5.5 – <12.2	<5.5	fasting	≥7.8	<7.8
				2h	≥12.2	8.9 – 12.2

Fig. 6.12 Diagnostic criteria for DM and IGT: (2) venous blood and capillary blood and plasma. The criteria for these samples differ slightly from those for venous plasma (see Fig. 6.10) which is the sample most commonly taken. (1.0mmol/l glucose is equivalent to 18mg/dl).

DIAGNOSTIC CRITERIA FOR GESTATIONAL DIABETES AND IGT

WHO:	same criteria as for non-pregnant adults		
NDDG (O'Sullivan and Mahan, 1964):	**100g OGTT criteria**		
		venous plasma glucose concentration	
	time of sample	diabetes	IGT
	0h (fasting)	≥ 5.8mmol/l (105mg/dl)	< 5.8mmol/l
	1h	> 10.6mmol/l (190mg/dl)	
	2h	> 9.2mmol/l (165mg/dl)	6.7–9.2mmol/l (120–165mg/dl)
	3h	> 8.1mmol/l (145mg/dl)	

Fig. 6.13 OGTT diagnosis of gestational DM and IGT. Unlike WHO, NDDG recommends the criteria of O'Sullivan and Mahan which require an oral glucose load of 100g and at least two of the values shown in the table to be exceeded.

DIAGNOSTIC CRITERIA FOR DIABETES AND IGT IN ASYMPTOMATIC CHILDREN

WHO:	same criteria as for adults
NDDG:	fasting, 2h and intermediate values as for adults
	if fasting < 7.8mmol/l, then 2h value ≥ 7.8mmol/l is IGT, including values ≥ 11.1mmol/l

Fig. 6.14 Diagnosis of diabetes and IGT in asymptomatic children.

Diagnosis of Diabetes in Children

In children, diabetes is usually of the classical type (IDDM), presenting with abrupt onset of symptoms such as thirst, polyuria and bedwetting, dehydration and varying degrees of ketoacidosis and of impaired consciousness. Diagnosis is easily confirmed with heavy glycosuria, ketonuria and gross elevation of the blood glucose concentration on a single sample at presentation. The recommended criteria for screening with OGTT are shown in Fig. 6.14.

NEW CLASSIFICATION OF DIABETES

The currently recommended classification of DM (Fig. 6.15) was developed by NDDG (1979) and adopted provisionally by WHO (1980). It is essentially a *clinical* classification but has attempted to combine this with aetiological factors (Fig. 6.16). WHO (1985) has subsequently modified the classification to include malnutrition-related diabetes mellitus (MRDM) as a major type in its own right (Fig. 6.17). The two systems of nomenclature used in the new classification (IDDM/NIDDM and Types I/II) originate from the use of either clinical or aetiological features to classify diabetes and there has been a tendency to use the two systems synonymously. It should be borne in mind, however, that a single aetiological mechanism may manifest itself with different clinical types of DM and that a single clinical type may arise from several different aetiologies. Thus, the correspondence between, for example, IDDM (clinical) and Type I (aetiological) is only approximate. The Type I process may also give rise to either NIDDM, IGT or no disturbance of glucose tolerance. Type II is a highly imprecise designation defined as any DM that is neither Type I nor 'other types' of DM. It does not describe any single known aetiological process. NIDDM is likely to arise from many different causal mechanisms.

Insulin dependency is largely a clinical judgement and is based upon a history of symptomatic onset, accompanied by ketonuria, ketoacidosis and a record of daily insulin injections, unbroken since diagnosis. This judgement may be supported by the absence of circulating C peptide either under basal conditions or after stimulation with food or glucagon injection. C peptide is a marker for endogenous insulin secretion. The onset of diabetes under the age of twenty years is almost always indicative of IDDM, although this clinical type may start at any age, even in the elderly.

NIDDM, though usually associated with diagnosis in the middle or later years of life, uncommonly occurs in the young and then is sometimes known as 'maturity onset diabetes of youth'

CLASSIFICATION OF DIABETES AND OTHER CATEGORIES OF GLUCOSE INTOLERANCE

clinical	statistical

diabetes mellitus:
  IDDM (Type I)
  NIDDM (Type II)
  MRDM
  other types
	previous abnormality of
	  glucose tolerance

impaired glucose
  tolerance
	potential abnormality of
	  glucose tolerance

gestational diabetes	

Fig. 6.15 Classification of diabetes and other categories of glucose intolerance (NDDG, 1979; WHO, 1980 and 1985).

CHARACTERISTIC FEATURES OF DIABETES SUBTYPES (1)

IDDM (Type I)	NIDDM (Type II)
ketosis prone	non-ketosis prone
insulin treatment mandatory	insulin treatment optional
acute onset	insidious onset
usually non-obese	obese or non-obese

typically onset in youth
  but any age possible
	onset usually over 50 yrs
	  but MODY is a variant

HLA-DR3 and DR4 common	HLA unrelated
islet cell antibodies	no islet cell antibodies

family history positive
  in 10%
	family history positive
	  in 30%

50% concordance in
  identical twins
	nearly 100% concord-
	  ance in identical twins

Fig. 6.16 Characteristic features of the subtypes of diabetes mellitus: (1) IDDM and NIDDM.

CHARACTERISTIC FEATURES OF DIABETES SUBTYPES (2)

malnutrition related DM	other types (secondary)

prevalent in tropical
  countries
	pancreatic disease e.g.
	  chronic pancreatitis

occurs in gross
  malnutrition
	endocrine disorders
	  e.g. acromegaly,
	  Cushing's disease

onset before 30 years	

hyperglycaemia without
  ketosis
	drug-induced
	  e.g. thiazides, steroids

insulin required for control	insulin receptor defect

subtypes with or without
  pancreatic duct calculi
  and diffuse fibrosis
  associated with high
  dietary cyanide
	genetic syndromes

	miscellaneous

Fig. 6.17 Characteristic features of the subtypes of diabetes mellitus: (2) MRDM and other types.

(MODY). Patients with NIDDM may receive insulin injections if they fail to respond adequately to diet or oral agents, but this does not justify the assumption of insulin dependency. Patients with NIDDM may, however, become insulin-dependent under the stress of infection, trauma or myocardial infarction. The IDDM may revert to NIDDM when the stress has passed. If NIDDM is a phase of the Type I process, it may progressively worsen to insulin dependency. In our opinion, it is advisable to use the descriptive terms 'IDDM' and 'NIDDM' and to reserve 'Type I' and 'Type II' for clearly defined, demonstrable aetiological processes. However, in order to meet the ambiguities of the two sets of terms, the WHO (1985) and the NDDG have recommended that if they are used at all, the terms Type I and Type II should be considered synonymous with IDDM and NIDDM respectively, without any aetiopatho-genic implication.

MRDM has been recognized in tropical countries for decades and has been described under many synonyms (tropical diabetes, J-type, Z-type, pancreatic diabetes and ketosis-resistant diabetes of the young). There is still considerable uncertainty about its reality as a single entity and subtypes with and without major fibrocalculous disease have been suggested. Its pathogenesis is also uncertain but protein malnutrition in the young and food toxins, particularly cyanogens, are thought to play a part.

In an era when primary prevention of diabetes and secondary prevention of some of its metabolic and tissue consequences are becoming possible, it is useful to consider classification of diabetes by its 'stage of evolution', starting at the state of unchallenged susceptibility in the totally 'normal' individual (Fig. 6.18).

IDENTIFYING FEATURES IN THE EVOLUTION OF DIABETES MELLITUS

stage	IDDM	NIDDM
1 unchallenged susceptibility	HLA-DR3 and DR4	DNA polymorphism on chromosome 11?
2 challenged susceptibility	islet cell antibodies? cell mediated immunity	changed insulin/glucose relationship
3 concealed dysfunction	low insulin release	IGT
4 minimal disease	stress glycaemia; IGT	labile DM
5 clinical disease	ketoacidosis	±DM symptoms
6 'early' complications	retinal/renal microvascular abnormalities; neuropathy	
7 organ failure	blindness; renal failure; tissue breakdown	

Fig. 6.18 Features of the various stages in the 'evolution' of diabetes mellitus. For each stage of DM from unchallenged susceptibility to clinical disease there are features which identify it as either IDDM or NIDDM.

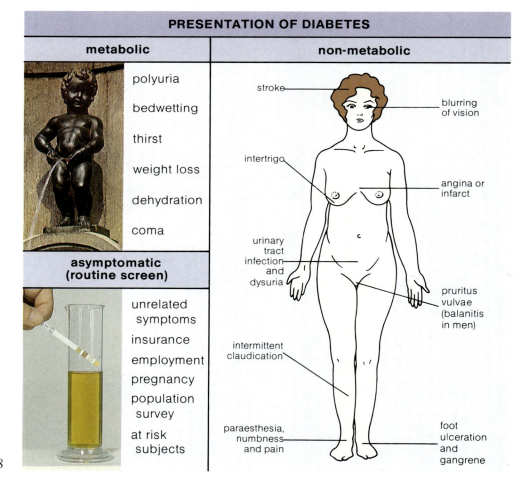

PRESENTATION OF DIABETES

metabolic

polyuria
bedwetting
thirst
weight loss
dehydration
coma

asymptomatic (routine screen)

unrelated symptoms
insurance
employment
pregnancy
population survey
at risk subjects

non-metabolic

stroke
blurring of vision
intertrigo
angina or infarct
urinary tract infection and dysuria
pruritus vulvae (balanitis in men)
intermittent claudication
paraesthesia, numbness and pain
foot ulceration and gangrene

Fig. 6.19 Presentation of diabetes. Diabetes may present in three ways: classical 'metabolic' symptoms are usually acute and severe in the younger and mild or moderate in the older patient; non-metabolic symptoms and asymptomatic glycosuria discovered on routine screening are also common modes of presentation in middle-aged and elderly patients.

PRESENTATION, SYMPTOMS AND SIGNS OF DIABETES

Diabetes may present in a variety of ways, ranging from abrupt onset of coma to asymptomatic glycosuria discovered on routine urine testing. The presenting clinical features depend on the degree of insulin lack, manifesting by the degree of hyperglycaemia, ketosis and wasting, and on the possible presence of tissue damage. Three types of presentation can be recognized: metabolic, non-metabolic and asymptomatic (Fig. 6.19).

Metabolic Presentation

Thirst and polyuria are the characteristic major presenting symptoms of IDDM and some cases of NIDDM, and are often associated with polyphagia, weight loss, ocular refractive change, pruritus vulvae and infection (Fig. 6.20). In IDDM, the gross hyperglycaemia greatly exceeds the renal threshold and results in heavy glycosuria; this, associated with heavy ketonuria, prompts a dramatic diuresis which continues day and night, with large volumes of pale urine of high specific gravity. Previously continent children may start bedwetting. Thirst is stimulated both by the raised plasma osmotic pressure and dehydration.

If the patient quenches his or her thirst with sugar-containing drinks, hyperglycaemia and its osmotic consequences will be aggravated. In severe cases, fluid intake may fall short of the polyuria; dehydration increases and severe hyperosmolarity may itself result in impairment of consciousness progressing from confusion and drowsiness to deep coma.

The hyperketonaemia and ketonuria of IDDM is the consequence of severe insulinopaenia. When ketone formation exceeds metabolic utilization and urinary disposal rates, keto-acidosis supervenes and results in hyperventilation (Kussmaul's breathing), detectable ketopnoea (smell of ketones on the breath), accelerated dehydration with drowsiness progressing to coma. The metabolic acidosis with depressed arterial blood pH (sometimes below pH 7.0) reduces plasma bicarbonate concentration (sometimes to 2–3 mmol/l). It is clinically important to note that vomiting, abdominal pain, pyrexia and polymorphonuclear leucocytosis may mimic a surgical emergency.

Severe dehydration, impaired consciousness and grossly elevated blood glucose levels with prerenal uraemia without ketosis constitute the syndrome of 'hyperosmolar non-ketotic coma'. Lowered plasma volume, increased blood viscosity and consequent slowing of the circulation may be complicated by arterial thrombosis, sometimes even affecting the aorta, and the patient may develop hemiplegic stroke or myocardial infarction.

In patients with classical metabolic symptoms, heavy glycosuria with or without ketonuria, and a plasma glucose level well above 11.1mmol/l (200mg/dl) confirms the diagnosis. In addition to careful clinical assessment, measurement of arterial pH, plasma osmolality and plasma bicarbonate, electrolytes and urea indicates the degree of severity of the metabolic disturbance. Precipitating or complicating factors such as infection or myocardial infarction should be sought and treated.

Non-Metabolic Presentation

The lesser degrees of hyperglycaemia and absence of heavy ketonuria typically encountered in NIDDM provoke milder thirst and polyuria; such symptoms may be completely absent. Patients may present with symptoms due to associated infection or to the tissue complications of diabetes.

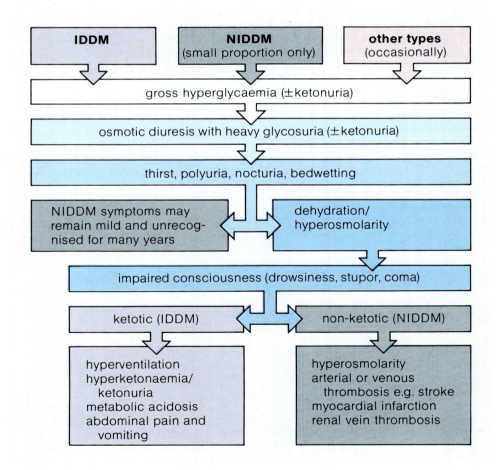

Fig. 6.20 The metabolic presentation of diabetes. Gross hyperglycaemia is the major pathogenic factor which leads to many of the matabolic symptoms of diabetes as shown here. These are aggravated by ketoacidosis in insulin-dependent diabetes.

Pruritus vulvae in women or balanitis in men (Fig. 6.21) sometimes bring the diagnosis to light in NIDDM; genital irritation by glycosuria is often aggravated by superadded *Candida* infection. Other infections may take the form of submammary or inguinal intertrigo (Fig. 6.22), boils, carbuncles, styes and urinary or respiratory infections. A proportion of patients presenting with diabetes indirectly, will admit on direct questioning to varying degrees of thirst and polyuria, sometimes over the previous months or years.

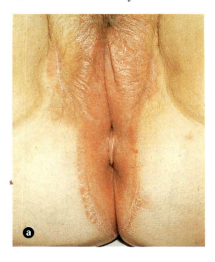 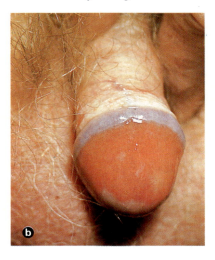

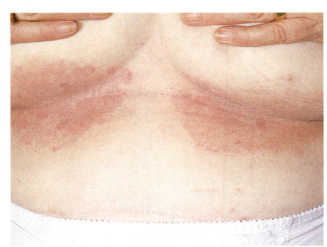

Fig. 6.21 Non-metabolic presenting features of NIDDM. Pruritus vulvae and ani (a) due to inflammation and *Candida* infection are common presenting features in women; in men, balanitis (b) may be the presenting symptom.

Fig. 6.22 Submammary intertrigo. This was the presenting feature of an elderly patient with newly diagnosed NIDDM.

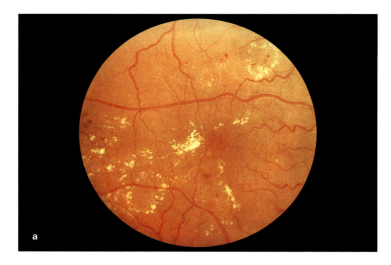

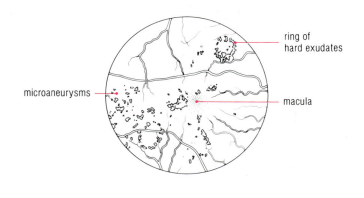

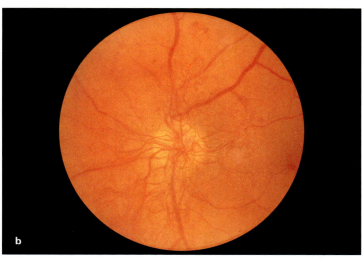

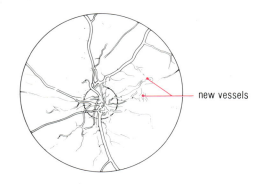

Fig. 6.23 Diabetic retinopathy. Although retinopathy at presentation in older patients is usually mild (microaneurysms and exudates mainly), it may be so severe that it is visual impairment which brings the patient to clinical attention and a diagnosis of diabetes. The two major causes of this are diabetic maculopathy (a) when retinal exudates, often circinate in form, encroach on the macular region and, less commonly, proliferative retinopathy (b) with new vessels which are prone to haemorrhages.

Diabetic microvascular complications

Although occurring in both major types of diabetes, only NIDDM may be brought to light by the vascular or neurological complications usually associated with long-standing diabetes. This strongly suggests a long prior period of unrecognized and untreated hyperglycaemia. Visual disturbance as a presenting symptom may be due to glucose-induced changes in refraction of the ocular media, although either characteristic diabetic retinopathy, often affecting the macular region (Fig. 6.23), or cataracts (Fig. 6.24) may be responsible. Photocoagulation treatment of the retinopathy may, in some cases, prevent further deterioration of vision. Surgical excision of cataract associated with unrecognized diabetes may precipitate postoperative metabolic problems.

Renal failure due to diabetic nephropathy is usually a late complication of diabetes but may uncommonly be a presenting feature. Proteinuria due to diabetic glomerulopathy may be detected at or soon after diagnosis of late-onset NIDDM. About twenty per cent of diabetic patients without clinical albuminuria exhibit raised urinary albumin excretion to a lesser degree, detectable only by immunoassay or other sensitive tests. Micro-albuminuria is of prognostic value since it is an early marker for diabetic nephropathy in IDDM patients. Hypertension accelerates microvascular and macrovascular complications in diabetic patients and should be vigorously controlled.

Macrovascular disease

Patients with NIDDM are particularly prone to atherosclerotic arterial disease (Fig. 6.25). Intermittent claudication due to arterial stenosis (Fig. 6.26), strokes or transient ischaemic attacks, foot

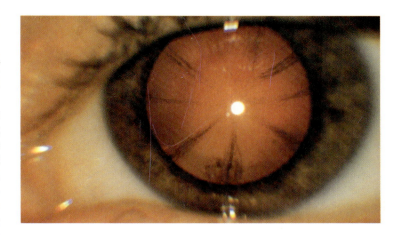

Fig. 6.24 Cataract in diabetes. Diabetes in older patients frequently presents with lenticular opacities; sometimes they are the cause of presentation. This picture shows early radiating spokes of opacity, indistinguishable from 'senile cataract', but occurring earlier and progressing more rapidly in the diabetic patient.

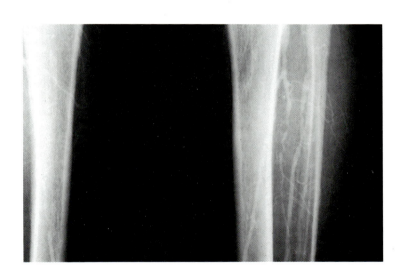

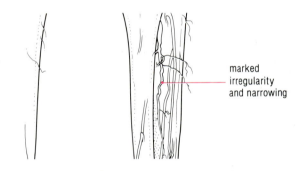

Fig. 6.25 Atherosclerotic arterial disease in NIDDM. Arteriogram of the left calf in a sixty-year-old man with newly diagnosed NIDDM, who presented with pre-gangrenous foot. Extensive irregularity and narrowing of arteries due to atherosclerosis can be seen.

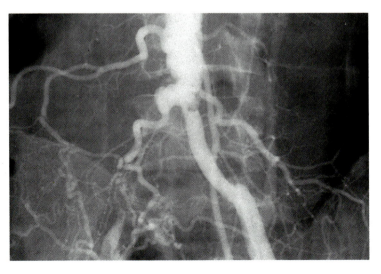

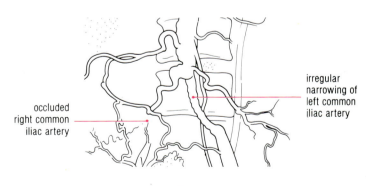

Fig. 6.26 Arteriogram of the pelvis and abdomen. This diabetic patient complained of intermittent claudication of the right leg.

Occlusion of the right common iliac artery can be seen. There is also irregular narrowing of the left common iliac artery.

ulceration or gangrene (Fig. 6.27), and angina or myocardial infarct (Fig. 6.28) may be present at, and sometimes prompt, diagnosis.

Neuropathy

This common complication of diabetes is occasionally a presenting feature. Subjective symptoms of paraesthesiae and pain in the feet and legs and occasionally in the hands and arms may be unaccompanied by objective neurological signs in the early, acutely manifesting form. In cases with insidious late NIDDM, however, touch, pin-prick and vibration sense may be symmetrically and irreversibly impaired and deep tendon reflexes are commonly absent. Neuropathic symptoms and signs may also

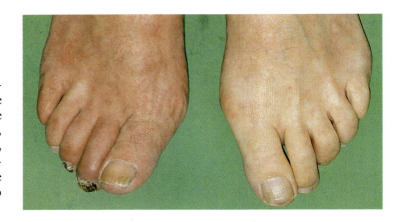

Fig. 6.27 Ischaemic gangrene of one toe and incipient gangrene of the foot. This fifty-eight-year-old man presented with previously undiagnosed diabetes; below-knee amputation was necessary later. Gangrene may be predominantly due to dense diabetic neuropathy with severe, advancing soft-tissue and bone destruction; local ablative surgery is often successful.

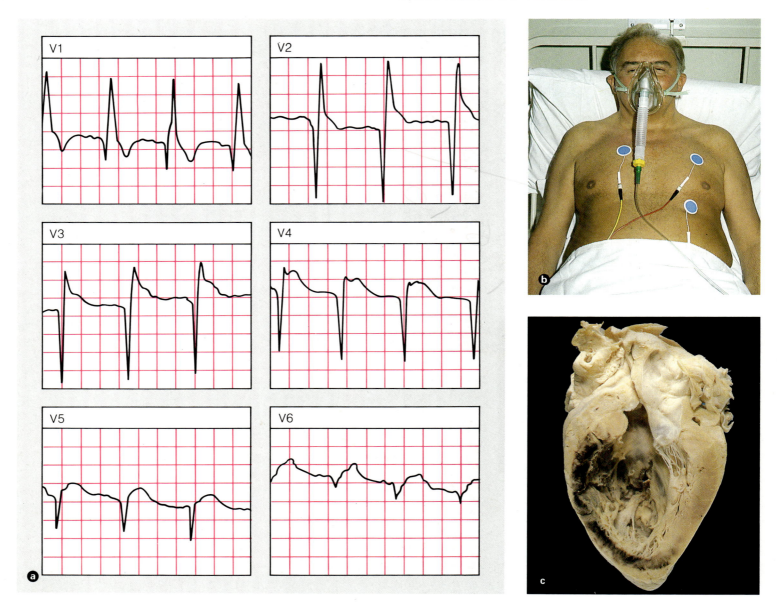

Fig. 6.28 Myocardial infarction in diabetes. A myocardial infarct is not infrequently the presenting feature of diabetes. Diabetes must be distinguished from the temporary loss of glucose tolerance, sometimes quite marked but remitting completely after recovery, which is associated with the acute stress of infarction. View (a) shows typical ECG changes of an acute myocardial infarct in a newly diagnosed diabetic patient (b), with elevation of ST segments, deep Q waves and T wave changes in the anterior chest leads. View (c) is a vertical section of the left ventricle of a heart showing extensive full thickness myocardial infarction (black discoloration) of the anterior wall, apex and septum.

include either mononeuropathies, for example, foot drop or isolated third or sixth nerve palsy, autonomic neuropathy causing impotence, hypotension or diarrhoea and diabetic amyotrophy with pain, weakness and wasting in the thighs and buttocks. Neuropathic ulceration or gangrene of the feet, with patent arteries, usually with gross infection can be extremely destructive.

Associated disorders
Diabetes associated with, or sometimes secondary to, other endocrine and metabolic disorders may present with diabetic symptoms or may be discovered when investigating patients with the primary disorder, for instance chronic pancreatitis (Fig. 6.29), acromegaly (Fig. 6.30), Cushing's syndrome or a glucagonoma (Fig. 6.31). Patients with postulated 'Type Ib' diabetes, that associated with autoimmune endocrinopathy, may rarely present with diabetes plus another endocrinopathy, such as hypothyroidism, hyperthyroidism (Fig. 6.32) or Addison's disease (Schmidt's syndrome). Alternatively, diabetes, usually IDDM, may develop

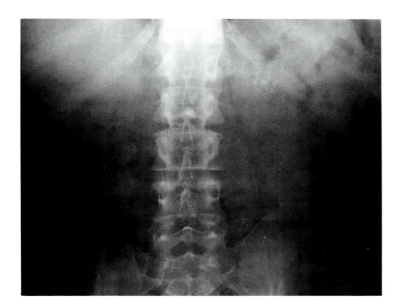

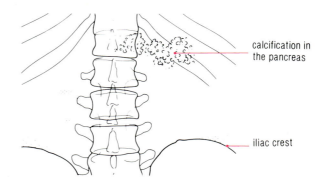

Fig. 6.29 Chronic pancreatitis and diabetes. This plain radiograph of a fifty-year-old male patient with diabetes mellitus, secondary to chronic pancreatitis, shows calcification in the region of the pancreas.

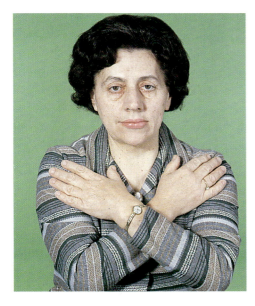

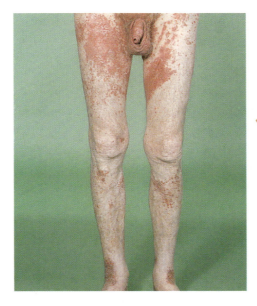

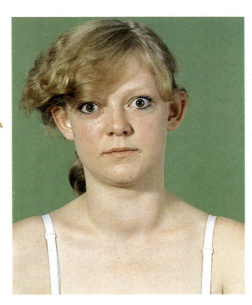

Fig. 6.30 Woman with acromegaly and associated diabetes mellitus. Note the coarse facial features and the broad hands characteristic of acromegaly.

Fig. 6.31 Patient with diabetes mellitus due to a confirmed glucagonoma. Note the characteristic widespread rash in this condition.

Fig. 6.32 Girl with IDDM and thyrotoxicosis due to Graves' disease. Both disorders were diagnosed simultaneously in this nineteen-year-old. Diffuse goitre and exophthalmos can be seen.

6.13

during the course of these endocrine disorders (Fig. 6.33). Obesity is so often linked with NIDDM that it is usually considered a major diabetogenic factor acting on susceptible persons rather than merely an associated phenomenon (Fig. 6.34).

Diabetes should be suspected in patients with the non-metabolic manifestations described above, with or without the promptings of thirst and polyuria. The urine should be tested for glucose and if positive, blood glucose should be measured. A high random value may establish the diagnosis and OGTT should be reserved for equivocal glycaemia or 'quantitation' of lesser degrees of glucose intolerance. The absence of glycosuria does not exclude diabetes. A high renal threshold for glucose as occurs in later life, particularly in women, may sometimes obscure marked degrees of glucose intolerance. A standardized test of a single blood sample measured two hours after 75g of glucose orally will often clarify the situation and full OGTT should be performed only if doubt still remains.

Asymptomatic Presentation (Routine Screening)
Diabetes (nearly always NIDDM) is often discovered in asymptomatic subjects when glycosuria is detected on urine testing, for example, during medical examination for insurance or employment purposes, pregnancy, an unrelated visit to the general practitioner or hospital or even before surgery. Diabetes

may also be detected on deliberate blood glucose screening of either asymptomatic subjects, such as in unselective population surveys, or high risk subjects, for example, the obese, those with a strong family history of diabetes, the elderly and the hyperlipidaemic.

It is in the asymptomatic, often aglycosuric, subjects that diagnosis requires to be established beyond doubt. Hyperglycaemia must be demonstrated and confirmed and OGTT may be necessary. Glycosuria may be shown to be due, not to diabetes, but either to a low renal threshold (renal glycosuria) or to rapid absorption of glucose (alimentary or lag storage glycosuria – see Fig. 6.7). Those people found to have IGT require annual follow-up and retesting with a search for, and where possible reversal of, risk factors for atherosclerosis. Glucose intolerance may be due to drugs like thiazide diuretics or corticosteroids. Withdrawal or replacement of these drugs may restore normal glucose tolerance, but when this is not possible or desirable, antidiabetic therapy with diet, oral agents or even insulin may be necessary.

CONCLUSION
The diagnosis of diabetes depends upon the demonstration of significant hyperglycaemia. Its classification and management depend upon the presence or absence of a set of accompanying symptoms, signs or investigative findings.

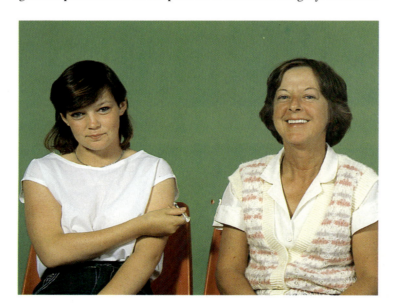

Fig. 6.33 Fifteen-year-old girl found to have primary autoimmune atrophic hypothyroidism four years after diagnosis of IDDM. Her mother had been treated for Graves' disease by subtotal thyroidectomy.

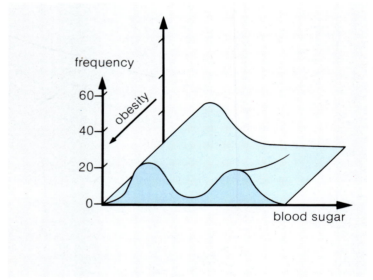

Fig. 6.34 Emergence of bimodality with obesity. This diagram illustrates one hypothesis for the emergence of a distinct subpopulation of diabetic blood glucose responses in obese populations (e.g. Pima Indians, Nauruans – see Fig. 6.9). As the overall prevalence of obesity in a population increases, individuals susceptible to its diabetogenic difference appear in increasing numbers, eventually rising to approximately half the population.

REFERENCES

Harris M, Hadden W, Knowler W & Bennett P (1985) International criteria for the diagnosis of diabetes and impaired glucose tolerance. *Diabetes Care*, **8**, 562–567.

Keen H & Ng Tang Fui S (1982) The definition and classification of diabetes mellitus. *Clinics in Endocrinology and Metabolism*, **11**, 279–305.

National Diabetes Data Group (1979) Classification and diagnosis of diabetes mellitus and other categories of glucose intolerance. *Diabetes*, **28**, 1039–1057.

Report of a World Health Organization study group (1985) Diabetes mellitus. *Technical Report Series*, **727**. Geneva: WHO.

World Health Organization Expert Committee on Diabetes Mellitus (1980) Second report. *Technical Report Series*, **646**. Geneva: WHO.

Aetiology and Pathogenesis of Type I Diabetes: Epidemiology

D Robert Gamble MB DipBact FRCPath

TWIN STUDIES AND ENVIRONMENTAL FACTORS

Several studies have shown that identical twins of patients with Type I (insulin-dependent) diabetes do not necessarily develop diabetes themselves (Fig. 7.1). Approximately fifty per cent of such twin pairs appear to remain discordant for diabetes. Thus, genetic factors cannot be the only determinant of Type I diabetes and environmental factors must also be involved.

Physical, chemical, infective and psychological factors have all been proposed as the responsible extrinsic agents. Since islet cell changes in Type I diabetes show specific destruction of B cells, infective agents or specific chemical poisons seem the most plausible candidates, acting either directly on B cells or indirectly by triggering an autoimmune process. Moreover, there is evidence that both viruses and chemical poisons induce specific B cell damage in both man and animals. Infections and intoxications have characteristic epidemiological features and the epidemiology of Type I diabetes should reveal important clues to the identity of the causative extrinsic factors.

PREVALENCE AND INCIDENCE

Estimates of prevalence of Type I diabetes vary widely. This is partly due to varying levels of ascertainment and, since prevalence rises steeply with age, differences in the age structure of study populations often make interpretations difficult. However, prevalence seems to be relatively high in parts of Scandinavia, less in countries of lower latitude and very low in Japan. It is also said to be very uncommon in Eskimos and in the tropics but data for these populations are very limited.

Estimates of incidence are more reliable and a pattern has emerged from many prospective investigations conducted over the last twenty years (Fig. 7.2). Incidence appears to be substantially higher in Finland, Sweden and Norway than

TYPE I DIABETES IN MONOZYGOTIC TWINS		
number of twin pairs	number of pairs concordant for diabetes	reference
12	6(50%)	Then Berg (1939)
20	15(75%)	Gottlieb & Root (1968)
64	32(50%)	Pyke & Nelson (1976)

Fig. 7.1 Prevalence of Type I diabetes in monozygotic (identical) twins. Approximately 50% remain discordant for diabetes.

SOME ESTIMATES OF INCIDENCE OF TYPE I DIABETES					
country	year	age (years)	M/F ratio	incidence per 100,000	reference
Finland	1970–79	0–14	1.07	28.6	Christau et al. (1981)
Sweden	1977–80	0–14	1.09	20.8	Christau et al. (1981)
Norway	1973–77	0–14	1.15	17.6	Christau et al. (1981)
U.S.A.	1965–80	0–20	1.10	14.7	LaPorte et al. (1981)
Denmark	1970–76	0–14	1.08	14.0	Christau et al. (1981)
Scotland	1968–76	0–18	1.09	13.8	Patterson et al. (1983)
New Zealand	1968–72	0–19	–	10.4	Crossley & Upsdell (1980)
Canada	1971–83	0–14	0.96	9.6	Siemiatycki et al. (1986)
Kuwait	1980–81	0–19	–	5.6	Taha et al. (1983)
Israel	1975–80	0–20	–	4.2	Laron et al. (1985)
France	1975	0–14	–	3.7	Lestradet & Besse (1977)
Japan	1974–80	0–18	0.70	0.8	Tajima et al. (1985)

Fig. 7.2 Some estimates of the incidence of Type I diabetes in different countries.

elsewhere, and lower than average in Kuwait, Israel, France and Japan. Whether these differences are due to genetic or environmental factors is uncertain but, at present, it seems likely that both play a part.

There is some evidence that incidence is related to racial differences within some countries. In Allegheny County, Pennsylvania, U.S.A., the incidence in Caucasians aged 0–20 years was fifteen per 100,000 compared with ten per 100,000 in non-Caucasians. In Israel, the incidence in the 0–20-year age group was 6.8 per 100,000 in Jews of Ashkenazi origin and 4.3 per 100,000 in Jews of non-Ashkenazi origin, while that for Arabs was

1.2 per 100,000. These observations suggest the existence of genetic factors which may protect against diabetes and thus explain the very low incidence in the Japanese. Migrant studies which could give a clear answer to this question have not yet been undertaken.

Conversely, the apparent relationship of high incidence with increasing latitude (see Fig. 7.2) may be related to either climatic or other environmental factors. Moreover, reports of secular changes in incidence clearly indicate that environmental factors affect incidence rates.

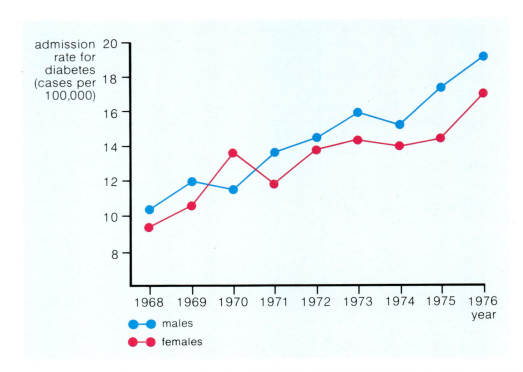

Fig. 7.3 Annual admission rates for Type I diabetes in Scotland over a nine-year period. From Patterson *et al.* (1983), by courtesy of Springer Verlag.

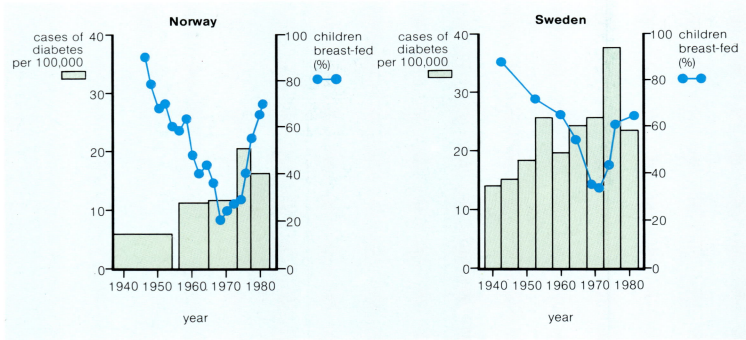

Fig. 7.4 Incidence of Type I diabetes in children aged 0–14 years in Norway and Sweden and breast-feeding frequencies. In the Norwegian study from Oslo, breast-feeding frequencies relate to children who were breast-fed for three or more months. In the Swedish study from Umeå, frequencies were calculated on the basis of two or more months breast-feeding. From Borch-Johnsen *et al.* (1984), by courtesy of the *Lancet*.

Secular Incidence

Several investigations have revealed secular changes in incidence. An increasing incidence has been reported in Norway, Sweden, Finland and Scotland. Data for Scotland (Fig. 7.3) show an increase from 10.0 per 100,000 to 18.3 per 100,000 subjects aged 0–18 years over a period of nine years. In Norway and Sweden (Fig. 7.4), the incidence has shown an increasing trend since 1940 but this was reversed in 1980 when the incidence declined. There may therefore be long-term cyclic changes over a period of many years. Borch-Johnsen and his colleagues (1984) speculated that

the rise in Norway and Sweden was associated with changes in breast-feeding frequency, but there has been no support for this idea from other countries where breast-feeding frequencies have also changed substantially in recent times. In Canada (Fig. 7.5) and the U.S.A. (Fig. 7.6), the incidence has fluctuated from year-to-year but with no consistent upward or downward trend. Indeed, one of the earliest attempts to estimate incidence of childhood diabetes in the U.S.A. (Fig. 7.7) suggested that the incidence sixty years ago may have been about thirteen per 100,000 which is close to the recent figure of 14.7 per 100,000.

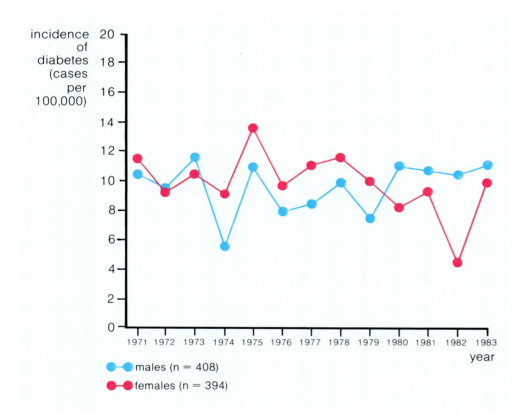

males (n = 408)
females (n = 394)

Fig. 7.5 Incidence of Type I diabetes in children aged 0–14 years in Montreal, Canada. From Siemiatycki *et al.* (1986), by courtesy of the *American Journal of Epidemiology*.

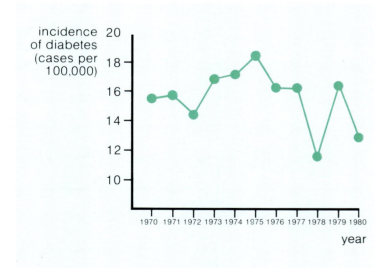

Fig. 7.6 Incidence of Type I diabetes in Pennslyvania, U.S.A. From Tajima *et al.* (1985), by courtesy of the American Diabetes Association.

ESTIMATE OF THE INCIDENCE OF DIABETES IN THE U.S.A.		
year	data	incidence rate
1922	1080 children died of diabetes each year in a population of 8 million	13.5 per 100,000
1932	1 child in 8000 became diabetic yearly	12.5 per 100,000

Fig. 7.7 Estimate of the incidence of childhood diabetes in the U.S.A. in 1922 and 1932 (White, 1932).

In view of the possible link with viral infection, evidence has been sought for outbreaks or 'epidemic years' of Type I diabetes and for clustering of cases in space and time, but results to date are inconclusive. In the U.K., notifications of childhood diabetes to the British Diabetic Association (BDA) Registry show no changing trend although year-to-year variation has occurred within a range of about twenty per cent (Fig. 7.8). This degree of annual fluctuation is small compared with the characteristic epidemicity of most childhood viral infections. For example, Fig. 7.8 shows the changing patterns of Coxsackie B and mumps virus infections, both of which have been speculatively linked with diabetes. They showed marked epidemicity over the years illustrated; a different Coxsackie B type predominated in each of the five epidemic years.

Most childhood infections follow a similar epidemic pattern and it is therefore unlikely that the onset of Type I diabetes is associated with infection by one particular virus such as mumps, Coxsackie or rubella in the period immediately preceding onset. However, it is still possible that either a number of different infections precipitate onset or one or more infections initiate the development of diabetes many years before its onset.

Seasonal Incidence

The seasonal distribution of new cases of Type I diabetes in the

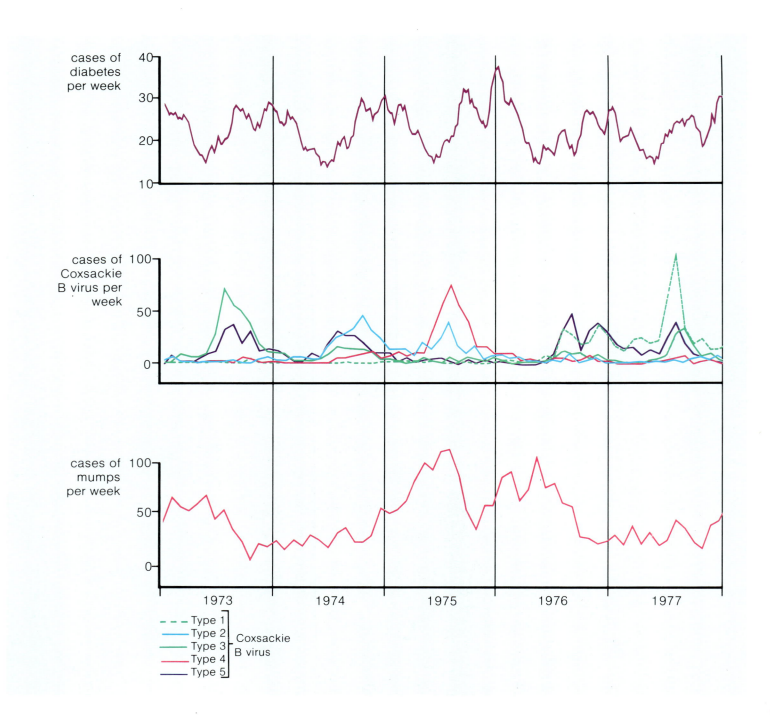

Fig. 7.8 Incidence of childhood diabetes and viral infections in the U.K. Data are from cases of diabetes notified to the BDA per week (five-week moving average) and viral infections notified to the Communicable Disease Surveillance Centre of the Public Health Laboratory Service, U.K.

U.K. (Fig. 7.9) shows a low incidence in May, rising through the summer to a peak in the autumn, followed by a second peak in winter. This pattern has been confirmed in a number of other countries in the northern hemisphere and in the southern hemisphere where the nadir occurs in December (Fig. 7.9). Seasonal variation tends to be less in females than in males and the seasonal pattern occurs in areas of both high (e.g. U.S.A.) and low (e.g. Japan) incidence (Fig. 7.10).

Seasonality clearly reflects environmental influence on the onset of some cases of diabetes. The similarity of this pattern to the autumn and winter prevalence of infectious illnesses of childhood suggests the possibility of an association. However, since the changes leading to diabetes often commence years before its clinical onset, the seasonal environmental factors which in some way provoke the onset of diabetes may act as non-specific precipitating factors rather than as primary causes of islet cell damage. Alternatively, the pathogenic process may comprise a series of environmentally induced attacks on the pancreas producing cumulative damage culminating in diabetes. If this is the case, the extrinsic factor that precipitates the onset of diabetes could be similar to, and act in the same way as, that which starts it.

Age Incidence
Most studies of the age of onset of Type I diabetes have been

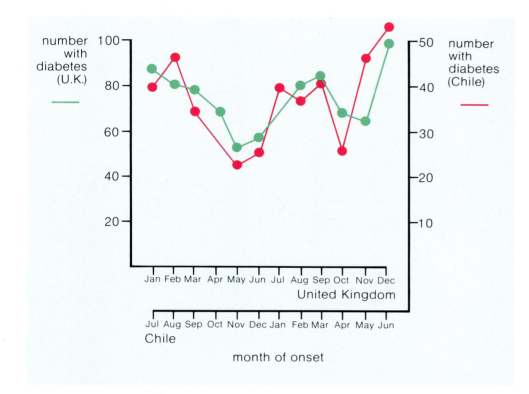

Fig. 7.9 Seasonal incidence of new cases of Type I diabetes in the U.K. and Chile. From Durruty *et al.* (1979) and Gamble (1980), by courtesy of Springer Verlag and John Hopkins University School of Hygiene and Public Health, respectively.

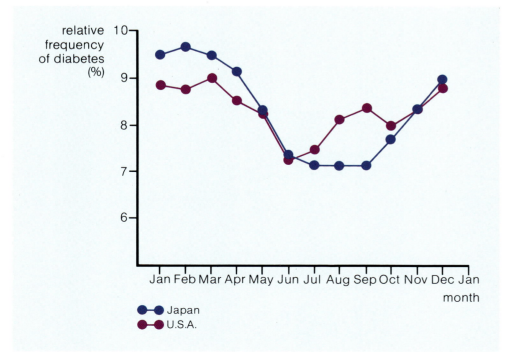

Fig. 7.10 Seasonal incidence of Type I diabetes in Japan and the U.S.A. Points are calculated from a five-month moving average. From Tajima *et al.* (1985), by courtesy of the American Diabetes Association.

restricted to children and little is known of the incidence in adults. In Fig. 7.11, data from several sources have been combined to give an estimate of age-specific incidence up to thirty-five years. The distribution shows a steep increase to a peak at about the age of puberty. The rate of increase is lower between 3–10 years of age forming a shoulder in the distribution and the decline in adolescence levels off to form a second shoulder in young adults. The incidence probably declines after thirty years of age. This overall pattern has been found in many countries.

Diabetes is rare in the first few months of life, its frequency increasing abruptly at about nine months of age (Fig. 7.12). This could have several explanations. If there is an association with infectious disease, this tends to be rare in the early months of life because of protection afforded by maternal antibodies and the relative isolation of young babies. The increase also coincides with increasing exposure to many dietary and other environmental factors. A latent period between initiation of diabetes and its clinical onset could also account for its rarity in the first nine months of life.

The age distributions in males and females show small differences which have been most clearly shown in surveys in children; an example from the U.K. is shown in Fig. 7.13. Most investigations have found an overall male preponderance of up to approximately twenty per cent but there is usually a female excess from 5–9 years of age and a male excess from 0–4 and 10–15 years of age. Minor peaks have often been found from 4–8 years of age, more in boys than girls, but these have varied in different surveys. These peaks may be due to either hormonal changes, which may increase susceptibility to diabetes at this age, or infections, which have their highest incidence in the first years at school.

The peak frequency of diabetes at about twelve years of age is later in boys than in girls, which suggests that it may be related to the hormonal changes of puberty. Indeed, the fact that it has proved such a regular feature of surveys in many countries over a long period suggests a link with intrinsic, rather than environmental, factors. However, the age of peak incidence in different surveys varies from age 11–15 years, which lacks the consistency of changes associated with puberty. The age distribution may thus be due to a combination of intrinsic and extrinsic factors.

The decline in incidence in adolescence and adult life is an interesting feature. It may be due to a decline in susceptibility to diabetes, although the incidence of autoimmune diseases generally increases with age. If the causative environmental factor is a chemical toxin, there is no obvious reason why exposure should diminish with age. However, if infection constitutes the extrinsic trigger, a declining incidence after childhood would be expected since most infections diminish as immunity is acquired with advancing age.

SOCIOECONOMIC FACTORS

Exposure to some environmental factors, particularly viruses, varies with social class and any effect of social class on the incidence of Type I diabetes would be of great interest. Unfortunately, published data are conflicting.

In Copenhagen, the incidence in children aged 0–14 years was significantly higher in the south of the county (20.0 per 100,000) than in the north (10.5 per 100,000). A number of socioeconomic indicators (Fig. 7.14) suggested that incidence was inversely related to social class in these areas.

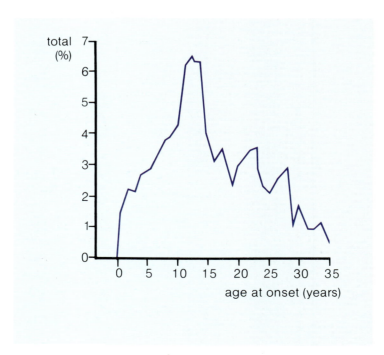

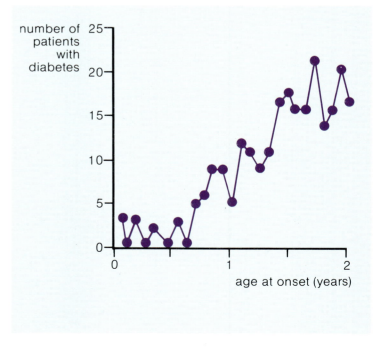

Fig. 7.11 Age at onset of Type I diabetes. 1460 cases have been combined from several sources to estimate age-specific incidence. From Gamble (1980), by courtesy of John Hopkins School of Hygiene and Public Health.

Fig. 7.12 Age at onset of Type I diabetes in infants under two years of age. From Gamble (1980), by courtesy of John Hopkins School of Hygiene and Public Health.

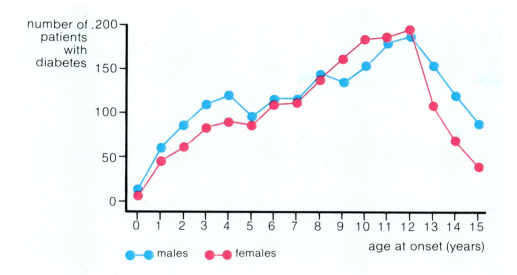

number of patients with diabetes / males / females / age at onset (years)

Fig. 7.13 Age at onset of Type I diabetes by sex in the U.K. From Gamble (1980), by courtesy of John Hopkins School of Hygiene and Public Health.

INCIDENCE OF TYPE I DIABETES AND SOCIOECONOMIC CHARACTERISTICS IN COPENHAGEN COUNTY

characteristic	area 1	area 2
incidence of juvenile diabetes mellitus (annual number per 100,000) in age groups 0–14 years	10.5	20.0
age group 0–14 years (% of total population)	23.9	27.9
five years growth rate of total population (%)	−2.27	+8.24
average number of persons per room	0.84	0.92
number of unskilled workers (% of total population)	9.7	13.6
population with school attendance ≥11 years (%)	7.6	3.6
women working away from home (%)	38.4	42.1
property according to assessment per family (Danish Crowns)	145,000	62,500

Fig. 7.14 Incidence of Type I diabetes and socioeconomic characteristics in two areas of Copenhagen County, Denmark. There is a negative correlation ($p < 0.05$) between the incidence and property assessment per family. From Christau *et al.* (1977), by courtesy of Springer Verlag.

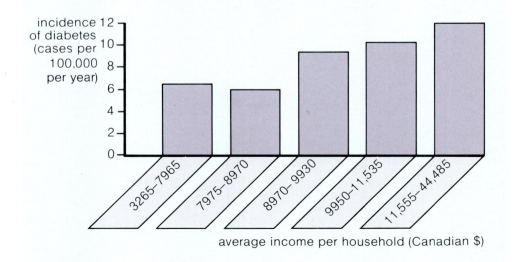

incidence of diabetes (cases per 100,000 per year) / average income per household (Canadian $)

Fig. 7.15 Incidence of Type I diabetes and average household income in Montreal, Canada. From West *et al.* (1979), by courtesy of the American Diabetes Association.

In Montreal (Fig. 7.15), the incidence of diabetes was examined in relation to average household income in the census tract of residence; a highly significant increase was found as income increased, the inverse of the relationship found in the Danish study. Further studies in Pennsylvania and Japan found no association with social class (Fig. 7.16).

Investigation of these social class effects is difficult. The classes tend to segregate in separate localities and social class effects may be confounded by geographical factors that also affect the incidence of diabetes. Further studies are required to resolve this important question.

SOCIOECONOMIC RELATIONSHIP TO PREVALENCE OF TYPE I DIABETES IN JAPAN AND ITS INCIDENCE IN U.S.A.			
Japan		**U.S.A.**	
yearly income per person (1979)	prevalence per 100,000	yearly income per family (1970)	incidence per 100,000
$5387	5.5	$8143	13.7
$5661	7.5	$9420	12.9
$6133	5.2	$10,463	14.9
$6425	4.7	$11,664	14.6
$6890	5.9	$15,208	15.5

Fig. 7.16 Prevalence of Type I diabetes in Japan and its incidence in the U.S.A. and their relationship to annual income per person. From Tajima *et al.* (1985), by courtesy of the American Diabetes Association.

REFERENCES

Bloom A, Hayes TM & Gamble DR (1975) Register of newly diagnosed diabetic children. *British Medical Journal*, **3**, 580–583.

Borch-Johnsen K, Joner G, Mandrup-Poulsen T, Christy M, Zachau-Christiansen B, Kastrup K & Nerup J (1984) Relation between breast-feeding and incidence rates of insulin-dependent diabetes mellitus: a hypothesis. *Lancet*, **2**, 1083–1086.

Christau B, Åkerblom HK, Joner G, Dahlquist G, Ludvigsson J & Nerup J (1981) Incidence of childhood insulin-dependent diabetes mellitus in Denmark, Finland, Norway and Sweden. *Acta Endocrinologica*, **98** (Suppl.245), 68–80.

Christau B, Kromann H, Ortved Anderson O, Christy M, Buschard K, Arnung K, Højland Kristensen I, Peitersen B, Steinrud J & Nerup J (1977) Incidence, seasonal and geographical patterns of juvenile-onset insulin-dependent diabetes mellitus in Denmark. *Diabetologia*, **13**, 281–284.

Crossley JR & Upsdell M (1980) The incidence of juvenile diabetes mellitus in New Zealand. *Diabetologia*, **18**, 29–30.

Durruty P, Ruiz F & Garcia de los Rios M (1979) Age at diagnosis and seasonal variation in the onset of insulin-dependent diabetes in Chile (southern hemisphere). *Diabetologia*, **17**, 357–360.

Gamble DR (1980) The epidemiology of insulin dependent diabetes with particular reference to the relationship of virus infection to its etiology. *Epidemiologic Reviews*, **2**, 49–70.

Gottlieb MS & Root HF (1968) Diabetes mellitus in twins. *Diabetes*, **17**, 693–704.

LaPorte RE, Fishbein HA, Drash AL, Kuller LH, Schneider BB, Orchard TJ & Wagener DK (1981) The Pittsburgh insulin-dependent diabetes mellitus (IDDM) registry. The incidence of insulin-dependent diabetes mellitus in Allegheny County, Pennsylvania (1965–1976). *Diabetes*, **30**, 279–284.

Laron ZV, Karp M & Modan M (1985) The incidence of insulin-dependent diabetes mellitus in Israeli children and adolescents 0–20 years of age: a retrospective study 1975–1980. *Diabetes Care*, **8** (Suppl.1), 24–28.

Lestradet H & Besse J (1977) Prévalence et incidence du diabète juvénile insulino-dependant en France. *Diabete et Metabolisme*, **3**, 229–234.

Patterson CC, Thorogood M, Smith PG, Heasman MA, Clark JA & Mann JI (1983) Epidemiology of Type 1 (insulin-dependent) diabetes in Scotland 1968–1976: evidence of an increasing incidence. *Diabetologia*, **24**, 238–243.

Pyke DA & Nelson PE (1976) Diabetes mellitus in identical twins. In *The Genetics of Diabetes Mellitus*. Edited by Creutzfeldt W, Köbberling J & Neel JV. pp. 194–202. Berlin: Springer Verlag.

Siemiatycki J, Colle E, Aubert D, Campbell S & Belmonte MM (1986) The distribution of type I insulin-dependent diabetes mellitus by age, sex, secular trend, seasonality, time clusters and space-time clusters: evidence from Montreal, 1971–1983. *American Journal of Epidemiology*, **124**, 545–560.

Taha TH, Moussa MAA, Rashid AR & Fenech FF (1983) Diabetes mellitus in Kuwait: incidence in the first 29 years of life. *Diabetologia*, **25**, 306–308.

Tajima N, LaPorte RE, Hibi I, Kitigawa T, Fujita H & Drash AL (1985) A comparison of the epidemiology of youth-onset insulin-dependent diabetes mellitus between Japan and the United States (Allegheny County, Pennsylvania). *Diabetes Care*, **8**, (Suppl.1), 17–23.

Then Berg H (1939) Zur frage der psychischen und neurologischen erscheinungen bei diabeteskranken und deren verwandten. *Zeitschrift Gesamte Neurologie und Psychiatrie Referate und Ergebrisse*, **165**, 278–283.

West R, Belmonte MM, Colle E, Crepeau MP, Wilkins J & Pourier R (1979) Epidemiologic survey of juvenile onset diabetes in Montreal. *Diabetes*, **28**, 690–693.

White P (1932) *Diabetes in Childhood and Adolescence*. Philadelphia: Lea & Febiger.

Aetiology and Pathogenesis of Type I Diabetes: Genetic Factors

Andrew N Gorsuch MA BM BCh MRCP

The classification and terminology of diabetes mellitus are still controversial. Diabetes seen in most patients in temperate zones has two broad clinical subdivisions. Fig. 8.1 shows the basis for this subdivision into Type I and Type II diabetes on biochemical, histological, genetic and immunological grounds. Fig. 8.2 shows the clinical features of the two types.

NOMENCLATURE

The terms 'juvenile-onset diabetes' (JOD) and 'maturity-onset diabetes' (MOD) are inadequate; 'insulin-dependent diabetes mellitus' (IDDM) and 'non insulin-dependent diabetes mellitus' (NIDDM) have the advantage of being self-explanatory and are generally satisfactory for clinical purposes. When considering the aetiology of diabetes, however, these terms have disadvantages. Even mild MOD may require insulin either at times of severe metabolic stress or after many years of diabetes, whereas in the tropics, diabetes may be intermittently insulin-dependent. Furthermore, some cases of mild diabetes not requiring insulin may actually represent an incomplete form of the juvenile-onset type, while on the other hand many patients treated with insulin are not truly dependent upon it. These considerations support the use of the terms Type I and Type II diabetes in a pathological sense, although it may be impossible to categorize some individual patients definitely.

CLASSIFICATION OF PRIMARY DIABETES	Type I	Type II
insulin secretion	deficient	present
size of pancreas	small	normal
pancreatic islets	B cell depletion and insulitis	B cells present hyalinosis
family history	Type I but not Type II	Type II but not Type I
genetic associations	HLA	none with HLA
autoimmunity	increased	normal

Fig. 8.1 Classification of primary diabetes.

CLINICAL HETEROGENEITY OF DIABETES features at onset	Type I	Type II
age	usually < 30 years	usually > 20 years
sex	M > F (children)	M < F
season	less in summer	any
body weight	usually lean	often obese
presentation	often acute	insidious
ketonuria (non-fasting)	heavy	absent
insulin dependence (unstressed)	yes	not in early years

Fig. 8.2 Features at the onset of Type I and Type II diabetes.

EARLY WORK ON GENETICS

Heredity in diabetes was suspected by ancient Hindu physicians, and by Rondoletius and Morton in sixteenth and seventeenth century Europe. In 1906, Naunyn stated that eighteen per cent of his diabetic patients had affected relatives. Pincus and White (1933) were the first of many to confirm a significant increase in diabetes in the parents and siblings of their patients. By the late 1930's it was reported that monozygotic twins were more often concordant for diabetes than dizygotic twins, implying that the familial occurrence of the disease was due, at least in part, to genetic factors.

Between 1900 and 1930, there were many attempts to determine the mode of inheritance of diabetes by inspecting individual pedigrees. By the early 1950's most groups favoured either a Mendelian recessive or a multi-factorial hypothesis, but the issue was hotly debated and Neel referred to diabetes as a 'geneticist's nightmare' (Fig. 8.3).

There were three main reasons for this nightmare: genetic heterogeneity between Type I and Type II diabetes (Fig. 8.4); incomplete (and age-related) 'penetrance' of the diabetic genotype; and an inability to identify individuals who possess the diabetic genotype but have normal glucose tolerance. Penetrance may be defined as the number of individuals in whom the genotype is actually expressed (i.e. the number with the disease or other characteristic), calculated as a proportion of the total number with the genotype.

Genetic heterogeneity of diabetes is strongly suggested by differences in patterns of inheritance between juvenile- and adult-onset cases. More recent evidence includes: a tendency for Type I and Type II diabetes to 'breed true to type'; a markedly lower concordance rate for juvenile-onset than for maturity-onset diabetes in identical twins; an excess of organ-specific auto-immunity in non-diabetic relatives of Type I diabetic patients; and, most importantly, different associations of the two types of diabetes with genetic markers. Thus, there are HLA associations with Type I but not with Type II diabetes (see below), whereas Type II diabetes may be associated with chlorpropamide-alcohol flushing and with blood group A rather than group O.

GENETIC SUSCEPTIBILITY

In any sufficiently large, unselected group of people, a small number with clinical Type I diabetes will be found (Fig. 8.5).

Typically, in young adults in a northern European population, the prevalence will be approximately one to three per thousand. Because of the increasing prevalence of Type I diabetes with age, it follows that some of the non-diabetic individuals also have the Type I diabetic genotype (i.e. they are genetically susceptible) since they are destined to develop diabetes in the future.

In addition, there is a group of genetically susceptible individuals which will never become clinically affected with diabetes. The most striking evidence for this is that when one of a pair of identical twins has Type I diabetes, in only about fifty per cent of cases does the co-twin become affected, even after many years of follow-up. Since such twins are genetically identical it follows that the genotype for susceptibility to Type I diabetes must have a low penetrance even when allowance is made for age; presumably environmental factors determine whether a susceptible person develops diabetes.

Some subjects who will develop diabetes in the future may already have immunological or other markers of pre-diabetic pathological changes, but, unless the susceptibility genotype can itself be detected, its penetrance cannot be determined and it is virtually impossible to distinguish between recessive and multi-factorial inheritance by quantitative genetic techniques. Identification of genetically susceptible children is important for accurate genetic counselling, for prediction of risk of future diabetes and for investigations of the nature of susceptibility and the mechanism by which it interacts with environmental factors to produce the disease. A major step in this direction was the discovery of HLA types as genetic markers for susceptibility.

HUMAN HISTOCOMPATIBILITY ANTIGENS AND OTHER MARKERS
The HLA System
Situated on the surface of animal nucleated cells is a mosaic of macromolecular histocompatibility antigens. In man, they are termed HLA (human leucocyte, series A) antigens and were first detected in transplantation experiments. Their biological role appears to be to facilitate certain types of cell-mediated immune interactions.

There are several series of HLA antigens including HLA-A, B, Cw, D and DR (Fig. 8.6). The overall mix of antigenic specificities (the pattern of shapes and colours in Fig. 8.6) is characteristic of an individual and can be recognized as 'self' by T lymphocytes.

DIABETES — 'A GENETICIST'S NIGHTMARE'

environmental factors	genetic factors
role? nature?	heterogeneous? singe gene or polygenic? mode of inheritance? penetrance?

↓ ↓

can individual with 'diabetes' genotype be identified?

Fig. 8.3 Understanding the genetics of diabetes; 'a geneticist's nightmare' (Neel, 1976).

GENETIC HETEROGENEITY OF DIABETES

	Type I	Type II
concordance in identical twins	<50%	100%
organ-specific autoimmunity increased in relatives	yes	no
association with genetic markers: HLA	yes	no
ABO blood groups	no	weak

Fig. 8.4 Genetic heterogeneity of diabetes.

GENETIC SUSCEPTIBILITY TO TYPE I DIABETES AND PENETRANCE

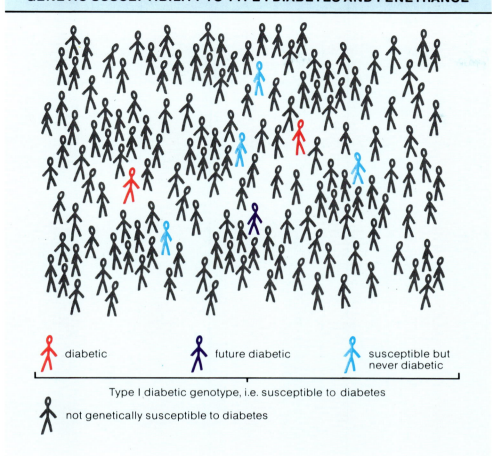

diabetic

future diabetic

susceptible but never diabetic

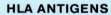
Type I diabetic genotype, i.e. susceptible to diabetes

not genetically susceptible to diabetes

Fig. 8.5 Genetic susceptibility to Type I diabetes.

HLA ANTIGENS

human nucleated cell

surface HLA antigens

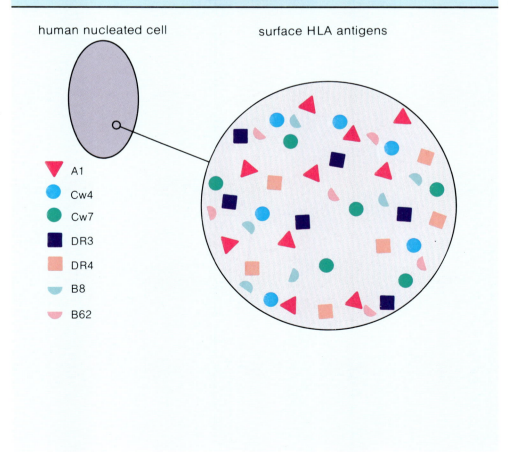

A1

Cw4

Cw7

DR3

DR4

B8

B62

Fig. 8.6 HLA antigens. The shapes indicate the series to which molecules belong and the colours indicate their specificity within a series.

HLA Typing (Tissue Typing) in the Laboratory

HLA-A, B and C typing is performed by adding live lymphocytes from the peripheral blood of the subject being typed to an array of sera containing antibodies against known HLA antigens obtained either from parous women or raised as monoclonal antibodies. Positive reactions are shown by cell killing in the presence of added complement.

HLA-DR typing is more difficult. B lymphocytes from the test subject are isolated or identified serologically and their binding of specific typing sera examined by immunofluorescence methods.

The HLA antigens are genetically coded by a complex of closely linked genetic loci (HLA-A, B, Cw, DP, DQ, and DR) on the short arm of chromosome 6 (Fig. 8.7). They are usually inherited together as Mendelian co-dominants, that is each allele appears to be expressed whatever other HLA alleles may be present, and they are inherited without sex linkage (Fig. 8.8). HLA-D types reflect various combinations of genes in the DP-DQ-DR complex and are determined by a complex immunological method. Recently, typing methods based not on serology but on recombinant DNA technology have come into use for the identification of some DR, DP and DQ DNA sequences.

Linkage Disequilibrium

A feature of the HLA system is that certain alleles tend to occur

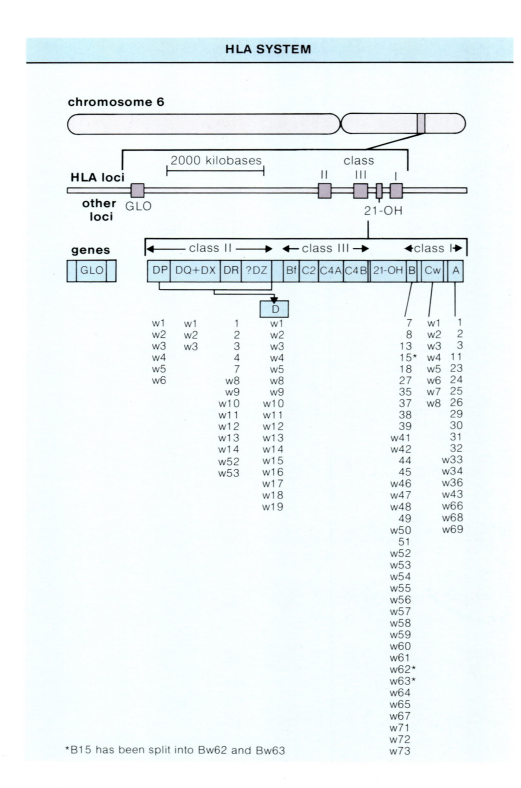

Fig. 8.7 Chromosome map of the HLA region. A, B, C, DP, DQ and DR are HLA loci. D is a series of immunological specificities determined by DR, DQ and DP genes. C4A, C4B and C2 are respectively the two loci for the fourth and second components of complement and Bf is factor B of the alternative complement pathway. Below the map are most of the HLA specificities recognized by the Ninth International Histocompatibility Workshop, 1984. The prefix w indicates that the specificity is provisionally recognized but has not been assigned a permanent number. At the C locus, however, w is always used to distinguish these specificities from C2 and C4. The map is approximately to scale. Class I antigens include A, B and C; class II include DP, DQ, DR and class III complement components. GLO is the enzyme glyoxylase.

*B15 has been split into Bw62 and Bw63

together in the same haplotype much more frequently than would be expected on the basis of random mixing by chromosome breakage and recombination over many generations. This phenomenon is called 'linkage disequilibrium'. Particularly common haplotypes in European Caucasoid populations include A1-B8-DR3, A2-Bw62-Cw3-DR4, A3-B7-DR2, B18-Cw5-DR3 and A29-B44-Cw4.

Relative Risk

Some genetic characters are more common in patients with certain diseases than in control subjects. The strength of such an association may be expressed as the relative risk (RR) or odds ratio. This is calculated from the numbers that are positive or negative for a particular phenotype in samples from the diseased and control populations (Fig. 8.9). A value greater than 1.0 suggests a positive association and less than 1.0 a negative one.

Since 1973, studies in various white Caucasoid populations have shown many positive and negative associations between Type I diabetes and different HLA phenotypes; none of them, however, is very strong. The overall picture may be simplified by taking into account the known linkage disequilibria within the HLA system.

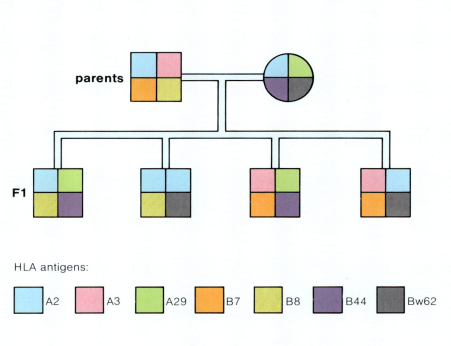

INHERITANCE OF HLA ANTIGENS

parents

F1

HLA antigens:

A2 A3 A29 B7 B8 B44 Bw62

Fig. 8.8 Inheritance of HLA-A and B phenotypes in a hypothetical family. No subject has more than two antigens of a single series. Each child inherits only one HLA-A and one HLA-B from each parent. Where two children inherit the same HLA-A from a given parent, they almost always inherit the same HLA-B as well; the two series are closely linked.

HLA AND DISEASE: RELATIVE RISK

subject	HLA antigen	
	positive	**negative**
diabetic	$h = 15$	$k = 12$
non-diabetic	$H = 12$	$K = 36$

$$\text{relative risk (odds ratio)} = \frac{h \times K}{H \times k} = \frac{15 \times 36}{12 \times 12} = 3.75$$

Fig. 8.9 Example of relative risk calculation. Each circle represents one individual.

8.5

Fig. 8.10 shows the haplotypes of HLA antigens in linkage disequilibrium with DR3, DR4 and DR2. It is now clear that it is the HLA-DR (or -D) specificities that have the strongest and therefore the primary associations with Type I diabetes; the disturbed frequencies of Bf, C4 and HLA-A, B and Cw antigens can all be explained by their known tendency to occur on the same haplotypes as DR3, DR4 and DR2 due to linkage disequilibrium. This is reflected in the progressively increasing deviation of RR from 1.0 as the region is traversed from right to left.

Cudworth (1978) suggested the concept of three apparently independent 'axes' or systems of alleles (Fig. 8.10). S1 and S2 were termed 'susceptibility axes' and emphasized earlier observations that coexistence of both in the same individual, giving the phenotype HLA-B8, w62, for example, appeared to carry an RR for Type I diabetes much higher than that from one axis alone. The R (resistance) axis, with an RR of less than 1.0, was so-called because of its postulated protective effect against diabetes.

Other Genetic Markers

Although susceptibility to Type I diabetes appears to be principally HLA-linked, a contribution from genes on other chromosomes cannot be excluded. The most rigorous investigations of this so far have failed to confirm some associations suggested earlier, but a significant excess of the fast acetylator phenotype was confirmed when published data were pooled. Further associations may occur with variable regions near the insulin gene on chromosome 11. This is suggested by work using restriction endonucleases and labelled complementary DNA probes to map the chromosome. The fragments created by the endonucleases are heritable and behave as a polymorphic system. A few reports suggest an association between restriction fragment length and Type II diabetes in some families, although not in others. There is also suggestive evidence for a weak association with Type I diabetes.

The complex HLA associations with Type I diabetes suggest that genetic susceptibility to this disease is probably determined by genes near the DR locus. For example, a susceptibility gene S1 is postulated to be in linkage disequilibrium (i.e. tending to occur in association) with the S1 axis specificities (Fig. 8.11).

Another implication of the HLA association concerns the mechanism of action of the HLA-associated susceptibility genes; it is likely that immunity is involved in some way (see Fig. 8.16).

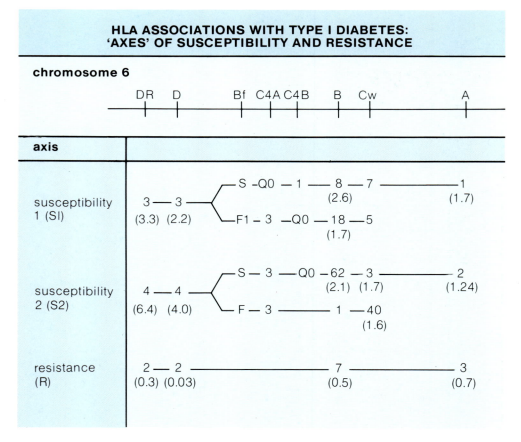

HLA ASSOCIATIONS WITH TYPE I DIABETES: 'AXES' OF SUSCEPTIBILITY AND RESISTANCE

Fig. 8.10 Haplotypes S1, S2 and R of HLA antigens in linkage disequilibrium with HLA-DR3, DR4 and DR2, respectively. A relative risk (RR) for the association of a specificity with Type I diabetes is given in parenthesis where available.

Family Studies: HLA Linkage

If genes in the HLA region of chromosome 6 do indeed determine susceptibility to Type I diabetes, then by HLA genotyping large numbers of families with two or more diabetic children it should be possible to demonstrate linkage between HLA and the disease. Fig. 8.12 shows a hypothetical family with two diabetic children who are HLA-identical by descent, that is, identical for both paternal and maternal haplotypes.

If it is assumed that inheritance by a child of one or the other parental HLA haplotype is random, then by the null hypothesis of no linkage, twenty-five per cent of pairs of diabetic siblings would be expected to be HLA-identical by descent, fifty per cent would share only one haplotype (a state termed haplo-identity) and twenty-five per cent would be non-identical (Fig. 8.13).

In the presence of linkage an excess of HLA-identical and maybe of haplo-identical pairs would be expected. The exact proportions would depend on several factors: closeness of linkage, mode of inheritance of susceptibility and the frequency of the susceptibility genes in the population and their penetrance.

HLA AND TYPE I DIABETES IN POPULATIONS

	HLA region	
	DR/D	B
S1 often with	3	8
S2 often with	4	15
R often with	2	7

Fig. 8.11 HLA and Type I diabetes in populations.

HLA AND TYPE I DIABETES IN FAMILIES: SIB PAIRS AND HLA GENOTYPES

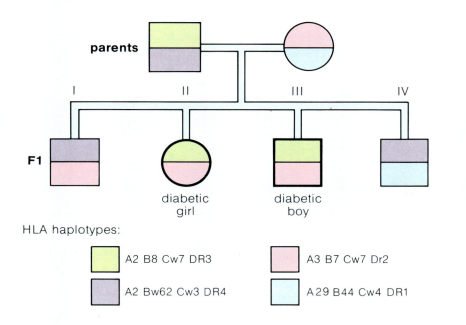

HLA haplotypes:

A2 B8 Cw7 DR3

A2 Bw62 Cw3 DR4

A3 B7 Cw7 Dr2

A29 B44 Cw4 DR1

Fig. 8.12 Linkage between HLA and Type I diabetes. In this hypothetical example, the two diabetic children are identical for both maternal and paternal HLA haplotypes.

HLA HAPLOTYPES IN PAIRS OF DIABETIC SIBLINGS: EXPECTED PROBABILITIES IF NO LINKAGE

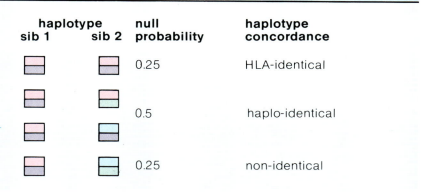

haplotype sib 1	haplotype sib 2	null probability	haplotype concordance
		0.25	HLA-identical
		0.5	haplo-identical
		0.25	non-identical

Fig. 8.13 Linkage between HLA and Type I diabetes. Probabilities if there were no linkage are given.

Fig. 8.14 incorporates pooled data from a large U.K. study and from several other sources. This shows that pairs of diabetic siblings are indeed far more likely to be HLA-identical than would be expected by chance. Evidently a non-diabetic sibling of an affected child is likely to be genetically susceptible if HLA-identical to the diabetic child, whereas haplo- and non-identical siblings are progressively less likely to be at risk. This argument does not depend on either the presence or absence of the 'high risk antigens' defined in population studies.

There are several possible modes of inheritance of HLA-linked susceptibility to Type I diabetes (Fig. 8.15). Data on haplotype concordance in diabetic sib pairs have been analysed and fitted to mathematical models based on the different possible modes of inheritance. Single-gene dominant inheritance has been excluded. Recessive inheritance (i.e. two copies of a single gene necessary for susceptibility) is possible, but fits only with an absurdly low penetrance.

Recently, a more sophisticated analysis has taken account of all affected and non-affected siblings in the families. Recessive inheritance with a penetrance of 0.75 has been shown to accord with the data very well. A good fit has also been obtained using a model based on intermediate inheritance (i.e. one copy of the single gene giving susceptibility with low penetrance and two copies giving high penetrance; a gene dosage effect).

However, it may be that none of these single-gene hypotheses represents the truth. The particularly high risk of Type I diabetes in individuals who are typed HLA-DR3, 4, that is positive both for S1-axis HLA specificities (-DR3) on one haplotype and for S2-axis specificities (-DR4) on the other, has already been mentioned. It is probable, although not incontrovertible, that this risk is greater than that in DR3, 3 or DR4, 4 homozygotes. If this is true, then there must be at least two different HLA-linked susceptibility genes, one tending to be associated with DR3 and the other with DR4; a high degree of penetrance would depend on the presence of both, while one alone could give either low-penetrance susceptibility or none at all.

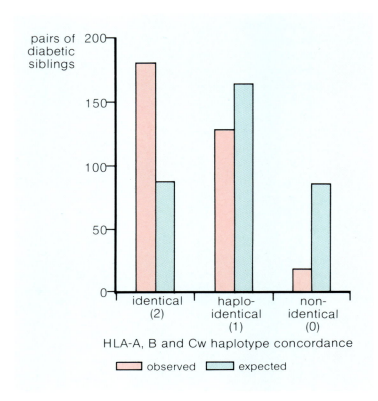

Fig. 8.14 Evidence for linkage between HLA and Type I diabetes in families. Pairs of diabetic siblings are grouped according to whether the two in each pair are identical for two, one or none of their HLA-A, B and Cw haplotypes. The difference between the observed and expected distributions is statistically highly significant.

INHERITANCE OF HLA-LINKED SUSCEPTIBILITY TO TYPE I DIABETES

inheritance	loci 'diabetes'	HLA-DR	occurrence
dominant			excluded
recessive			possible
intermediate			possible
2 or more inter-acting genes			probable

Fig. 8.15 Possible modes of inheritance of HLA-linked susceptibility to Type I diabetes. A state of susceptibility is indicated by a completed circle at the 'diabetes' locus; the larger the circle the greater the penetrance. By the intermediate hypothesis, penetrance depends upon the number of appropriate genes present (a gene dosage effect); the small dark circles represent the low penetrance associated with a single copy of the gene, while the combined effect of two copies (large circle) gives higher penetrance.

Is There a Protective Gene?

All the HLA-DR antigens, except 3 and 4, are less frequent in diabetic patients than in non-diabetic subjects. This is because such a high proportion of haplotypes in diabetic patients is occupied by DR3 or DR4 that the proportion available for the remainder is substantially reduced. However, HLA-DR2 is excessively rare in Type I diabetes, a consistent finding usually held to indicate the existence of a gene near the HLA locus which protects against diabetes.

GENE ACTION
Action of the Postulated Susceptibility 1 (S1) Gene

Most of the genes in the HLA region code either for cell surface and therefore immunologically important components or for other molecules involved in immune reactions, and it is inherently likely that one or more of the hypothetical diabetes susceptibility genes in this region should have a similar function. This means that such genes could be directly responsible for some of the immunological abnormalities commonly found around the time of onset of clinical Type I diabetes (see *Chapter 9*). Alternatively, the immunological changes might be secondary to the disease process itself, rather than being causative.

In non-diabetic relatives of Type I diabetic patients, organ-specific autoimmunity is more common than in non-diabetic control subjects, suggesting either a common susceptibility gene (not necessarily HLA-linked) or a haplotypic association due to linkage disequilibrium between an 'autoimmunity' gene and a different diabetes susceptibility gene.

Injected exogenous insulin is antigenic and the immune response has been extensively studied in man. There is probably an association between low insulin antibody response and the S1 axis. Other antigen-response systems showing evidence of HLA-linked or associated variation include leprosy, influenza vaccination and various allergies.

In animals, there is more evidence in favour of immune response genes in the major histocompatibility complex (MHC) which corresponds to the human HLA region. This has been shown, for example, in breeding experiments. Genes of this type may be important in certain animal models of Type I diabetes, including the low-dose streptozotocin model and the BB rat. Fig. 8.16 summarizes the evidence for a susceptibility gene which could modify the immune response.

The possibility that one of the HLA-linked diabetes susceptibility genes enhances organ-specific autoimmunity generally has been examined in HLA-genotyped siblings of one hundred and fifty-six Type I diabetic children (probands). Fig. 8.17 shows the prevalence of autoantibodies in the non-diabetic siblings, grouped according to HLA haplotype concordance with their respective probands. If the hypothesis were true, positive tests for thyroid or gastric parietal-cell antibody (TGA), or both, would be most common in the HLA-identical siblings, since they would be highly likely to carry the gene, and least common in the non-identical siblings. The observed prevalences show no such deviation from a random distribution.

Interestingly, the same applies to islet cell antibody tested by the conventional immunofluorescence technique (see *Chapter 9*). By contrast, complement-fixing ICA (CF-ICA) does appear to segregate with HLA-linked susceptibility. Thus, if there is a common genetic basis to Type I diabetes and to serological organ-specific autoimmunity, the common gene is not HLA-linked.

On balance it seems likely, although not proven, that HLA-linked immune response genes exist in man. Comparable genes may indeed contribute to susceptibility in animal models of human Type I diabetes, but the extrapolation from animal model to human disease is not justified at present.

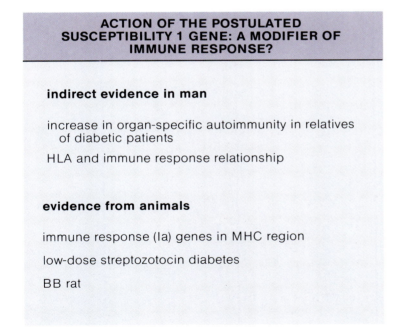

Fig. 8.16 Evidence for the action of the susceptibility 1 gene which could modify the immune response.

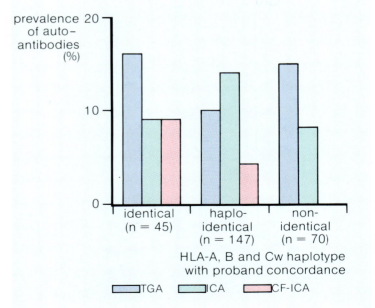

Fig. 8.17 Organ-specific autoantibodies and HLA-linked susceptibility to Type I diabetes in non-diabetic siblings of diabetic probands. The only statistically significant segregation ($p<0.013$) with HLA haplotypes is that of complement-fixing islet cell antibody (CF-ICA).

Action of the Postulated Susceptibility 2 (S2) Gene

Animal models of diabetes may help the understanding of the role of the susceptibility 2 (S2) gene. Virus-induced diabetes in laboratory animals depends upon the genetic background or strain of the host. The inheritance of suceptibility in mice to diabetes induced by encephalomyocarditis virus behaves as a recessive trait in cross-breeding experiments. However, if this does have any bearing on human Type I diabetes, it can have little to do with the postulated HLA-linked S2 gene, since there is no evidence of linkage to the homologous H-2 system in the mouse.

The mechanism of variation in susceptibility of mice to viral diabetes probably involves general host responses to viral infection (e.g. interferon production) rather than more specific islet B cell effects. It has been postulated that, in man, genetically-determined abnormalities of complement components might be important in HLA-linked genetic susceptibility to Type I diabetes. This idea arose because the unexpressed allelomorphs of C4, now termed C4-AQ0 and BQ0, showed increased relative risks for the disease in certain populations (see Fig. 8.10). Some support for this concept comes from the report that not only Type I diabetic patients but also their non-diabetic identical twins have abnormally low levels of circulating C4. Fig. 8.18 summarizes the evidence for a gene determining susceptibility to environmental agents.

So far, the mode of action of the S2 diabetes gene remains unresolved. The only other condition known to be associated with HLA-DR4 is seropositive rheumatoid arthritis, the aetiology of which remains equally obscure.

It can be postulated that two HLA-linked genes, S1 and S2 each in linkage disequilibrium with HLA-DR3 and HLA-DR4, respectively, interact to produce susceptibility to Type I diabetes. Such interaction is termed 'co-dominance' if the genes concerned are allelomorphic (at the same locus) and 'epistasis' if they are not.

Epistasis between two genes is the simplest example of multifactorial inheritance. It is possible that susceptibility results from interaction between a number of genes in the HLA region (some in linkage disequilibrium with HLA-DR3 and some with DR4) and perhaps elsewhere. Indeed, the HLA and complement alleles may themselves jointly determine, or contribute to, susceptibility, suggesting a direct role for abnormal C4 gene products. Such a mechanism, similar to that proposed in the BB rat model, would be very difficult to disprove and could explain the distributions of HLA phenotypes and genotypes observed in populations and families. As yet, however, the simpler hypothesis shown in Fig. 8.19 is sufficient to explain the data available in man.

ACTION OF THE POSTULATED SUSCEPTIBILITY 2 GENE: SUSCEPTIBILITY TO ENVIRONMENTAL AGENTS

viral diabetes in mice
strain-dependent
'recessive' pattern
not H-2-linked

human Type I diabetes
role of abnormal complement?

Fig. 8.18 Evidence for the action of the susceptibility 2 gene which could make the individual susceptible to environmental agents.

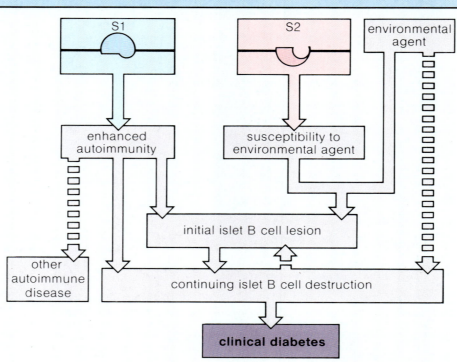

ACTION OF HLA-LINKED TYPE I DIABETES SUSCEPTIBILITY GENES

Fig. 8.19 Hypothesis for the action of HLA-linked Type I diabetes susceptibility genes.

Practical Applications

Whatever the details, certain further questions arise in relation to genetic counselling: (i) Does susceptibility to Type I diabetes always have the same genetic basis or is there further genetic heterogeneity within it? (ii) Can susceptible, but not yet diabetic, individuals be identified? (iii) Given that an individual is genetically susceptible, what is the risk of future diabetes? (iv) What is the time course of the destructive process? Does a single initiating event lead inexorably to diabetes or are there cumulative episodes of self-limiting insulitis, each initiated by a separate event? The last question is considered further in *Chapter 9*. The first three questions are considered next.

Genetic Heterogeneity within Type I Diabetes

Even within the accepted definition of Type I diabetes (insulin-dependent and ketosis-prone) the clinical picture of the disease, the seasonal pattern in its onset and particularly the rate of its progression, appear to vary with the age at onset. Does this reflect genetic heterogeneity, or is there merely a shorter time course of a single disease process in children compared to adults, for non-genetic reasons?

It has been shown that Type I diabetes in patients with other manifestations of organ-specific autoimmunity seems to be different from isolated cases of Type I diabetes, in that these patients tend to be female and adult (often middle-aged) at the onset of diabetes. This 'Type Ib' diabetes is associated only with 'S1-axis' HLA specificities (e.g. DR3) whereas 'Type Ia' (the majority of young-onset cases without coexistent autoimmune disease) shows increased frequencies of both S1 and S2 specificities (Fig. 8.20). The differences between Type Ia and Type Ib are too great to be explained by differences in the way the autoimmune and the juvenile-onset diabetic patients were ascertained and have been confirmed in several populations. There is thus no real doubt that they are genuine and that the two subtypes are not genetically identical. Type Ib diabetes is a rather uncommon variant. More controversial is the question whether the common juvenile form, Type Ia, is itself completely homogeneous.

One possible explanation for the heterogeneity is that susceptibility to Type I diabetes is determined by one or more genes, perhaps recessive and not necessarily HLA-linked, their expression being modified by the HLA-complex gene products themselves. Something of this nature appears to underlie spontaneous insulin-dependent diabetes in the BB rat.

Identification of Susceptible Individuals

Only a small minority of individuals who possess a 'high risk' antigen, such as HLA-DR4, is susceptible to Type I diabetes. HLA-identity with a diabetic sibling carries greater risk.

Risk of Diabetes in Siblings of Diabetic Children

In a large U.K. series of identical twin pairs, each including at least one Type I diabetic patient (see *Chapter 12*), a little over fifty per cent of the pairs ascertained were or became concordant for diabetes (i.e. both twins diabetic). Because of ascertainment bias the true concordance rate is likely to be less than fifty per cent.

The concordance rate in HLA-identical siblings of diabetic children is comparable, with a risk for diabetes about forty times greater than that in children of similar age in the general population, representing a cumulative incidence of diabetes of about twenty per cent by thirty years of age. In haplo-identical siblings the risk is lower but probably increased by a factor of about ten with five per cent diabetic by thirty years of age. This is similar to that estimated in U.K. siblings of diabetic children irrespective of HLA genotype. The risk in HLA-non-identical siblings has not been shown to exceed that in the general population.

A common question today concerns the risk of diabetes in children of Type I diabetic parents. It seems probable that in a northern European family where one parent has the disease about 2–5% of the offspring will develop it by thirty years of age. Obviously the risk is higher where both parents are affected, but is unlikely to exceed thirty per cent even if recessive inheritance proves to be true. Diabetes in a child is more likely if the father has diabetes rather than the mother.

If a child genetically at risk of Type I diabetes is found to be positive for CF-ICA as well, the development of clinical disease is more likely but not certain; at present, it does not justify potentially harmful attempts at prophylactic intervention.

GENETIC HETEROGENEITY WITHIN TYPE I DIABETES	Type Ia		Type Ib
age at onset	<15	>15	often >30
diabetes in sibs	++	+	
HLA-DR associations	3?,4	3,4	3,(4?)
BfF1 associations	+	?	
sex	M > F		M < F
persistent ICA	uncommon		common
polyendocrine autoimmunity	+		+++

Fig. 8.20 Evidence for genetic heterogeneity within Type I diabetes.

REFERENCES

Cudworth AG (1978) Type I diabetes. *Diabetologia*, **14**, 281–291.
Gorsuch AN (1987) Immunogenetics of diabetes. *Diabetic Medicine*, **4**.
Neel JV (1976) Diabetes mellitus — a geneticists's nightmare. In *The Genetics of Diabetes Mellitus*. Edited by Creutzfeldt W, Kobberling J and Neel JV. pp.1–11. Berlin: Springer Verlag.
Pincus G & White P (1933) On the inheritance of diabetes mellitus. I. An analysis of 675 family histories. *American Journal of Medical Sciences*, **186**, 1–14.

9 Aetiology and Pathogenesis of Type I Diabetes: Immunology

Kate M Spencer MD MRCP ● **Gian Franco Bottazzo** MD MRCP MRCPath

IMMUNE SYSTEM

Our understanding of the characteristics and functions of the immune system has increased enormously over the last three decades.

All lymphocytes have common precursor cells and the characteristics of the mature lymphocytes depend upon the site of differentiation (Fig. 9.1). In the thymus, cells acquire the characteristics of T lymphocytes, whereas cells migrating to the liver or bone marrow become B lymphocytes. These mature cells express a number of cell surface markers which distinguish individual types.

Specific receptors for antigens have only recently been identified on human T cells, but the methods for *in vitro* separation of these cells still take advantage of their specific receptors for sheep erythrocytes (E-rosette; Fig. 9.2). T cells are primarily involved in delayed hypersensitivity reactions, allograft rejection, graft-versus-host disease, direct killing of tumour cells and the lysis of viral-infected cells. B lymphocytes have the capacity to synthesize immunoglobulins which become membrane receptors for the binding of foreign antigens (Fig. 9.3). B lymphocytes differentiate further into plasma cells, whose main function is the production of circulating antibodies.

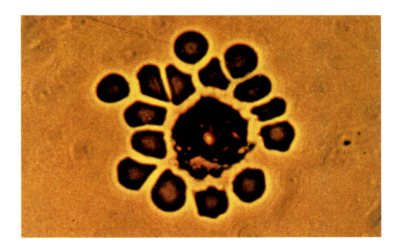

Fig. 9.2 E-rosette formation. Typical 'rosette' appearance of sheep erythrocytes (E) around a T lymphocyte viewed by phase contrast microscopy. This is a practical *in vitro* assay for separation of T lymphocytes which have receptors for red cells. By courtesy of Dr P.M. Lydyard.

LYMPHOCYTE DEVELOPMENT

common lymphoid lineage precursor cell

committed progenitor cells

thymus

fetal liver

post-natal bone marrow

inductive microenvironments

T lymphocytes

B lymphocytes

Fig. 9.1 Lymphocyte development. The process of lymphocyte maturation and differentiation from precursor cells to mature T and B lymphocytes.

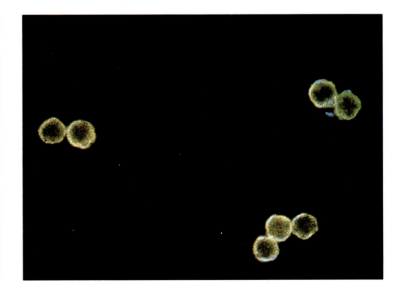

Fig. 9.3 B lymphocytes. Peripheral blood lymphocytes showing immunoglobulins on their surface. Anti-human Ig serum stain. By courtesy of Dr P.M. Lydyard.

Killer (K) cells are another subset of lymphocytes which possess membrane receptors for the constant fragment (Fc) of circulating immunoglobulins. The interaction between K cells and antibodies takes part in the phenomenon known as 'antibody-dependent cellular cytotoxicity' (ADCC; Fig. 9.4). Natural killer (NK) cells are a more primitive defence mechanism and do not require the presence of antibodies attached to the target in order to produce cytotoxicity. Certain virus-infected cells are eliminated by a more

KILLER LYMPHOCYTE ACTION

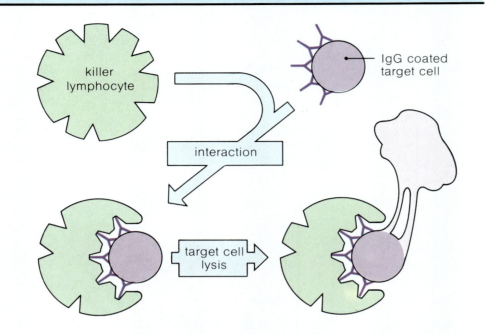

killer lymphocyte

IgG coated target cell

interaction

target cell lysis

Fig. 9.4 Killer lymphocyte action. A killer lymphocyte interacts with the Fc portion of antibodies bound to the antigens expressed on the membrane of a target cell. When contact is made, cytotoxic factors are released from the K cell, resulting in the lysis of the foreign cell.

HLA REGION IN MAN

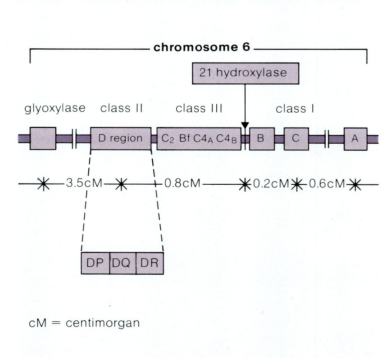

chromosome 6

21 hydroxylase

glyoxylase   class II   class III   class I

D region   C2 Bf C4A C4B   B   C   A

—✳—3.5cM—✳— —✳—0.8cM——✳✳0.2cM✳—0.6cM—✳—

DP DQ DR

cM = centimorgan

Fig. 9.5 HLA region in man. Approximate distances between different loci are given in centimorgans (cM). The central region encodes class III (complement) proteins including C2, C4 and factor B (Bf).

HLA CLASS I MOLECULE

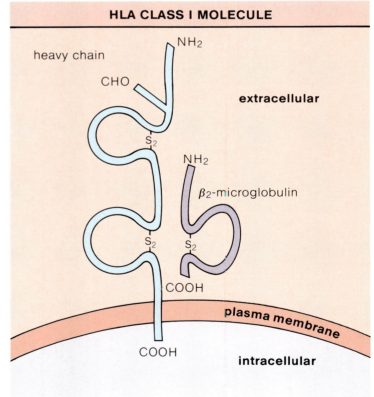

heavy chain NH_2

CHO

extracellular

S_2

NH_2

β_2-microglobulin

S_2 S_2

COOH

plasma membrane

COOH

intracellular

Fig. 9.6 HLA class I antigens. Schematic representation of the HLA class I molecule. The molecule consists of a 44,000 dalton glycoprotein, the heavy chain, which bears polymorphic determinants, which is non-convalently associated with a 12,000 dalton non-polymorphic protein, β_2-microglobulin.

complex defence mechanism involving cytotoxic T cells. These lymphocytes can eliminate viruses on infected cells only by recognizing the foreign antigen in association with HLA-A, -B and -C (class I) molecules of the major histocompatibility complex (MHC). The HLA (human leucocyte antigen) region is located in the short arm of chromosome 6 in man (Fig. 9.5) and class I products (Fig. 9.6) are expressed on the surface of virtually all nucleated cells in the body.

An immune response involves a complex interplay of positive and negative regulatory processes. If a foreign antigen enters the body, it is first recognized by macrophages which process it and present it to precursor helper T cells which are, in turn, activated. The presentation of the processed foreign antigen by macro-phages is made possible by the presence of another of the MHC products on the macrophage surface, the HLA class II molecules (DP, DQ and DR in man). It should be emphasized that class II products (Fig. 9.7) have a peculiar physiological cellular restriction, being expressed only on antigen-presenting cells (APC), such as macrophages, B lymphocytes, activated T cells, certain capillary epithelial cells and epithelium-lined cavities, for example, the gut and lung. While cytotoxic T cells recognize antigens in association with class I molecules, helper T lymphocytes interact with the antigen via co-recognition of class II molecules. These specific recognition and antigen-presenting processes involving HLA class I (Fig. 9.8) and class II antigens (Fig. 9.9), are known as the 'MHC restriction' phenomena.

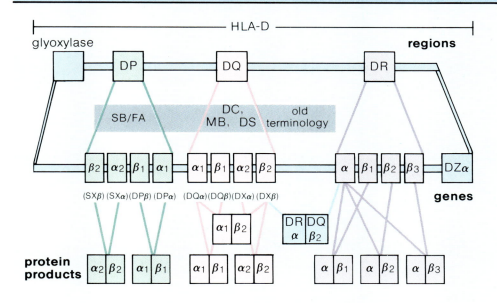

HLA CLASS II GENES AND PROTEIN PRODUCTS

Fig. 9.7 HLA class II antigens. The genes and protein products of the HLA-D region.

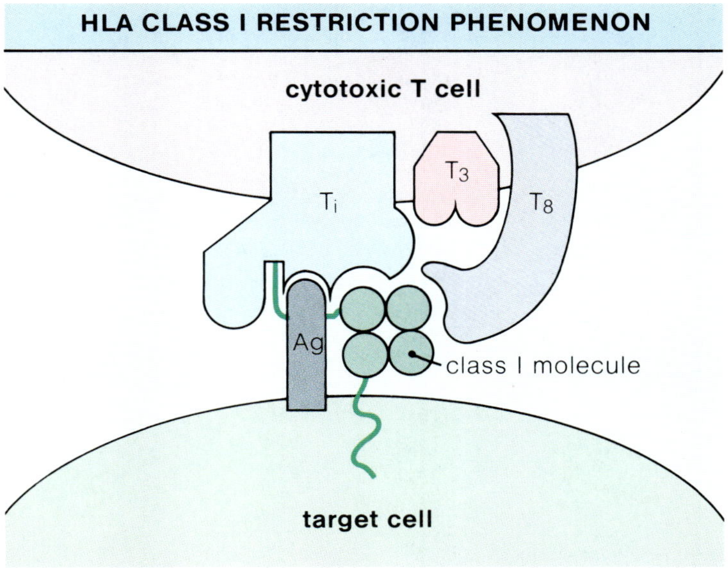

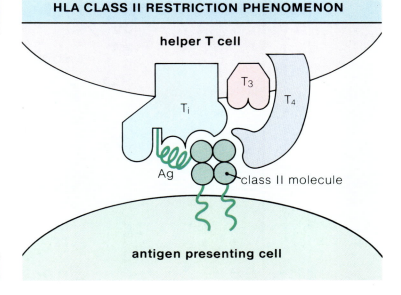

HLA CLASS I RESTRICTION PHENOMENON

Fig. 9.8 HLA class I restriction phenomenon. The cytotoxic T cell, through its surface expressed molecules (T_i, T_3 and T_8), recognizes and subsequently eliminates the antigen (Ag) only by recognizing HLA class I molecules. By courtesy of Dr R. Pujol-Borrell.

HLA CLASS II RESTRICTION PHENOMENON

Fig. 9.9 HLA class II restriction phenomenon. The helper T cell, through its surface expressed molecules (T_i, T_3 and T_4), recognizes the antigen (Ag) only in the context of HLA class II molecules expressed on the surface of an antigen-presenting cell such as a macrophage. By courtesy of Dr R. Pujol-Borrell.

MODEL OF PANCREATIC B CELL AUTOIMMUNITY

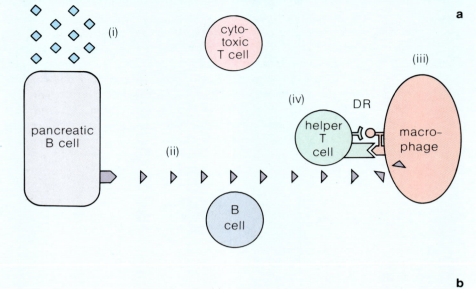

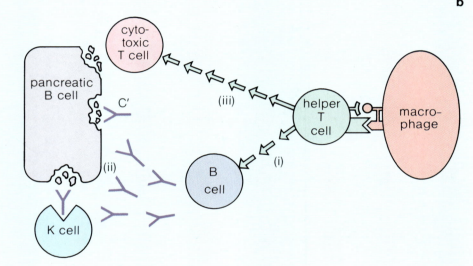

Fig. 9.10 Model of autoimmunity. One of the hypothetical schemes leading to the initial activation of the immune system against a target cell which could be a pancreatic B cell. (a) the process is started by: (i) environmental attack of a pancreatic B cell; (ii) release of autoantigens from the damaged cell; (iii) processing of the autoantigens by a macrophage, which inserts them on its surface membrane, and presentation by HLA class II molecules of the target autoantigens to the helper T lymphocyte; and (iv) activation of the helper T lymphocyte. (b) the cycle is completed by: (i) activation of B lymphocytes by the sensitized helper T cell; (ii) production of autoantibodies followed by antibody-dependent complement (C') and killer-cell-mediated cytotoxicities; and (iii) activation of the cytotoxic T lymphocyte. Death of the target cell follows.

Fig. 9.11 Evidence for heterogeneity in islet cell antibody (ICA) response. Cross-sectional study showing a high prevalence of ICA at diagnosis which tends to decrease with time. Persistent ICA are found in approximately 10–15% of Type I diabetic cases. These cases tend to have similar clinical and immunological characteristics to patients with primary autoimmune endocrine disorders. The number of patients sampled at each point is indicated.

When helper T cells are activated, they stimulate, in turn, both B lymphocytes, to secrete specific antibodies to the particular antigen, and cytotoxic T cells, the other effector mechanism against external assaults. Suppressor T cells, another of the T cell sub-populations, are important in regulating any given immune response and ultimately they are involved in stopping antibody production and cell-mediated immune reactions as soon as the antigen has been eliminated.

This carefully modulated defence system protects against foreign organisms and toxins but in normal circumstances does not respond to autologous self-antigens. However, in some individuals the regulatory mechanisms of tolerance to self molecules break down and cells in the body are mistakenly recognized as foreign, leading gradually to a process of spontaneous rejection. This is the concept which defines an 'autoimmune' disease.

Evidence accumulated over the last decade has strongly suggested that Type I or insulin-dependent diabetes mellitus has an autoimmune pathogenesis. How the autoimmune attack against insulin producing B cells in the pancreas is initiated and carried out remains at present unresolved. Among the several hypotheses put forward, one in particular supports the concept that sensitization against the autoantigens expressed on the pancreatic B cells follows a similar series of combined events to those indicated above for the elimination of environmental antigens (Fig. 9.10). The role of the suppressor T lymphocyte is not at present clearly understood and it is not represented in Fig. 9.10. There is growing evidence, however, which indicates that organ-specific T cells may exist, leading to de-repression of autoreactive T cells, B cells and cytotoxic T lymphocytes.

IMMUNOLOGY OF TYPE I DIABETES
Humoral Immunity

Islet cell antibodies (ICA) were first described in insulin-dependent diabetic patients who had other coexistent autoimmune endocrine disorders. Later, ICA were found in juvenile diabetic patients without other endocrine disorders when the test was performed within a few weeks of diagnosis. In contrast to the former group, ICA tend to disappear rapidly after a few weeks or months in the latter group (Fig. 9.11).

ICA are exclusively of IgG class and are demonstrated by a conventional indirect immunofluorescence (IFL) technique (Fig. 9.12). The antibodies react with the cytoplasm of glucagon (A) and somatostatin (D) cells as well as B cells, suggesting that the endocrine cells in the pancreas have a common autoantigen. If insulin, glucagon or somatostatin are added to sera containing ICA, the intensity of IFL reaction on the islet is not affected, indicating that ICA must bind to intracellular antigens other than pancreatic hormones. The autoantigens with which ICA react are not yet precisely identified but a protein of 64 kilodaltons (kd) has been precipitated from islets. It is likely that there are several relevant antigens in the islets, some of which are common to all endocrine cells and some specific to pancreatic B cells only.

Some ICA are able to fix complement (CF-ICA; Fig. 9.13) and these specificities have been found predominantly in newly diagnosed diabetic patients, their relatives who are genetically predisposed to diabetes and in patients who have other associated autoimmune endocrine diseases. Some CF-ICA are pancreatic B cell specific and at present are considered the most useful detectable marker of progressive B cell damage in subjects genetically susceptible to diabetes.

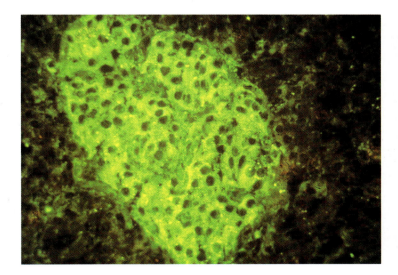

Fig. 9.12 Conventional islet cell antibodies (ICA). Cryostat section from a blood group O human pancreas stained by the indirect immunofluorescence (IFL) technique. The section was first incubated with a serum from a Type I diabetic patient and subsequently stained with anti-human IgG fluoresceinated serum. All cells within the islet are strongly positive. Orange granules scattered in the islet and in the exocrine portion of the gland are naturally occurring lipofuscin/lipid granules.

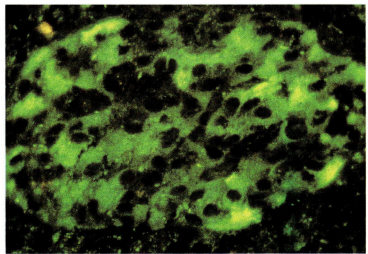

Fig. 9.13 Complement-fixing islet cell antibodies (CF-ICA). Section from the same pancreas as in Fig. 9.12. After incubating the patient's serum, fresh normal human serum is added to the section as a source of complement. An anti-complement-C3 fluoresceinated serum is subsequently used to reveal the positive reaction. CF-ICA react more selectively than conventional ICA with cells within the islets. In some instances, CF-ICA specifically stain B cells.

Some sera from diabetic patients contain antibodies specific for glucagon (Fig. 9.14) or somatostatin cells. Such sera may also contain other organ- and non-organ specific autoantibodies, including antibodies to pituitary cells (Fig. 9.15).

Islet cell surface antibodies (ICSA) have been detected using viable cultured human fetal or adult rat islet cells (Fig. 9.16). There are separate specificities for A, B and pancreatic polypeptide (PP) cells. Some CF-ICA which selectively stain B cells may recognize cytoplasmic antigens which are also represented on the cell surface. However, surface islet cell staining is found in about thirty per cent of diabetic sera that are negative for cytoplasmic ICA by conventional IFL techniques. This suggests that there is an additional antigen which is expressed only on the plasma membrane of B cells. CF-ICA and ICSA are cytotoxic to cultured islet cells and interfere with glucose-stimulated insulin release. It must be stressed that these are *in vitro* effects and their relevance to the actual killing mechanisms *in vivo* remains conceptually attractive but is still speculative.

More recently, spontaneous autoantibodies to insulin (IAA) have been described in untreated newly diagnosed diabetic patients and the same phenomenon has been detected in a proportion of unaffected first degree relatives using either radioimmunoassay (RIA) or enzyme-linked immunoabsorbent assay (ELISA). A good correlation has been found between the presence of IAA and CF-ICA and the subsequent progression to overt diabetes.

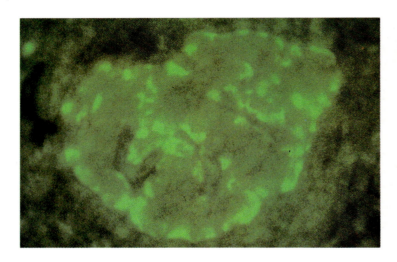

Fig. 9.14 A cell antibodies. Section of pancreas stained as in Fig. 9.12 showing selective reactivity in discrete cells at the periphery of the islet. A four layer IFL technique using a specific anti-glucagon serum has confirmed that the patient's autoantibodies react only with A cells. A similar IFL pattern is obtained with some human diabetic sera containing antibodies to somatostatin (D) cells. Also, in this case, specificity to D cells of the initial IFL reaction is confirmed by the use of the corresponding anti-hormone serum which specifically identifies D cells.

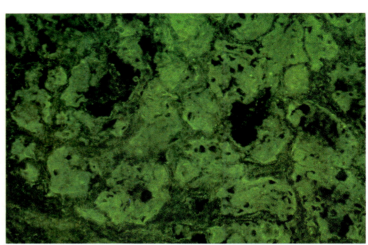

Fig. 9.15 Pituitary antibodies and Type I diabetes. Section of human pituitary stained by indirect IFL with a serum of a pre-diabetic ICA positive family member. The antibodies react with several pituitary cells and this so-called multiple IFL pattern is typically found in Type I diabetic patients whose condition is not complicated with other endocrine autoimmune diseases. Pituitary antibodies detected in patients with endocrine autoimmune disorders react preferentially with prolactin-secreting cells.

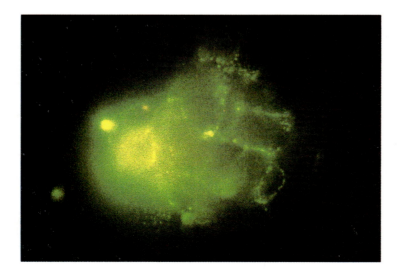

Fig. 9.16 Islet cell surface antibodies (ICSA). Human fetal islets in a monolayer culture were stained by an indirect IFL technique with serum from a diabetic patient. There is a typical granular pattern of antibodies recognizing autoantigens expressed on the plasma membrane of cells.

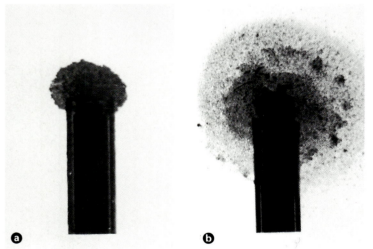

Fig. 9.17 Leucocyte migration inhibition test (LMIT). Peripheral blood leucocytes from patients are placed in a capillary tube which is sealed at one end. Migration of cells from the tube is studied in a medium (a) containing or (b) lacking antigen. In the presence of antigen, factors causing inhibition of the leucocyte migration are produced indicating previous sensitization of these cells to the antigen. Leucocytes from subjects unsensitized to the antigen migrate freely into the medium. By courtesy of Dr J. Brostoff.

Cell-mediated Immunity

Much research has been done on the cell-mediated immune processes involved in the autoimmune destruction of the islets. The leucocyte migration inhibition test (LMIT; Fig. 9.17) has shown that peripheral blood leucocytes from newly diagnosed Type I diabetic patients are sensitized to pancreatic antigens (Fig. 9.18). Lymphocytes from Type I patients can produce cytotoxicity to various islet cell targets *in vitro*. However, it is likely that these cells recognize different pancreatic B cell antigens to those reacting with ICA.

Conflicting results have been obtained in Type I diabetic patients when total numbers of peripheral T and B lymphocytes are counted. Similarly, responses to phytohaemagglutinin and other mitogens are variable. These variabilities are probably explained, at least in part, by differences in metabolic control of

patients at the time of study and the choice of techniques. Several abnormalities of lymphocyte subsets have been found in newly diagnosed diabetic patients. These include raised K cell levels (Fig. 9.19), increased numbers of circulating activated T cells, reduced suppressor T cell function and enhanced natural K cell activity for xenogenic islet cells. Some cell-mediated immune abnormalities noted in newly diagnosed diabetic patients have also been detected in non-diabetic subjects genetically susceptible to diabetes, together with humoral responses against islet cells.

INSULITIS

The majority of cells constituting the architecture of islets of Langerhans are insulin-producing B cells (Fig. 9.20). In Type I diabetes, the number of B cells is dramatically decreased to approximately ten per cent of normal (Fig. 9.21). The pancreas

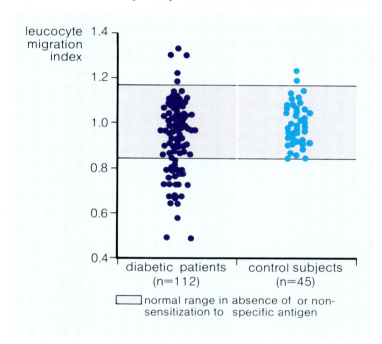

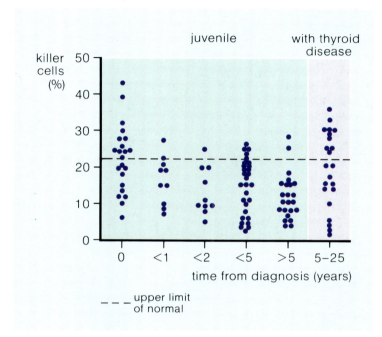

Fig. 9.18 Impaired cell-mediated immunity in Type I diabetes: (1). Results of an LMIT in newly diagnosed Type I diabetic patients. One-third are sensitized to pancreatic antigens (positive migration index <0.82). From Nerup *et al.* (1974), by courtesy of the Royal Society of Medicine.

Fig. 9.19 Impaired cell-mediated immunity in Type I diabetes: (2). K cell levels are raised in Type I diabetic patients at diagnosis with subsequent disappearance. A similar trend is also observed for ICA (see Fig. 9.11). Elevated K cell numbers persist in patients with associated autoimmune thyroid disease. From Pozzilli *et al.* (1979), by courtesy of the *Lancet*.

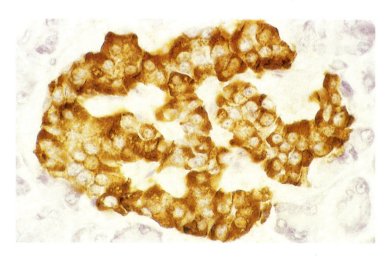

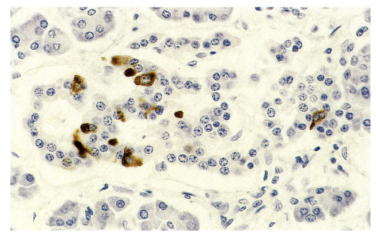

Fig. 9.20 Islet of Langerhans. View of an islet from the glucagon-rich lobe of the pancreas of a non-diabetic individual. The majority of brown cells in the islet are B cells. From Bottazzo (1986), by courtesy of Dr A. Foulis and John Wiley & Sons.

Fig. 9.21 A diabetic islet. View of an islet from a child who died in ketoacidosis at presentation with acute onset of diabetes. Note the striking reduction in the number of insulin-containing B cells. Immunoperoxidase stain for insulin. From Bottazzo (1986), by courtesy of Dr A. Foulis and John Wiley & Sons.

of a Type I diabetic patient contains pseudoatrophic and hyperactive islets. The former are predominant, are almost deprived of B cells and are composed of small cells with dense nuclei which by immunocytochemical techniques have been shown to be mainly glucagon- and somatostatin-secreting cells (Fig. 9.22). It should be emphasized that A and D cells are spared by the destructive process which affects B cells exclusively.

Lymphocytes, macrophages and plasma cells are found in tissues undergoing active autoimmune destruction. A similar histopathological pattern can also be seen in sections of pancreas from insulin-dependent diabetic patients dying soon after diagnosis, but plasma cells are rarely detected by conventional histological staining; Von Meyenberg referred to the mononuclear cell infiltration of the islets of Langerhans in diabetes as 'insulitis' (Fig. 9.23).

Classical histological examination of fixed pancreatic tissue does not allow the precise characterization of the various lymphocyte sub-populations infiltrating the islet. Recently, examination of frozen blocks of a fresh pancreas taken from a diabetic child who died shortly after diagnosis has given new information. By using various monoclonal reagents for immunofluorescence with single or double fluorochrome techniques, it was shown that the majority of mononuclear cells in the inflammatory infiltrate were T lymphocytes (Fig. 9.24a). Cytotoxic/suppressor (CD8) lymphocytes formed the majority of these T cells (Fig. 9.24b), but all the other lymphocyte subsets were also present. A large proportion of these T lymphocytes expressed HLA class II molecules and a lesser number were positive for interleukin-2 receptors (Fig. 9.24c), thus showing that the infiltrating T cells were activated and suggesting a specific immune response directed against islet autoantigens.

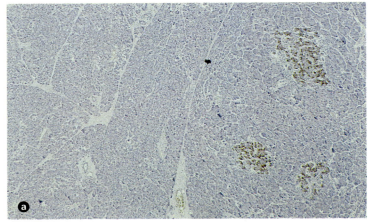

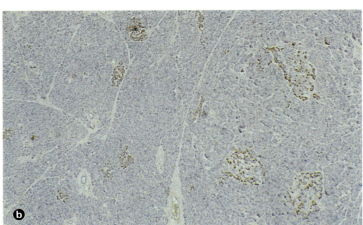

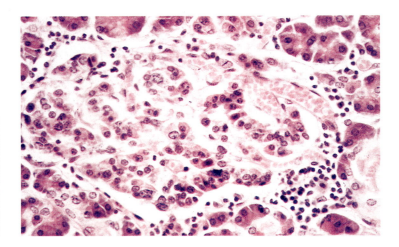

Fig. 9.22 Histological evidence of heterogeneity in the diabetic pancreas. (a) section of a pancreas from a Type I diabetic patient who died shortly after diagnosis. In the large pancreatic lobe on the right there are well-preserved islets still containing numerous B cells (hyperactive islets). This is in contrast to the view of the pancreatic lobes on the left where few B cells can be identified. Immunoperoxidase stain for insulin.

(b) serial section of the same pancreas. There is a normal distribution of A cells in the hyperactive islets (the right lobe) and the re-appearance of 'ghost' islets in the lobes on the left. A similar pattern was observed when anti-somatostatin antibody was applied to a section. This provides evidence that A and D cells are unaffected by the inflammatory process which selectively destroys B cells. Islets greatly deprived of B cells, but still containing A and D cells, are classified as pseudoatrophic islets. By courtesy of Dr A. Foulis.

Fig. 9.23 Insulitis. Section of a pancreas from a newly diagnosed diabetic child displaying the characteristic pattern of a mononuclear cell infiltration around the islet. H and E stain. From Bottazzo *et al.* (1985), by courtesy of the *New England Journal of Medicine.*

When antisera to human IgG were applied to other sections of the same diabetic pancreas, it was seen that many B lymphocytes were present around individual islets (Fig. 9.25a). This is of particular interest because, as previously explained, conventional histological techniques have failed to detect mature plasma cells in the insulitis process. IgG was also demonstrated around (Fig. 9.25b) and within (Fig. 9.25c) islet cells, thus proving penetration by antibodies following injury to the cell membrane. In most cases, the islets showed complement deposition (Fig. 9.25d).

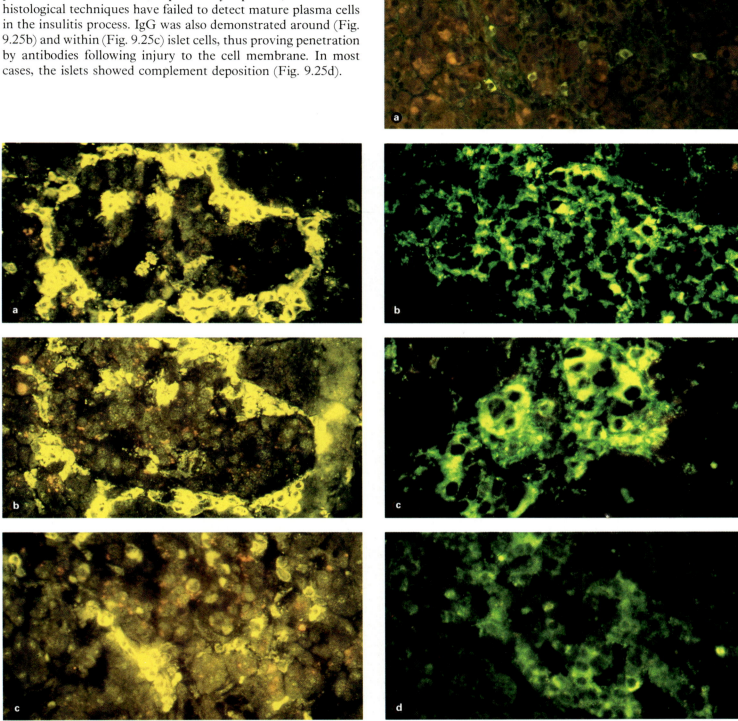

Fig. 9.24 Characterization of invading T lymphocytes. Serial sections from the same pancreas as in Fig. 9.23. (a) indirect IFL technique using a monoclonal antibody which defines all leucocytes. The majority of mononuclear cells infiltrating the islet were T lymphocytes. (b) a monoclonal antibody stain which defines CD8 (?cytotoxic) T cells. CD8+ cells predominate in the insulitis process. Other serial sections of the same islet showed that helper T cells and natural killer/killer lymphocytes were also present in the mononuclear cell infiltrate, though to a lesser extent. (c) section stained with monoclonal antibodies to interleukin-2 receptors, indicating that a proportion of the infiltrating T cells are activated. Staining with monoclonal antibodies to HLA class II molecules detected an even greater number of T cells expressing this particular marker of cell activation. From Bottazzo et al. (1985), by courtesy of the New England Journal of Medicine.

Fig. 9.25 Evidence of immunoglobulins attacking islet cells. Serial sections from the same pancreas as in Fig. 9.23. (a) unfixed sections stained by an indirect IFL technique with an antiserum to human IgG, showing numerous Ig-bearing immunocytes (?pre-plasma cells) around an islet. (b) another large islet, stained as in view (a), showing IgG deposition around and inside endocrine cells. (c) a diseased islet in which the abnormal internalization of antibodies is more pronounced. (d) islet stained for complement (C9), suggesting deposition of antigen–antibody complexes on islet endocrine cells. (b) and (c) from Bottazzo et al. (1985), by courtesy of the New England Journal of Medicine; (d) from Bottazzo (1986), by courtesy of John Wiley & Sons.

GENETICS OF TYPE I DIABETES

The short arm of chromosome 6 in man contains genes coding for the HLA antigen system. By analogy with the corresponding region in mice (Ia), the major histocompatibility complex is likely to contain immune response (Ir) genes. Apart from genes coding for HLA class I and class II products, the HLA region contains genes coding for some components of the complement cascade, that is, C2, C4A and C4B of the classical complement pathway, and Bf of the alternative complement pathway (see Fig. 9.5). The HLA system is highly polymorphic in nature and individuals possess a particular combination of HLA antigens expressed on the surface of their cells.

Every child inherits one chromosome 6 from each parent and the alleles are co-dominant, so that both maternal and paternal gene products are expressed. The individual parental HLA regions are referred to as 'haplotypes' and this region is relatively stable with recombination being unusual. Because of this, the number of possible haplotype combinations from a given mating is usually limited to four. Any child will have a one-in-four chance of being HLA-identical (both haplotypes in common) with a sibling, a one-in-two chance of being haplo-identical for HLA (one haplotype in common) with a sibling and a one-in-four chance of being HLA non-identical (no haplotype in common) with a sibling.

There is a tendency for some specificities within the HLA system to occur together on the same haplotype more often than would be expected by chance in an outbred population; for example, HLA-A1, B8 and DR3. This phenomenon is described as 'linkage disequilibrium'. Certain diseases are associated with particular HLA specificities. Type I diabetes is associated with HLA-DR3, like many other autoimmune endocrine disorders, but also with HLA-DR4. The risk of developing Type I diabetes is

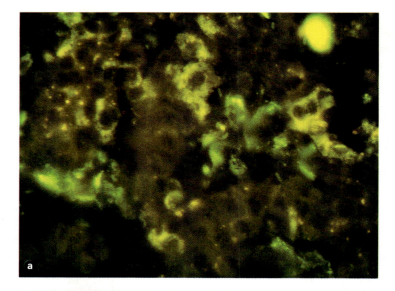

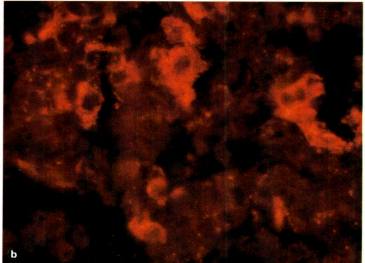

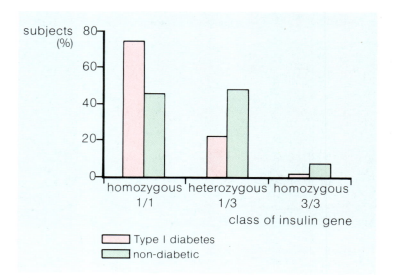

Fig. 9.26 Insulin gene polymorphism and Type I diabetes. Combined data from Denmark, California and the U.K. showing that more than 70% of Type I diabetic patients (n = 233) are homozygous for class I insulin gene alleles. From Bottazzo (1986), by courtesy of Dr G. Hitman and John Wiley & Sons.

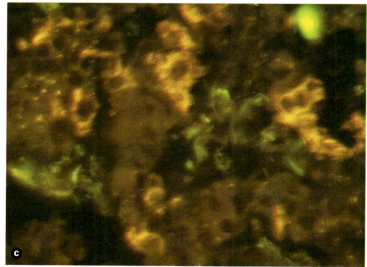

Fig. 9.27 Inappropriate HLA class II molecule expression on diabetic B cells. Sections from the same pancreas as in Fig. 9.23. (a) indirect IFL staining with monoclonal antibodies to HLA class II molecules. There are few large epithelial-like cells which are strongly positive for class II products. (b) the same section as in (a) stained with antibodies to C peptide, proving that the few class II positive epithelial cells are indeed still functioning B cells. (c) double exposure photograph of (a) and (b) together. The typical yellow-orange colour finally confirms that the HLA class II positive cells in the islet are B cells. (a) and (b) from Bottazzo *et al.* (1985), by courtesy of the *New England Journal of Medicine*.

greater for individuals who are heterozygous for HLA-DR3 and DR4 than for individuals who are homozygous for either HLA-DR3 or DR4. This suggests that there is more than one susceptibility gene for diabetes and that these operate in an interactive way. HLA-DR2 is rarely detected in diabetic patients and this antigen, or a gene in linkage disequilibrium with it, appears to confer resistance to Type I diabetes. (For more detail see *Chapter 8*.)

Apart from the HLA region, genes on other chromosomes possibly increase the genetic susceptibility for Type I diabetes. Chromosome 11, which contains the gene coding for insulin, has been studied in detail. The 5′ flanking region of the insulin gene is also polymorphic in nature. By using restriction enzymes and DNA probes and analysing different fragments by Southern blotting, it has been found that more than seventy per cent of Type I diabetic patients are homozygous for class I insulin gene alleles (Fig. 9.26). This pattern is present in forty-five per cent of non-diabetic Caucasoid individuals. The contribution to the genetics of Type I diabetes of chromosome 14, which contains the heavy chain of human immunoglobulins, and chromosome 2, which contains the light chain of human immunoglobulins and the Kidd blood group antigen system, remains controversial.

HLA System and Its Relationship to the Pathogenesis of Diabetes

As previously described, physiological immune responses are initiated by HLA class II positive cells, such as macrophages, which present antigens to helper T lymphocytes which then trigger a chain of immune reactions. Recently, class II molecules have been found to be inappropriately expressed on a variety of cells which are the targets of autoimmune attack, including B cells of diabetic islets (Fig. 9.27). A and D cells do not express class II products in these islets which is consistent with the sparing of these cells in the killing process (Fig. 9.28).

The exact role of the aberrant expression of class II molecules in the pathogenesis of autoimmune diseases is not yet fully understood. Nevertheless, it provides a clue to the association of autoimmune diseases with certain HLA specificities, including Type I diabetes. It has been postulated that still unrecognized agents, which could be environmental, are responsible for triggering class II expression on cells, such as B cells, which subsequently undergo an autoimmune destruction. If this phenomenon occurs in genetically susceptible individuals, who,

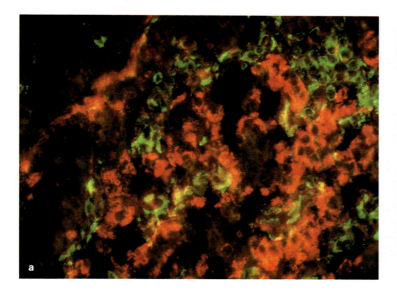
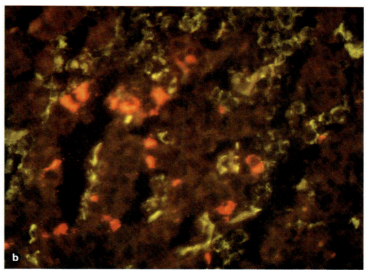

Fig. 9.28 Lack of HLA class II molecule expression on A and D cells. (a) double exposure photograph of a second cryostat section showing A cells stained bright red and class II positive capillaries and lymphocytes stained separately green. The section was stained by a four layer fluorochrome technique with the corresponding antisera. There are no yellow-orange cells indicating that A cells do not express class II products. (b) a similar double exposure photograph to (a), showing that in a consecutive section of the same islet, D cells are also stained bright red and class II positive capillaries and lymphocytes stained separately green. The D cells do not express class II products and, like A cells, are not affected by the killing process which selectively destroys B cells in the islets. From Bottazzo *et al.* (1985), by courtesy of the *New England Journal of Medicine*.

for example, develop Type I diabetes, the configuration of certain class II products (HLA-DR3 or DR4 or both, but not HLA-DR2; Fig. 9.29a) may present the set of autoantigens which are normally expressed on the surface of B cells (Fig. 9.29b). As for macrophages, this initial event could lead to activation of helper T cells which, in turn, stimulate effector B and cytotoxic T cells. Whether the induction of autoimmune T cells leads to clinical autoimmune disease may depend upon the activity of regulatory mechanisms within the immune system such as suppressor T cell activity and production of anti-idiotypic antibodies (antibodies directed against particular clones of autoreactive lymphocytes).

Lymphokines, for example, interferons and tumour necrosis factor, produced by invading lymphocytes and macrophages and which are known to be potent modulators of class II product expression in some cells, would then be responsible for perpetuating the cycle of inappropriate HLA gene activation. External agents or leucocyte products, or both, could also act in enhancing HLA class I expression, another new phenomenon recently detected in diabetic islets (Fig. 9.30). This latter observation may now explain the abundant presence of cytotoxic T cells among infiltrating lymphocytes at the time of diagnosis. Cytotoxic T cells seem to play a key role in the final selective destruction of B cells. This conclusion comes from data obtained after an *in vivo* 'accidental'

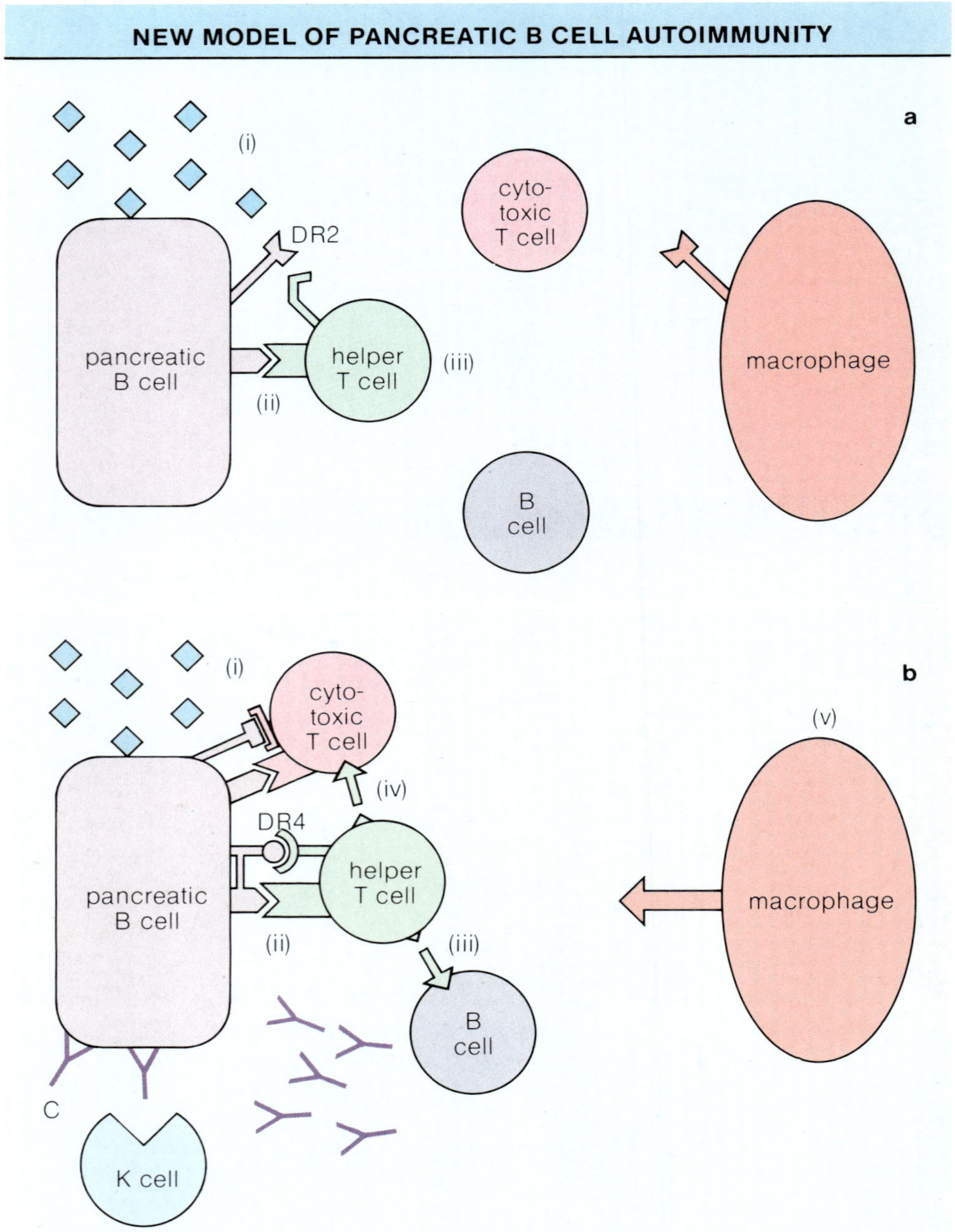

NEW MODEL OF PANCREATIC B CELL AUTOIMMUNITY

Fig. 9.29 New model of autoimmunity. The hypothetical steps leading to the activation of the B cell which in turn attracts autoreactive immunocytes.

(a) the wrong presentation: (i) unidentified environmental agents may lead to the induction of HLA class II molecules in the B cell; (ii) the phenomenon occurs in an HLA-DR2 individual who may be protected against developing Type I diabetes; (iii) the helper T cell is attracted but the HLA-DR2 complex is not ideal for the presentation of the surface autoantigen on the B cell and the interaction does not occur.

(b) the right presentation: (i) similiar initial events as described in (a); (ii) the phenomenon leads to an inappropriate expression of HLA class II molecules in an HLA-DR3/DR4 susceptible individual. These particular D/DR products are now ideal for the presentation of the surface autoantigen on the B cell. Helper T cells recognize the complex, interact with it and become activated. (iii) B lymphocytes are activated and produce islet cell antibodies. Partial cell damage follows via complement (C) and cell activation. (iv) finally, the signal is sent to cytotoxic T lymphocytes which are attracted by an enhanced expression of HLA class I molecules on the B cells. (v) macrophages obey their physiological function and intervene by clearing the scene of damaged cells.

experiment when a long-standing diabetic twin was transplanted with part of the pancreas donated by the unaffected identical co-twin. Unexpectedly, diabetes recurred after a few weeks in the transplanted diabetic twin. Only B cells were destroyed (Figs 9.31a and b) and cytotoxic T cells were the predominant lymphocyte sub-population present in the inflammatory infiltrate (Fig. 9.31c).

Interestingly, capillary endothelial cells around diabetic islets were hypertrophied and strongly positive for class II expression (Fig. 9.32). This phenomenon is at present under active investigation but these structures could represent the openings which allow the invasion of autoreactive immunocytes.

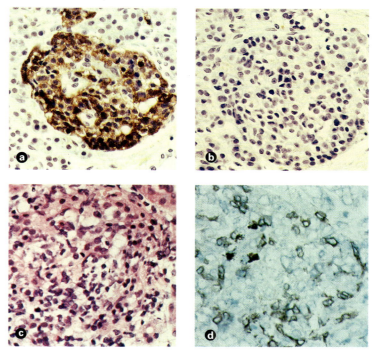

Fig. 9.31 Role of cytotoxic T lymphocytes in Type I diabetes. Sections of a pancreas which was transplanted from an unaffected identical twin to the long-standing diabetic co-twin.

Before transplantation: (a) the islet shows the expected number of B cells as in a normal pancreas. Immunoperoxidase stain for insulin.

After transplantation: (b) after a few weeks, Type I diabetes recurred and the islet shown here is now deprived of B cells. A and D cells were unaffected and, as in the original disease process, did not decrease in number (immunoperoxidase stain for insulin). (c) the mononuclear cell infiltration resembles the pattern of insulitis. (d) the positive infiltrating mononuclear cells are cytotoxic T cells. They predominate in the inflammatory process, resembling the pattern detected in the pancreas of Type I diabetic patients at the time of diagnosis. (d) was incubated with the same monoclonal antibody as in Fig. 9.24b, but stained with the immunoperoxidase technique. By courtesy of Dr R. Sibley.

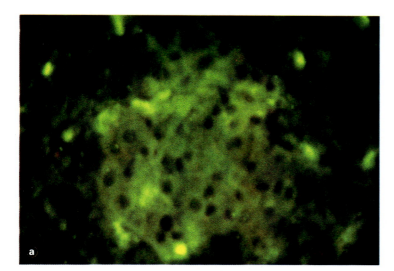

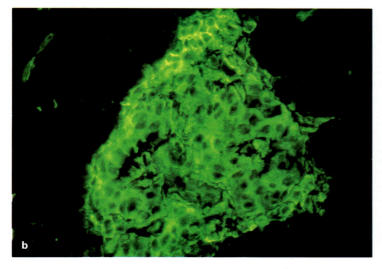

Fig. 9.30 Enhanced expression of HLA class I molecules in diabetic islets. (a) normal pancreas stained by an indirect IFL technique with a monoclonal antibody to HLA class I molecules showing the expected weak positive reaction. The brighter dots and lines around the islet represent capillaries. (b) islet from the same pancreas as in Fig. 9.23, stained as in (a), showing strong fluorescence of a diabetic islet. The phenomenon is present in most islets regardless of the presence of lymphocytic infiltration. From Bottazzo *et al.* (1985), by courtesy of the *New England Journal of Medicine.*

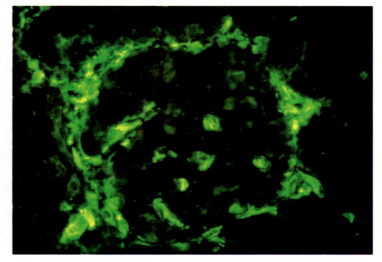

Fig. 9.32 Capillary cells in Type I diabetes. Section of a diabetic pancreas showing a dilated crown of capillary cells around the islet strongly positive for HLA class II molecules. In this islet the endocrine cells are unstained. Indirect IFL staining with monoclonal antibodies to HLA class II molecules. From Bottazzo *et al.* (1985), by courtesy of the *New England Journal of Medicine.*

PROSPECTIVE STUDIES IN TYPE I DIABETES

The 'Bart's–Windsor Family Study' was initially organized to follow the events leading to Type I diabetes in a group of genetically susceptible individuals. All families with an insulin-dependent diabetic child and at least one unaffected sibling under the age of twenty within a given area were ascertained and invited to join the study. By HLA genotyping the families, it has been possible to identify susceptible individuals, that is, those with one or two haplotypes in common with the diabetic proband (Fig. 9.33). The study has recently been enlarged by including families from the nearby Oxford area.

Surprisingly, conventional ICA were found in siblings who were HLA non-identical with the proband as well as HLA-identical and haplo-identical siblings and in some parents. However, CF-ICA were only found in the genetically susceptible groups and diabetes has developed in approximately fifty per cent of them to date (Fig. 9.34). Unexpectedly, these antibodies were present for many months before the onset of clinical diabetes. Type I diabetes was previously thought to have an acute onset but the insulitis is clearly present for a long time before the abrupt symptoms of diabetes become manifest. There are still several relatives in the study with CF-ICA who remain euglycaemic. Furthermore, some relatives with ICA have shown fluctuations in the presence of these antibodies and have not, so far, become diabetic.

It is possible that regulatory mechanisms within the immune system are able to restrict autoimmune damage in some individuals. Alternatively, the continuing presence of environmental agents may be necessary for the continuation and expansion of the autoimmune process. Within family members,

ICA, including CF-ICA, have been seen to reappear in some diabetic probands who had previously lost these antibodies. It seems likely that this could also occur in some of those non-diabetic relatives who were previously positive and have then lost ICA.

As mentioned previously, cell-mediated immune abnormalities and insulin autoantibodies are also detectable in these susceptible individuals and, like ICA, they preceded diabetes in some cases by many months or years.

VIRUSES AND TYPE I DIABETES

Viruses have been incriminated in the aetiology of Type I diabetes for many years. There is good evidence that certain viruses can cause diabetes in some susceptible animals. In humans, a direct causal link between viruses and diabetes has not been fully proven. Circumstantially, the pattern of age of onset of Type I diabetes (Fig. 9.35) and the seasonal variations in its incidence (see *Chapter 7*) are consistent with and most easily explained by a viral aetiology. However, the incidence of particular viral infections varies from one year to the next, whereas the incidence of diabetes is more constant and it is therefore unlikely that one particular virus or group of viruses is directly responsible for diabetes.

There is an increased incidence of both Coxsackie and mumps infection in the months preceding the onset of clinical diabetes. However, since B cell destruction is now recognized to occur gradually and to antedate clinical diabetes by months and even years, the role of common viruses in initiating B cell damage has been questioned. The problem is illustrated by a young boy who

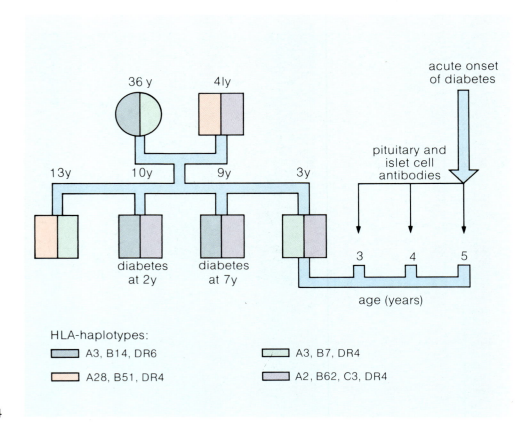

Fig. 9.33 Example of immunogenetic linkage in Type I diabetes. Representative multiplex family from the 'Bart's–Windsor Prospective Family Study' of diabetes. Diabetes is linked to possession of the A2, B62, C3, DR4 haplotype. The younger brother was discovered to have CF-ICA at the age of three years and, two years later, he developed acute Type I diabetes. His serum was also positive for pituitary antibodies (see Fig. 9.15). The age of each family member is indicated. From Gorsuch *et al.* (1981), by courtesy of the *Lancet*.

developed diabetes three months after an episode of mumps. Six months before the mumps infection, he had another mild viral illness and at that time his serum did not contain anti-mumps antibodies but was already positive for ICA (Fig. 9.36).

It seems likely that in cases such as this the virus is simply acting as a non-specific precipitant of metabolic decompensation or, alternatively, causes additional B cell damage in individuals with active insulitis. So far, there is no evidence from prospective family studies to incriminate any particular virus at the time when CF-ICA first appears. However, the number of subjects who have developed CF-ICA during the years of observation is still very small and it is only by prolonged follow-up of susceptible individuals that this important point will be clarified.

PREVENTION OF TYPE I DIABETES

Several attempts have been made to arrest Type I diabetes soon after diagnosis. Partial success has been obtained with massive immunosuppressive therapy and more recently with cyclosporin A treatment. However, all these studies have been carried out in patients who are already diabetic and whose B cell mass is greatly reduced. It must be remembered that the 'honeymoon' period in Type I diabetes, during which B cell function tends temporarily to improve, is well recognized and that the apparent success in about thirty per cent of patients treated with various immunosuppressive regimens may be explained, in part, by this.

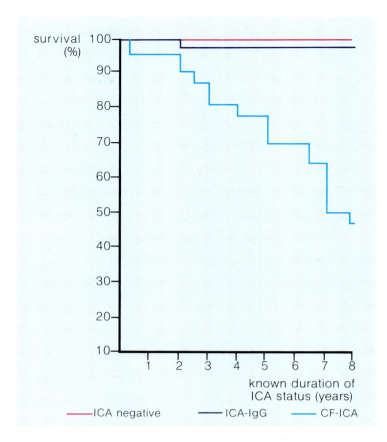

Fig. 9.34 Evidence for a long prodromal period in Type I diabetes. Curve of B cell survival in family members in the 'Bart's–Windsor Prospective Family Study'. The curve is calculated as a percentage of first degree relatives who have developed diabetes during the nine year period of observation according to their ICA pattern. More than 50% of individuals possessing CF-ICA became diabetic. Those remaining are, at present, still symptom-free. The risk of contracting the disease for relatives who either do not have ICA or are only positive for conventional ICA is minimal. By courtesy of Dr A. Tarn.

Fig. 9.35 Incidence of Type I diabetes according to age of onset. Combined data from studies carried out in Denmark, the U.S.A., Canada and Chile. The major peak occurs at puberty but the disease can develop in the first few months of life and its frequency increases abruptly at about nine months of age. In juvenile diabetes, there is a trend for males to be more affected than females. By courtesy of Dr R. Gamble.

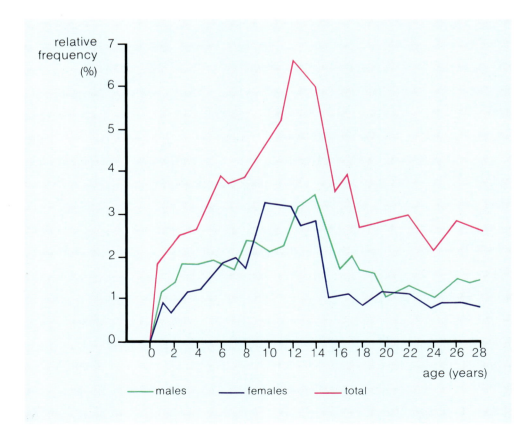

The long latency period before Type I diabetes becomes established lends itself to the possibility of immunosuppression at an earlier stage before there is substantial damage to the islet B cells. However, if immunosuppression has to be prolonged, then the treatment itself is not without danger. The hope for the future relies in a better understanding of the various components of the autoimmune response against islet cells so that selective immunosuppressive agents can be employed. Any therapeutic manoeuvre will have to take account of the evidence that autoimmune destructive processes may fluctuate, indicating natural protective mechanisms against B cell damage. This re-emphasizes the importance of prospective studies in genetically susceptible individuals for a better understanding of the natural history of the disease.

HISTORY OF VIRAL INFECTION IN A 4-YEAR OLD BOY		
1983	**condition**	**ICA**
January	mild viral infection	+
July	mumps	not tested
September	Type I diabetes	+

Fig. 9.36 Do common infectious environmental agents initiate or precipitate Type I diabetes? Example of a retrospective clinical, virological and immunological study of a young child who became diabetic a few months after he suffered from a mumps infection. A stored serum sample collected eight months prior to diagnosis was analysed and showed the presence of ICA. Clearly, the destructive immunological process against B cells was already under way in this child and mumps could only have been a potential precipitating and damaging agent of already injured B cells. From Bodansky *et al.* (1984), by courtesy of the *Lancet*.

REFERENCES

Bodansky JH, Littlewood JM, Bottazzo GF, Dean BM & Hambling MH (1984) Which virus causes the initial islet lesion in Type I diabetes. *Lancet*, **1**, 401–402.

Bosi E, Todd I, Pujol-Borrell R & Bottazzo GF (In press) Mechanisms of autoimmunity and relevance to the pathogenesis of Type I diabetes. *Diabetes / Metabolisme Reviews*.

Bottazzo GF (1986) Death of a beta cell: homicide or suicide? *Diabetic Medicine*, **3**, 119–130.

Bottazzo GF, Dean BM, McNally JM, McKay EH, Swift PGF & Gamble DR (1985) *In situ* characterization of autoimmune phenomena and expression of HLA molecules in the pancreas in diabetic insulitis. *New England Journal of Medicine*, **313**, 353–360.

Bottazzo GF & Doniach D (1980) Autoimmunity in diabetes mellitus. In *Secondary Diabetes: the Spectrum of the Diabetes Syndrome*. Edited by Podolsky S & Kiswanathan M. pp. 391–408. New York: Raven Press.

Bottazzo GF, Pujol-Borrell R & Gale EAM (1985) Etiology of diabetes: the role of autoimmune mechanisms. In *The Diabetes Annual, Volume 1*. Edited by Alberti KGMM & Krall LP. pp. 16–52. Amsterdam: Elsevier Science Publishers B.V.

Bottazzo GF, Pujol-Borrell R & Gale EAM (1986) Autoimmunity and diabetes progress, consolidation and controversy. In *The Diabetes Annual, Volume 2*. Edited by Alberti KGMM & Krall LP. pp. 13–29. Amsterdam: Elsevier Science Publishers B.V.

Bottazzo GF, Pujol-Borrell R & Gale EAM (1987) Autoimmunity and Type I diabetes: bringing the story up to date. In *The Diabetes Annual, Volume 3*. Edited by Alberti KGMM & Krall LP. pp.15–38. Amsterdam: Elsevier Science Publishers B.V.

Bottazzo GF, Todd I, Mirakian R, Belfiore A & Pujol-Borrell R (1986) Organ-specific autoimmunity — a 1986 overview. *Immunological Reviews*, **94**, 137–169.

Gorsuch AN, Spencer KM, Lister J, McNally JM, Dean BM, Bottazzo GF & Cudworth AG (1981) The natural history of Type I (insulin-dependent) diabetes mellitus: evidence for a long pre-diabetic period. *Lancet*, **2**, 1363–1365.

Nerup J, Andersen O, Bendixen G, Egeberg J, Gunnarsson R, Kromann G & Poulsen JE (1974) Cell mediated immunity in diabetes mellitus. *Proceedings of the Royal Society of Medicine*, **67**, 506–513.

Pozzilli P, Sensi M, Gorsuch A, Bottazzo GF & Cudworth AG (1979) Evidence for raised K-cell levels in Type I diabetes. *Lancet*, **2**, 173–175.

Roitt IM (1984) *Essential Immunology*. 5th edition. Oxford: Blackwell Scientific Publications.

Roitt IM, Brostoff J & Male D (1985) *Immunology*. Edinburgh: Churchill Livingstone. London: Gower Medical Publishing.

Scherbaum WA, Mirakian R, Pujol-Borrell R, Dean BM & Bottazzo GF (1986) Immunochemistry in the study and diagnosis of organ-specific autoimmune disease. In *Immunocytochemistry, Modern Methods and Applications*. Edited by Polak JM & Van Norden S. pp. 456–476. Bristol: J Wright & Son.

10 Aetiology and Pathogenesis of Type I Diabetes: Viruses

Antonio Toniolo MD ● **Giovanni Federico** MD
Italo Manocchio DVM ● **Takashi Onodera** PhD

INTRODUCTION: THE ASSOCIATION BETWEEN VIRAL INFECTION AND TYPE I DIABETES

The pathogenic destruction of islet B cells in Type I (insulin-dependent) diabetes may result from either organ-specific autoimmunity or a mixture of autoimmune and environmental factors, or from environmental factors alone. Which of these pathogenic pathways is actually the cause of diabetes is unknown, but in different individuals the relative importance of each may vary.

Until recently, because of the sudden clinical onset of this condition, it was considered that the pathogenic process was relatively short. In contrast, current epidemiological, immunological and pathological studies clearly suggest that a long prodromal period of between several months and several years precedes the clinical onset in most cases.

Evidence for the role of environmental factors in the aetiology of Type I diabetes has been provided by twin studies, where approximately fifty per cent of identical twin pairs ascertained for the presence of Type I diabetes are concordant for the condition. This implies that factors other than inherited ones, and hence presumably environmental, are involved.

Experiments on animals have shown that diabetes can be produced by exposure to both chemical and viral agents and much work has been done in the hope of identifying naturally occurring agents which may be involved in the pathogenic process in human diabetes.

Although the available epidemiological evidence can only be considered to be circumstantial, several observations are in favour of an infectious, rather than a toxic, aetiology: infants under nine months of age tend to be spared, as is seen with many viral diseases where maternal antibody confers passive protection; the world-wide incidence peak lies between ten and fifteen years of age and onset after thirty-five years is less common; in pairs of siblings where both are diabetic, the interval between clinical onset is usually less than one year, suggesting that the causative agent had a relatively short period of action, acting simultaneously on both members of the pair; and the peak onset of diabetes is in the autumn and winter, coinciding with the majority of viral infections. The latter was originally interpreted as suggesting an acute viral cause for Type I diabetes, although the current concept of a long prodromal period has altered this view. Viral infections may still be important, either by triggering the initial B cell damage, leading to an autoimmune reaction, or by precipitating metabolic decompensation in previously damaged islets. Alternatively, the development of diabetes might either require cumulative insults to islet B cells, or be due to infections with long-acting or 'slow' viruses.

As early as 1864, an association between diabetes and recent mumps infection was noted by the Norwegian physician J. Stang. In 1924, Gundersen reported that epidemics of parotitis in Norway were followed four years later by an increased number of deaths from juvenile-onset diabetes. This finding is consistent with the current concept of a long prodromal period. Gamble, however, concluded that recent antecedant mumps infection was uncommon in Type I diabetic children.

Diabetes has also been reported to follow an epidemic of infectious hepatitis in Nigeria, but virtually nothing is known about the agent responsible for this epidemic. Reports of diabetes following other viral diseases, such as influenza, infectious mononucleosis and Coxsackie B infections, have been published sporadically from all over the world. Except for mumps, the only firm epidemiological connection between viruses and Type I diabetes concerns the congenital rubella syndrome. However, there are no data suggesting that diabetes can be triggered by postnatal infection with the rubella virus.

VIRAL ANTIBODIES IN TYPE I DIABETES

Gamble and colleagues reported in 1969 that higher mean antibody titres to Coxsackie virus B4 were present in patients tested at the onset of acute diabetes than in patients with diabetes of longer duration or in non-diabetic subjects. A later study confirmed this observation only in those cases with a later onset, while younger patients up to nine years of age had a lower prevalence of Coxsackie virus B4 antibodies compared to age-matched non-diabetic subjects. Virus-specific IgM antibodies, a serological sign of recent infection, were detected in about one-third of the cases and were predominantly directed to Coxsackie virus B4 and B5.

Evidence of the role of other viruses is limited. Fig. 10.1 shows data from published reports of viruses potentially linked to human diabetes. In general, antibodies to Coxsackie virus B4 and specific IgM to the Coxsackie B virus group have been detected more frequently in diabetic than in non-diabetic subjects. The same is probably true for both cytomegalovirus (CMV) and mumps virus. In contrast, the antibody response to reovirus types 1 and 3, and to the rubella virus, appears to be significantly reduced in the patients studied so far. Reports from the U.S.A., Venezuela and Italy indicate that both the prevalence and the mean titres of antibodies to other agents such as encephalomyocarditis (EMC) virus, Venezuelan equine encephalomyelitis (VEE), measles and BK virus are not significantly different in diabetic and non-diabetic subjects.

Although different conclusions were drawn in individual reports, it appears that alterations of the antibody response to several viruses are present in a significant proportion of patients with Type I diabetes, even though serum immunoglobulin levels at the onset of the disease are approximately normal.

In general, an increased response to a given virus has been interpreted as though patients were infected with this agent more frequently than normal. In contrast, when a lower than expected frequency has been found in diabetic patients, it has been postulated that people developing diabetes early in life have some defects in their immune response to certain viruses. This interpretation has been reinforced by a recent study showing alterations in the cell-mediated immune response to mumps and Coxsackie B4 viruses in HLA-DR3 positive individuals. Thus, selective defects in the immune defence against infection might place certain individuals at increased risk of developing diabetes.

It is not surprising, however, that no firm conclusions can be drawn from the serological studies performed so far. These have been concerned with common viruses to which approximately half the population are exposed at some time in life and there are cases of diabetic patients lacking antibodies to most of the candidate viruses. Therefore, it is possible that any of several different viruses may act as a triggering agent in diabetes; one particular virus has not been definitely implicated.

MAJOR PATHOGENIC MECHANISMS IN VIRUS-INDUCED DISEASE
Factors Affecting Viral Entry and Passage to Target Organs

The initial entry of a virus into the animal host is impeded by a series of natural anatomical barriers, which include the skin and the mucosal surface of the respiratory, gastrointestinal and genitourinary tract. After penetration of these barriers, viruses causing systemic disease undergo limited replication in peripheral tissues and reach the blood stream either directly or via the

PREVALENCE OF VIRAL ANTIBODIES IN TYPE I DIABETES OF RECENT ONSET			
virus		diabetic patients (% positive)	healthy controls (% positive)
family	species		
Picorna	Coxsackie B1	26.1	23.6
	Coxsackie B2	46.3	44.9
	Coxsackie B3	45.3	47.2
	Coxsackie B4	62.8*	56.0
	Coxsackie B5	36.1	41.0
	Coxsackie B6	7.2	7.3
	Coxsackie B-group IgM (age group 0.5–15y)	40.7*	22.7
	encephalomyocarditis (EMC)	12.1	6.0
Paramyxo	mumps	66.7*	50.9
	measles	60.3*	40.6
Toga	rubella	76.5†	85.4
	Venezuelan equine encephalomyelitis (VEE)	10.4	7.1
Herpes	cytomegalovirus (CMV)	41.7	32.0
Reo	reovirus-1	23.9†	56.7
	reovirus-2	51.0†	66.3
	reovirus-3	83.3†	98.0
Papova	BK	76.6	76.6

* significantly more prevalent in diabetic subjects
† significantly less prevalent in diabetic subjects

Fig. 10.1 Viruses and diabetes. The prevalence of viral antibodies in Type I diabetes of recent onset. Data are from a number of published reports.

lymphatic system. Through this primary viraemia, which is often limited, viruses can reach primary target organs and, after multiplication, produce a secondary viraemia of larger magnitude which is followed by infection of a fresh set of tissues. The protection of tissues from penetration by circulating viruses depends, to some extent, on the anatomical nature of the blood–tissue junction. In addition, one of the most important barriers to the spread of viruses into a tissue is a layer of non-susceptible cells, either the capillary endothelium itself or a mantle of other extravascular cells.

In the islets of Langerhans, the afferent arterioles enter at discontinuities of the peripheral mantle of non-B cells, then divide into capillaries that traverse the B cell core and coalesce into collecting venules at the other side of the islet. Islet capillaries have fenestrated gaps in their endothelium and, in these spaces, only the two basement membranes separate the endocrine cells from blood. The mechanism by which viruses cross endothelial cells and basement membrane is unknown, but it is known that the capillary blood flow in the islets is regulated by the innervation and by the metabolic activity of the endocrine cells. Thus, transient changes of blood flow and of capillary permeability might favour the penetration of viruses into islets.

Factors Affecting Viral Entry into Cells

Once a virus has reached a tissue, its tropism is mediated by the interaction of specific viral polypeptides with specific cell receptors on the plasma membrane. Both these structures are under genetic control and are thus highly variable. This concept is very relevant for the pathogenesis of viral diseases and gives an idea of: (i) how variants of the same virus may exhibit different degrees of tropism; (ii) how the expression of cell receptors for viruses may vary among different individuals and different cell types in the same host; and (iii) how the expression of receptors may vary in relation to the physiological state of the cell. Experimental studies indicate that cultured islet B cells are highly susceptible to a number of viral infections, but nothing is known about the *in vivo* expression of virus receptors on these cells. Thus, the presence of increased numbers of virus receptors on islet cells might expose certain individuals to an increased risk of diabetes.

Cellular factors other than receptors may also be important. These range from the genetically determined presence or absence of a cellular enzyme vital to the multiplication of the virus, to differences in the physiological state of the cell. For instance, the vulnerability of cells to parvovirus infection depends upon their mitotic state. It has been shown that a human parvovirus produces only a mild self-limiting disease in normal individuals (erythema infectiosum), while the same agent leads to aplastic crisis in patients with erythropoietic defects, since in the latter, large numbers of erythropoietic cells are continuously dividing and, as a consequence, are susceptible to this agent.

Other Factors Affecting the Outcome of Viral Disease

A variety of other factors influence the outcome of viral infections; among these are the interferon system and the immune response to the infecting agent. Not only can different individuals produce different amounts of interferon in response to the same virus, but also the antiviral effect of these molecules is variable in different subjects. In addition, individuals with a genetically determined poor immune response to a given viral antigen, especially the critical surface antigen, would theoretically have difficulty in controlling infection with that particular virus. Thus, the development of a viral disease is dependent to a significant extent upon individual factors.

Conclusion

Viral pathogenesis is an intriguing multifactorial process, and current understanding of the factors involved is very incomplete. *In vitro* and *in vivo* studies, however, have clearly established that viruses can injure cells in at least four distinct ways. First, the virus itself may directly destroy the cell with toxic products of the viral genome or by disruption of regulatory functions needed for cell survival. Secondly, both cytopathic and non-cytopathic viruses may either produce antigens foreign to the host or alter host antigens on the cell surface, indirectly inducing the immune system to kill such modified cells. Both these mechanisms yield similar results and cause fairly rapid pathological consequences. Thirdly, infection with certain viruses may trigger the production of autoantibodies that react with antigens of normal cells, thus also injuring cells that have not been infected previously. As a consequence, tissue injury is considerably delayed with respect to the initial infection. Finally, some variants of non-cytopathic viruses cause persistent infection *in vivo* without altering either the viability or antigenicity of infected tissues. These viruses, however, may induce functional disorders in infected cells that are reflected in a reduced synthesis of hormonal products or of other 'luxury' functions. In this case, the disease is characterized by an insidious onset and by the lack of inflammatory changes in infected tissue. A summary of the major events leading from infection with a virus to the development of disease is presented in Fig. 10.2.

When relating a particular disease to an infection, the relatively short incubation periods of most common viral diseases is familiar. In contrast, it should be remembered that both animal and human studies have shown that the time between infection and the development of overt disease may range from only a few hours to several decades (Fig. 10.3). In addition, chronic diseases such as Type I diabetes, rheumatoid arthritis, rheumatic fever, multiple sclerosis, subacute sclerosing panencephalitis and Reiter's syndrome, to name just a few, may represent unusual host responses to a microorganism. Therefore, even if these diseases were of infectious origin and were caused by widespread agents, their prevalence would necessarily be low. Even aggressive agents, such as polioviruses, cause paralysis in only one in 100–500 infected individuals. With this background information, the fragmentary knowledge of the link between viral infection and diabetes will be examined.

THE PANCREAS AS A TARGET FOR VIRUSES

Clinical and experimental observations indicate that the pancreas is involved in a variety of viral infections. The symptoms of pancreatic involvement in man are quite variable and, due to the difficulty of clinical diagnosis, it is likely that mild forms of pancreatic damage are more common than is clinically recognized. As shown in Fig. 10.4, many viruses have been associated with pancreatic disease and, in a number of cases, it has been possible to establish the main target cell for each agent. Although target tissues may vary in different animal species, it appears that most pancreatotropic viruses replicate in acinar cells; in contrast, ductal epithelial cells seem to be infected infrequently.

Endocrine cells appear quite resistant to infection under natural conditions and knowledge of their involvement mostly comes from animal models and the study of rare human cases. It is noteworthy that islet cells are usually spared by infection, even in the course of massive viral replication in exocrine tissue. Undoubtedly, this reflects the existence of unknown mechanisms which protect islets from viral invasion. Thus, the involvement of islet cells either is due predominantly to infection with particular variants of common viruses, which usually spare the acinar tissue, or occurs in the course of overwhelming viral infections.

The mechanism of pancreatic damage due to viral infection is incompletely understood, but it seems that the initial step in the process is the focal infection of acinar tissue, followed by cell necrosis and release of zymogen enzymes into the tissue. Autoactivation of enzyme precursors certainly potentiates virus-induced damage. Eventually, massive necrosis of acinar tissue occurs in the absence of gross damage to the islets of Langerhans. The progression of acute pancreatitis produced by Coxsackie B

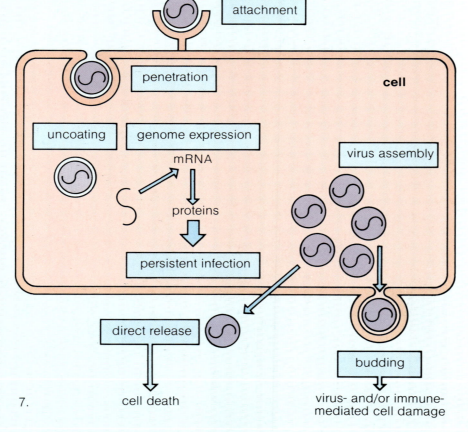

MAJOR PATHOGENIC MECHANISMS IN VIRUS-INDUCED DISEASE

human body

1. entry into host (respiratory or enteric tract, inoculation)

2. primary multiplication (respiratory or enteric mucosa, subcutaneous tissue or muscle, lymph nodes)

3. spread through host (most frequently by viraemia)

4. crossing from blood to target organs (favoured by replication in endothelial cells)

5. cell and tissue tropism (binding to specific virus receptors on target cells)

6. immune defence mechanisms (specific and non-specific)

intracellular events

attachment

penetration

cell

uncoating

genome expression

mRNA

proteins

virus assembly

persistent infection

direct release

budding

7.   cell death

virus- and/or immune-mediated cell damage

8. elimination or persistence of virus

Fig. 10.2 Stages in the pathogenesis of virus-induced disease.

viruses is a typical example of these events (Fig. 10.5). In contrast, other agents, such as rubella virus, apparently fail to destroy acinar tissue and induce only an interstitial pancreatitis.

Experimental studies have also shown that the pancreas may be a target for the replication of viruses which fail to destroy target cells and to induce inflammatory changes. Among these are viruses responsible for chronic asymptomatic infections such as endogenous or exogenous retroviruses and lymphocytic choriomeningitis virus. The role of these agents in pancreatic disease is presently unknown, but they may cause functional alterations at the cellular level.

INCUBATION PERIOD OF SOME VIRAL DISEASES

disease	time
Rift Valley fever (mouse)	6 hours
influenza	1–2 days
common cold	2–4 days
poliomyelitis	5–14 days
measles	8–12 days
rubella	10–14 days
varicella	14–21 days
mumps	18–21 days
hepatitis A	25–80 days
CMV mononucleosis	30–40 days
rabies	14–140 days
hepatitis B	50–180 days
AIDS	1 to >5 years
subacute sclerosing panencephalitis (measles variant)	2–20 years
progressive rubella panencephalitis	10–20 years
kuru	5–30 years
Creutzfeldt–Jakob	months to years
certain unconventional viral diseases (calculated)	50 to >100 years

Fig. 10.3 Incubation period of some viral diseases.

THE PANCREAS AS A TARGET FOR VIRUSES

virus	host	main target cell		
		acinar	ductal	endocrine
Coxsackie B-group	human, mouse	+	–	+
foot-and-mouth disease	cattle	+	–	+
encephalo-myocarditis	mouse, hamster, guinea pig, marmoset	+	–	+
reovirus	mouse	±	+	+
mumps	human	+	–	+
varicella–zoster	human	+	–	+
cytomegalovirus	human, mouse	+	+	+
Venezuelan encephalitis	hamster	+	–	+
retrovirus	chick, mouse	+	+	+
murine hepatitis	mouse	+	–	–
rubella	human, hamster	?	?	±
lymphocytic choriomeningitis	mouse	?	?	±
Epstein–Barr	human	?	?	?

Fig. 10.4 Main target cells of viruses associated with pancreatic disease.

10.5

ANIMAL MODELS OF VIRAL DIABETES
Betatropic Cytolytic Viruses
Foot-and-mouth disease virus (FMDV)

During the 1960 epidemic of foot-and-mouth disease in Italy, over 1000 cattle in the Perugia area developed clinical disease. Within two months of infection, many of the surviving animals developed either cardiomyopathy or a syndrome resembling diabetes without myocardial involvement. In some cases, the diagnosis of diabetes was confirmed by histology which revealed a marked reduction in the number of pancreatic islets. The few islets spared by infection were reduced in size and their B cells were degranulated and frequently had pyknotic nuclei. In contrast to the histology seen in human cases, however, mononuclear cell infiltrates in the islets were rare. The exocrine tissue, although remarkably spared, showed a proliferation of small ducts and small blood vessels.

To confirm that FMDV was indeed responsible, adult cattle were inoculated with different serotypes of the virus (O2, C, A7). Within five to fourteen days, approximately a quarter of the animals developed overt diabetes and several of them showed transient hyperglycaemia. The main histopathological change in the experimental animals consisted of an acute necrosis of the islet cells (Fig. 10.6). This effect was probably a direct consequence of the cytopathological effect of the virus; insulitis was again a rare finding. Comparable results were obtained in animals which had

been inoculated with either the FMDV type C responsible for the original epidemic or other isolates of the C or O2 types. This is in agreement with very limited observations of diabetes induced in cattle and goats by natural infection with FMDV type A; the anterior pituitary was also involved in the rare cases described.

Taken together, these studies represent the only available evidence that, under natural conditions, viruses can cause epidemics of diabetes in animals. Sporadic reports have also suggested that spontaneous diabetes in wild and domesticated animals may be a consequence of viral infection; in a few cases, parvoviruses and CMV have been identified in the islet B cells of diabetic cats and rodents, respectively.

Encephalomyocarditis virus (EMC)
The most convincing evidence supporting a viral aetiology of diabetes comes from work by Craighead and colleagues in 1968 on the myocardiotropic (M) variant of EMC. EMC belongs to the genus Cardiovirus of Picornaviridae and infects primarily rodents, although almost identical agents, such as Mengovirus, have been occasionally isolated from humans.

In experimentally infected mice, EMC multiplies in a variety of tissues, but causes specific lesions in islet B cells. During the early stages of infection, the pancreatic insulin content decreases markedly leading to hyperglycaemia (Fig. 10.7). A few days after infection, mononuclear cell infiltrates are found in and around the

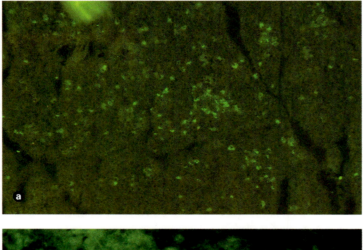

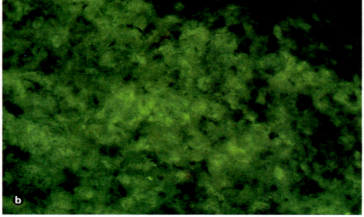

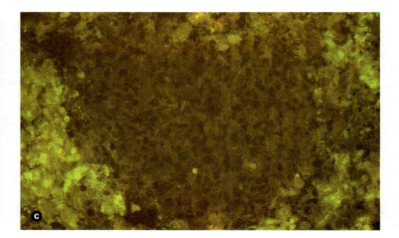

Fig. 10.5 Progression of pancreatitis induced by Coxsackie virus B3 in mice. (a) initial focal distribution of viral antigens in the exocrine tissue eighteen hours after infection. (b and c) massive involvement of exocrine tissue seventy-two hours after infection. The pancreatic islet seen in (c) is completely spared by infection. Viral antigens were detected by immunofluorescence with antiviral antibody.

islets; this insulitis is transient, however, for it is rarely observed after the second or third week. As in acute viral infections, the early infiltrate consists predominantly of macrophages disposing of necrotic cells, while in the later stages small numbers of lymphocytes are present.

EMC-induced diabetes in mice appears to be under genetic control as only certain inbred strains are susceptible. For example, SJL, SWR and CD-1 mice are susceptible to EMC-induced diabetes, while C57BL/6, CBA, and AKR are not. When diabetes-prone SWR mice were crossed with diabetes-resistant C57BL/6 mice, the F1 offspring were completely resistant to viral diabetes. More than twenty per cent of the F2 offspring, however, developed diabetes when exposed to the virus, indicating that susceptibility was inherited as an autosomal recessive trait. Backcross of the resistant F1 progeny to the resistant C57BL/6 parents also gave resistant offspring. In contrast, when the resistant F1 progeny were backcrossed to the susceptible SWR parents, approximately fifty per cent of the offspring developed

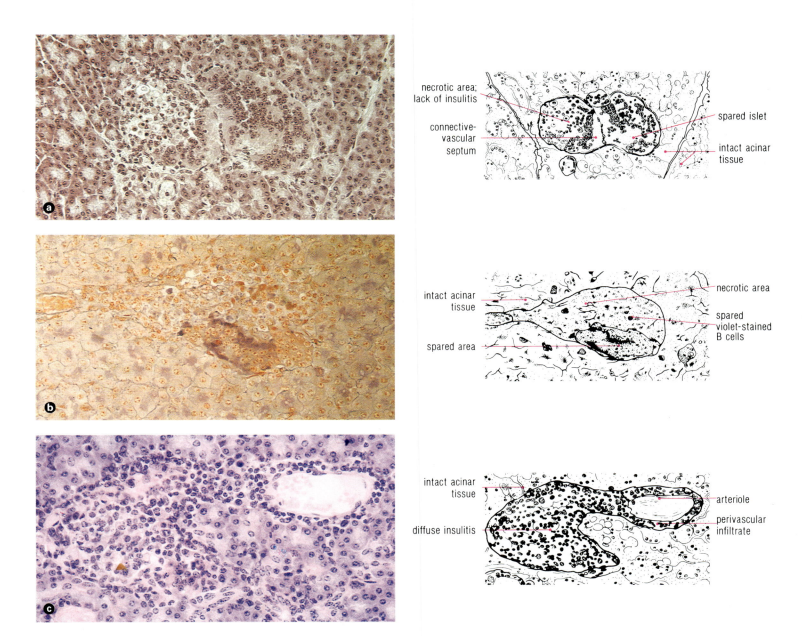

Fig. 10.6 Histopathology of bovine pancreas one week after infection of the animal with FMDV type C. (a) adjacent islets divided by a connective-vascular septum; acute necrosis of islet cells is seen in one islet, while the other appears normal (H and E stain). (b) some A and B cells are apparently spared in an islet partially destroyed by acute necrosis (aldehyde fuchsin–toluidine stain). (c) rare incidence of insulitis in the same case. There is a perivascular mononuclear cell infiltrate consisting predominantly of lymphocytes. In all cases the acinar tissue is essentially spared by infection. H and E stain.

diabetes. Although the situation may be more complex, these data are consistent with the idea that EMC-induced diabetes shows Mendelian inheritance and that susceptibility is probably controlled by a single locus. It should be noted that, in contrast to human Type I diabetes, the major histocompatibility complex of the mouse (H-2) has no influence on EMC-induced diabetes. In addition, it has been found that Mengovirus, which is antigenically indistinguishable from, but more virulent than EMC, escapes this genetic restriction and causes diabetes even in strains of mice resistant to EMC.

Thus, it appears that the genetic control of viral diabetes does not apply to all diabetogenic viruses, even if mouse strains susceptible to EMC-induced diabetes are always more susceptible than other strains to viral diabetes. Resistance, however, is not absolute, since small numbers of islet B cells are infected even in those mouse strains which do not develop hyperglycaemia (Fig. 10.8). In addition, other factors in the host, such as age, sex and hormonal status influence viral diabetogenesis. Since production of diabetes by the M-variant of EMC is variable and tends to diminish after passage of the virus in mouse embryo cell cultures, EMC-M might itself consist of different variants, some of which are diabetogenic and some not. In fact, by repeated plaque-purification of the original virus stock, Yoon and Notkins showed that at least two populations of virus, one diabetogenic (D) and the other non-diabetogenic (B), were present in the M

variant of EMC. EMC-D causes severe diabetes in susceptible mice, while EMC-B does not. Yet B and D variants can neither be distinguished antigenically nor by other physicochemical properties, with the exception of genomic analysis; an oligonucleotide of approximately twenty-five bases is missing from the RNA of the B-variant, which is present in EMC-D. Thus, a loss of less than 0.003% of the genomic RNA can abolish the diabetogenic effect of this virus.

How does EMC virus cause diabetes? In general, Picornaviridae cause acute infections and the resultant pathology is a balance between the direct lytic effect of the virus and the extent that spared target cells are capable of regeneration. Thus, it is likely that in the course of systemic infection EMC virus reaches the islets of Langerhans via the blood stream and infects B cells which are directly killed by intracytoplasmic viral replication. This is probably what happens in susceptible mice exposed to highly diabetogenic variants of EMC. However, experiments with partially resistant mouse strains infected with mildly diabetogenic variants have suggested that cell-mediated immunity may be involved in the completion of B cell destruction. This may be the case when the numbers of B cells directly killed by the virus are relatively small, but are still sufficient to induce inflammatory changes which amplify the initial damage. Thus, the primary pathogenic event is undoubtedly the direct lysis of infected cells, while the occasional immune potentiation of islet cell damage must be regarded as a complementary pathogenic factor.

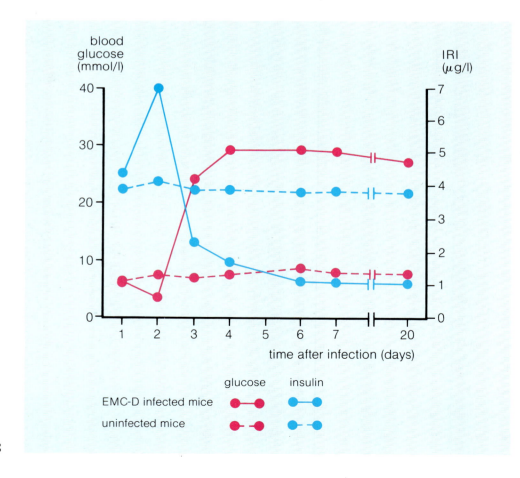

Fig. 10.7 Blood glucose and immuno-reactive insulin (IRI) levels in mice infected with the D-variant of encephalomyocarditis virus. Data from uninfected mice are shown for comparison. The transient hypoglycaemia seen on day two is related to the abrupt release of insulin from the infected pancreas.

If the long-term effects of EMC-induced diabetes are compared with the chronic complications of human diabetes, striking similarities emerge. First, glucagon levels and A cell numbers are higher than normal in diabetic animals; the pancreatic insulin reserve is reduced and new endocrine cells are formed from the exocrine tissue adjacent to islets. Secondly, the basement membrane in the capillaries of renal glomeruli, pancreatic islets, the central nervous system and the retina shows a two- to fourfold increase in thickness. Thirdly, endochondral bone formation and mineralization are greatly impaired in diabetic mice and fourthly, the mortality rate of diabetic animals is increased four- to sixfold. Thus, this animal model of diabetes is complete in that it reproduces both the early metabolic changes and many of the long-term complications of human diabetes.

The EMC model has also been used in studies of the prevention of diabetes. After inoculation with the B-variant, susceptible mice become resistant to the induction of diabetes by EMC-D. Thus, an attenuated live vaccine can prevent viral diabetes in mice, exactly as the live Sabin vaccine prevents poliomyelitis in humans.

Group B Coxsackie viruses (CBV)

The possible role of CBV in the aetiology of diabetes has been the subject of intensive investigations since Gamble and others found that patients with Type I diabetes had increased titres of antibody to them. Coxsackie, like FMDV and EMC viruses, belongs to the family Picornaviridae and infects almost exclusively humans, usually producing a mild infection, but, on occasion, causing severe meningitis, encephalitis, myocarditis or fulminant infection in neonates. There are six different types of CBV and their pathological effects can be studied conveniently in mice. All these agents replicate very efficiently in the exocrine pancreas of adult mice, virtually sparing the endocrine cells. Subtle insular changes, however, can be detected occasionally by electron microscopy in infected mice, showing that even common strains of CBV have a tropism for the endocrine pancreas.

The most common consequence of infection is acute pancreatitis accompanied by a marked rise in blood amylase concentration. Nevertheless, when these agents are serially passaged in mouse islet B cell cultures, or in pancreatic tissue *in vivo*, their tropism for the exocrine pancreas is very much reduced and variants emerge which are capable of infecting large numbers of islet cells. Thus, as in the case of EMC virus, natural strains of CBV probably consist of mixtures of different variants each endowed with a different tissue tropism.

For unknown reasons, variants found in human infections are predominantly tropic for the nervous system and for the heart; the existence of possible diabetogenic variants, however, has been suggested indirectly by rare cases of CBV-induced diabetes and by the relatively frequent finding of insulitis in infants with fatal CBV infections.

With the possible exception of rare diabetogenic strains of CBV-4, CBV are far less effective than EMC virus in producing diabetes in mice. In general, the distribution of viral antigens in the islets of Langerhans is restricted to a small proportion of B cells and occurs only during the early phase of infection. Virus-induced damage is, however, sufficient to induce insulitis, hypoinsulinaemia and glucose intolerance. Overt hyperglycaemia rarely develops. Although the data are far from complete, it is believed that the same genetic factors controlling the susceptibility of mice to EMC-induced diabetes also operate in the case of CBV infection. In addition, it seems likely that, as in the case of EMC, the primary event in CBV-induced diabetes is the direct destruction of B cells during viral replication. This does not preclude a contribution by the immune system as in the case of CBV-induced cardiomyopathy

Conclusion

Taken together, the studies on diabetogenic picornaviruses (i.e., FMDV, EMC and CBV) consistently indicate that pathogenic B cell-tropic viral variants can occasionally emerge from natural pools. This is probably due to the high mutation rate observed in these single-stranded RNA viruses and their fast circulation rate in animal and human populations.

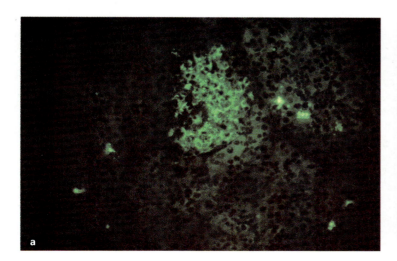 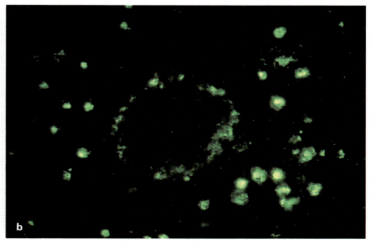

Fig. 10.8 Sections of pancreas from (a) susceptible SJL mice and (b) resistant C57BL/6 mice three days after infection with EMC virus. A high proportion of the islet cells of susceptible mice contains viral antigens, whereas only a few islet cells of resistant mice are infected. Viral antigens were detected by immunofluorescence with antiviral antibody. Little fluorescence is present in the acinar tissue.

Viruses Inducing Autoimmunity and Endocrine Disease
Reoviruses

The three serotypes of mammalian reoviruses are widely distributed in humans and in a number of animal species. These agents were identified in the 1950's and, although frequently isolated from the respiratory and enteric tracts, they have not been associated with any distinct human disease; in fact, the prefix 'reo' stands for respiratory enteric orphan. These agents offer an excellent system for the study of molecular aspects of viral pathogenesis as reovirus genetics has provided information about the role of specific viral components involved in the disease process. In addition, reoviruses have a prominent position in experimental viral diabetogenesis since they are the only known agents capable of inducing both endocrine disease and organ-specific autoimmunity.

In newborn mice, reovirus types 1 and 3 (reo-1 and reo-3) can infect several organs, but show differences in tissue tropism which are related to the structure of the viral haemagglutinin, that is, the sigma-1 outer-capsid protein which binds to cell receptors. After passage in islet B cell cultures, variants capable of infecting islet cells *in vivo* can be easily selected. Infection of newborn mice with B cell-passaged reo-1 and reo-3 produces mild transient hyperglycaemia and marked glucose intolerance with a depressed insulin response to a glucose load.

Viral antigens are easily detected in islet cells by immunofluorescence and intracellular viral particles can be demonstrated by electron microscopy where they can be seen developing in a reticulogranular matrix or in a crystalline array within the endocrine cells (Fig. 10.9). In contrast to reo-3 infection, mice exposed neonatally to reo-1 develop a runting syndrome characterized by retarded growth, alopecia and steatorrhoea. Histopathological changes are produced in the islets of Langerhans and also in the anterior pituitary, where viral antigens can be found in cells producing growth hormone (GH). As a consequence, insulin and GH blood levels are reduced in infected mice, whereas glucagon levels are a little increased.

Infected tissues show inflammatory infiltrates consisting of both lymphocytes and large numbers of plasma cells. This finding, together with histopathological and functional changes of lymphoid organs, suggests that the immune system may be involved in reo-1-induced polyendocrinopathy. In fact, serum autoantibodies reacting with normal pancreatic islet cells (Fig. 10.10), the anterior pituitary, gastric parietal cells and T lymphocytes are produced by most reo-1-infected mice, particularly during the first month of infection. As has been found in some patients with recently diagnosed Type I diabetes, these mice also produce autoantibodies to endogenous hormones including GH and insulin.

To clarify the pathogenic role of these autoantibodies, infected mice were subjected to various immunosuppressive regimens. As shown in Fig. 10.11, the administration of either anti-lymphocyte serum, anti-thymocyte serum or cyclophosphamide was about

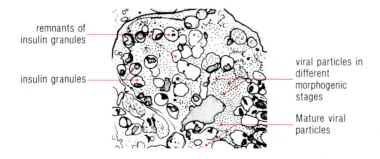

remnants of insulin granules

insulin granules

viral particles in different morphogenic stages

Mature viral particles

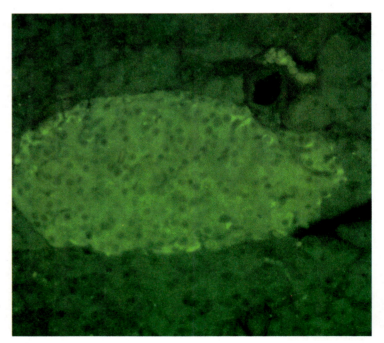

Fig. 10.9 Electron-microscopic changes in islet B cells of suckling mice five days after infection with reovirus type 1. Reovirus particles are interspersed among altered insulin granules. EM × 14,000.

Fig. 10.10 Autoantibodies to endocrine cells produced by mice neonatally infected with reovirus type 1. This agent produces diabetes and an autoimmune polyendocrinopathy. The serum autoantibody to islet cells used here resembles human islet cell autoantibody (ICA) since it reacts with unfixed frozen sections of normal pancreas and stains all islet cells. Indirect immunofluorescence technique.

equally effective in preventing the development of hyperglycaemia. In addition, these treatments reduced the mortality rate and almost suppressed autoantibody formation without influencing viral replication kinetics. This finding shows that autoimmunity plays a central role in reo-1-induced polyendocrine disease and indicates that timely immunosuppression, introduced in the early phase of infection, may prevent viral-induced autoimmunity and arrest the progression of the disease.

As far as is known, reo-1-infected mice produce only organ-specific autoantibodies, usually against those tissues which have been previously infected. In contrast, monoclonal autoantibodies which can be easily obtained from infected mice are both organ-specific (Fig. 10.12) and multiple-organ reactive. It appears, therefore, that this virus can trigger a vast repertoire of autoreactive B lymphocytes to secrete autoantibodies, but that *in vivo* only part of these clones is allowed to expand. For unknown reasons, the sigma-1 protein of reo-1 is essential for the induction of autoimmunity, because neither reo-3 nor a recombinant virus containing nine genes from reo-1 together with just one from reo-3 (the gene coding for the sigma-1 protein) can trigger autoantibody production. Thus, once again, subtle structural properties of a virus are responsible for the production of diabetes and autoimmunity.

Precisely how reoviruses cause polyendocrinopathy in mice is unknown, but it probably results from the cumulative injury to endocrine cells produced by a direct lytic effect of the virus and the effect of autoantibodies against normal cells and hormonal products.

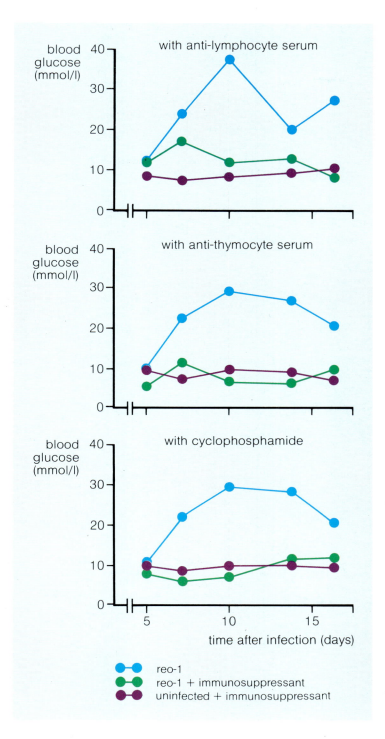

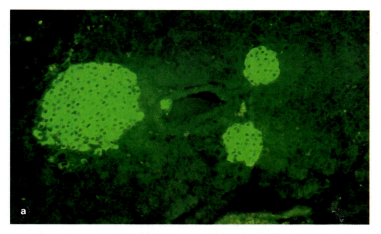

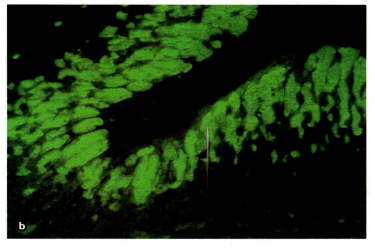

Fig. 10.11 Reversal of reovirus-induced diabetes by immunosuppression. Effect of immunosuppressive agents on glucose tolerance tests in mice neonatally infected with reovirus type 1. Mice were given either anti-lymphocyte serum, anti-thymocyte serum or cyclophosphamide in the early phase of infection. Infected mice treated with these agents consistently failed to develop hyperglycaemia and showed glucose levels similar to control animals.

Fig. 10.12 Organ-specific monoclonal antibodies obtained from reovirus-infected mice. (a) cytoplasmic staining of cells in the central areas of islets is produced by a monoclonal autoantibody against insulin. (b) strong fluorescence of the deeper parts of the gastric mucosa is seen with a monoclonal autoantibody to the stomach wall. Indirect immunofluorescence technique.

Viruses Perturbing Endocrine Functions by Unknown Mechanisms

Other viruses, primarily slightly cytopathic or non-cytopathic enveloped viruses (so-called because of the lipid membrane surrounding them), may cause a diabetes-like syndrome by means other than direct islet B cell damage. Enveloped viruses, due to peculiarities of their replication and maturation processes, produce subtle alterations of cell membranes which, though frequently compatible with cell survival, are reflected in either altered cellular physiology or reduced synthesis of certain products, or both. When such agents cause persistent infections, the host suffers long-term consequences. Two interesting animal models of virus-induced diabetes will be described.

Venezuelan equine encephalitis virus (VEE)

In 1976, Rayfield and colleagues reported that both a virulent and an attenuated (vaccine) strain of VEE could replicate in the pancreas of golden Syrian hamsters; this virus induced focal necrosis in some islets of Langerhans which subsided within three weeks of infection. Metabolic studies showed that the animals had a transient impairment of glucose tolerance and a persistent reduction of glucose-stimulated insulin release. Comparable results were also obtained in C57BL/KS mice and in young monkeys. Although viral particles can be detected in islet B cells during the early phase of infection, the late phase is characterized by a lack of morphological changes on light and electron microscopy; pancreatic insulin content is not reduced during the late phase of infection.

Experiments *in vitro* on isolated perfused islets from chronically infected hamsters confirmed that although basal insulin secretion was normal, glucose-stimulated release was greatly reduced. In this *in vitro* system, analogues of cyclic AMP and the phosphodiesterase inhibitors, tolbutamide and theophylline, can correct the B cell response to glucose stimulation. This suggests that VEE infection somehow induces persistent alterations of post-receptor

events (Fig. 10.13). The reduced insulin secretion that occurs in VEE-infected hamsters thus provides a potential model for the insulin-deficient form of Type II diabetes.

Lymphocytic choriomeningitis virus (LCMV)

In another viral model, Oldstone and colleagues showed that inoculation of newborn mice with various strains of LCMV resulted in a persistent infection with little or no associated pathology. This virus, however, can replicate continuously in a variety of cells including pituitary and islet B cells. When BALB/WEHI mice were inoculated at birth with a small dose of LCMV, all mice became persistently infected despite mounting anti-viral immune responses. Three to six months after infection, LCMV could be demonstrated in the islets of Langerhans by electron microscopy, immunohistochemical methods and by looking for viral genomes. Over fifty per cent of islet cells from persistently infected mice contained viral nucleoprotein, a gene product expressed during the intermediate phase of viral replication. Just a few cells expressed viral glycoproteins on their surface, that is, 'late' proteins associated with viral maturation and budding.

Generally, mature virions in islet cells are infrequently found on electron microscopy. The restricted expression of LCMV glycoproteins in the presence of abundant nucleoproteins probably accounts for the virtual absence of necrosis and inflammatory infiltrates in the islets, since viral glycoprotein must be expressed in sufficient quantity on the surface of infected cells for recognition and successful assault by the host's immune system. Thus, pancreatic endocrine tissues appear normal and do not provide morphological clues to the hidden but partially replicating virus within. The majority of persistently infected mice show abnormal glucose tolerance, but both basal insulin blood levels and the *in vitro* production of insulin by B cells are normal. Therefore, the final result of persistent LCMV infection resembles the metabolic and morphological aspects of the early stages of Type II diabetes.

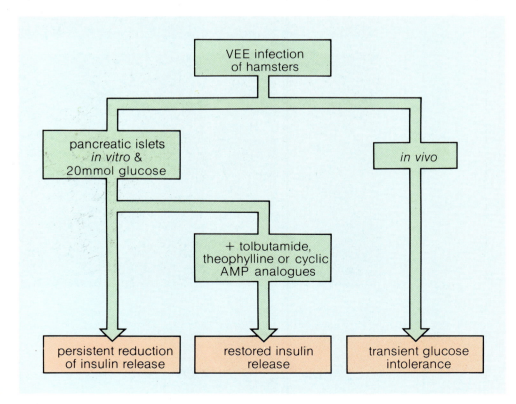

Fig. 10.13 Venezuelan equine encephalitis (VEE) virus-induced alterations of insulin release. The infection of golden Syrian hamsters with VEE causes transient alterations of the response to a glucose load. Persistent alterations of the B cell response to glucose, however, can be detected in islets isolated from chronically infected hamsters. When pancreatic islets from these animals are incubated *in vitro* with glucose their insulin release appears significantly reduced. The response is restored by the addition of tolbutamide, theophylline or cyclic AMP analogues.

Though the mechanisms by which VEE and LCMV alter glucose homoeostasis are poorly understood, these animal models challenge the current opinion that viral infections are only of importance in Type I diabetes.

Cumulative Environmental Insults as a Cause of Diabetes
In strains of mice resistant to EMC-induced diabetes, insufficient B cells are damaged to alter glucose homoeostasis. Diabetes, however, can be produced in many species by a variety of highly specific B cell toxins, such as, alloxan and streptozotocin. When mice are exposed to a small dose of streptozotocin, hyperglycaemia does not result, although there is a persistent reduction of B cell reserve. When the same animals are subsequently infected with EMC virus, diabetes develops in a high proportion of mice of the

resistant strains. Conversely, pre-treatment of susceptible strains with streptozotocin followed by EMC infection does not result in an increase of diabetes prevalence, but causes a conspicuous rise in blood glucose levels. Thus, severe diabetes can be produced by the additive effects of the two agents.

A similar synergy has been observed in mice neonatally infected with either reo-1 or murine cytomegalovirus and given streptozotocin one month later. Subdiabetogenic doses of streptozotocin can also potentiate the capacity of weakly diabetogenic viruses to alter glucose homoeostasis, as in the case of the six members of the Coxsackie B virus group (Fig. 10.14), but such doses do not allow the production of diabetes following infection with non-diabetogenic agents such as the B-variant of EMC virus.

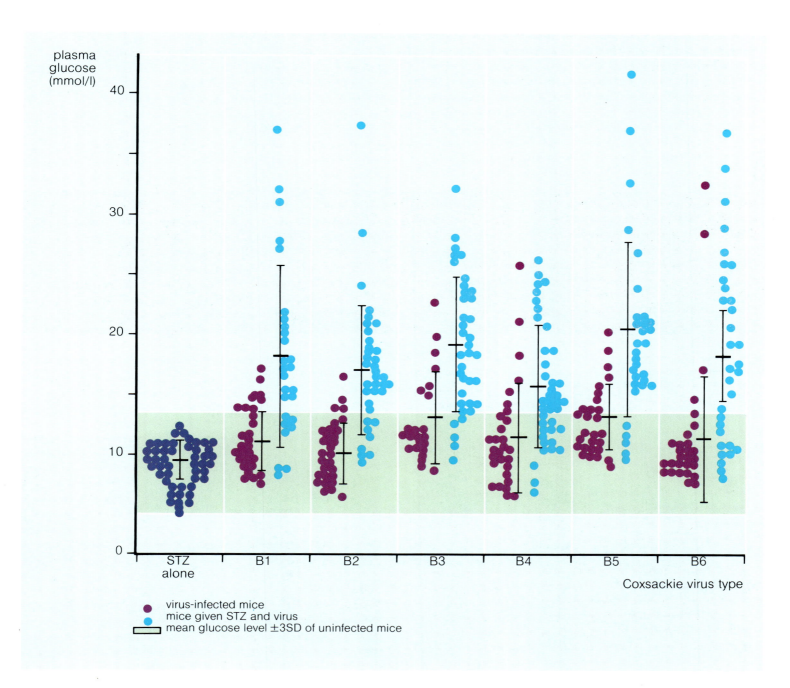

Fig. 10.14 Glucose abnormalities induced by the six members of the Coxsackie B virus group (B1–B6) enhanced by depletion of islet B cell reserve with subdiabetogenic doses of streptozotocin (STZ). Mice were given STZ and infected twelve days later with virus.

Results for mice given only STZ, only virus, and both STZ and virus are shown. Each point represents an individual animal and the means ±SD are also shown.

Experimental evidence indicates that streptozotocin does not act by causing a non-specific increase in the susceptibility of islet cells to infection, but by irreversibly damaging a proportion of B cells. Therefore, viral infections have only to complete previously initiated damage to trigger overt diabetes. Severe diabetes can also result from sequential infections of mice with two or more related viruses. For example, neonatal infection of mice with murine cytomegalovirus followed by EMC virus infection at the adult stage is followed by a more severe metabolic disturbance than by either agent alone.

It should be emphasized that, in addition to direct B cell damage, a variety of factors may contribute to any alteration in glucose homoeostasis: exposure to chemicals and viruses may induce hormonal changes, and autoimmunity and pre-existing islet pathology may influence the regenerative capacity of damaged B cells. Mention should also be made of the mysterious role of endogenous retroviruses, which are vertically transmitted to the progeny predominantly as proviruses integrated in parental chromosomes and which could play a part in genetic, and perhaps viral, diabetogenesis.

It has been shown that many diabetes-prone mouse strains carry genomic information for the production of type C or type A retrovirus particles. In these strains, retrovirus particles or viral components are produced in islet B cells when subjected to a variety of physiological or pathological stimuli, such as elevated blood glucose levels or streptozotocin treatments. It has been suggested that the expression of retroviral products on the B cell membrane can initiate an immune response against B cell-associated viral antigens. In addition, it has been proposed that during this response local conditions may favour the development of B cell-specific autoimmunity.

Whatever role, if any, these endogenous viruses play in diabetogenesis, these studies in mice point to the possibility that a variety of interactions can occur among environmental agents at the cellular level and that many different insults, occurring together or sequentially, may predispose the animal to develop diabetes.

VIRUS-INDUCED DIABETES IN HUMANS
Viral Infection of Human Islet B Cells in Culture
Since it is difficult to determine whether human cells are susceptible to viral infections *in vivo*, an *in vitro* system has been developed to determine which viruses are capable of infecting these cells in culture. Due to the difficulty of obtaining large

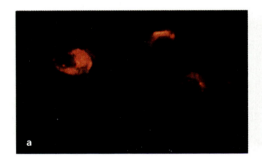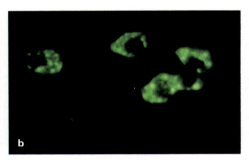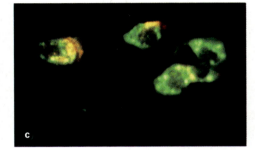

Fig. 10.15 *In vitro* infection of human islet B cells by reovirus type 3. Thirty hours after infection, the cultures were stained with rhodamine-labelled antibody to insulin and with fluorescein-labelled antibody to reovirus. (a) three insulin-containing cells (red); (b) the same area taken with fluorescein filters showing reovirus-infected cells (green); and (c) double exposure showing three cells (orange) that contain both insulin and reovirus antigens. By this double-label immunofluorescent staining technique, it is possible to ascertain whether a virus can replicate in insulin-producing cells.

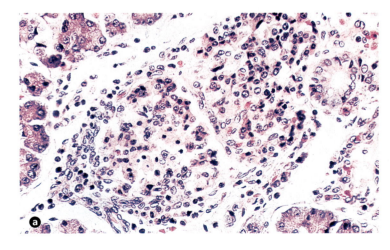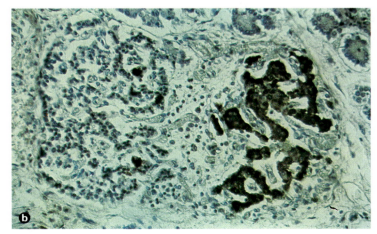

Fig. 10.16 Histopathology of pancreatic islets from a neonate who died of disseminated Coxsackie virus B4 infection without evidence of diabetes. (a) degeneration and necrosis without lysis of islet cells is characterized by pyknotic nuclei of varying size and condensed eosinophilic cytoplasm (H and E stain). (b) immuno-chemical staining of an islet for insulin; insulin-containing cells are marked by the dark brown staining. More than half of the islet is completely degranulated of insulin (peroxidase–antiperoxidase stain). By courtesy of Dr A.B. Jenson.

quantities of functionally active B cells, these studies have been rather limited in scope. Since these cultures are not composed of B cells alone, a double-label immunofluorescent antibody technique has been used to show unequivocally that B cells and not other contaminating cells have been infected (Fig. 10.15).

By this method, Notkins and colleagues have shown that B cells from seven human donors allowed the replication of mumps virus. This agent caused direct lysis of most B cells in about six days, but also infected a sizeable proportion of non-B cells. In a series of similar experiments, Yoon and colleagues showed that CBV-3, CBV-4 and selected strains of reo-3 caused rapid B cell lysis and a remarkable decrease of intracellular immunoreactive insulin. In contrast, reo-3 strains which had not been passed through B cell cultures replicated in only a small percentage of B cells without reducing the insulin content of the culture. It has also been shown that BK virus (a Papova virus which may cause insulinoma in hamsters and intra-uterine infection in humans) may infect and destroy human B cells *in vitro*.

In most cases, human donors were not typed for their human leucocyte antigen (HLA), thus precluding any conclusions with regard to the influence of the genetic make-up of the host on virus susceptibility. Although it is known that viral susceptibility *in vitro* does not necessarily reflect the situation *in vivo*, further studies in this direction may help to identify naturally occurring betatropic viruses.

Post-mortem Studies: Viruses Capable of Infecting Pancreatic Islets in the Living Host

The finding that many viruses which are widely disseminated in humans may induce diabetes in experimental animals and may infect human B cells *in vitro*, raises the question of whether and how frequently viral infections of islet cells occur *in vivo* in humans.

Theoretically, this problem should be approached by looking for histological damage of pancreatic islets in the course of clinical viral infections. Since pancreatic biopsies cannot be obtained from patients, the only available information has come from studies of rare cases of patients dying of severe viral infections. Thus, when interpreting these data, it should be remembered that these findings result from unusual clinical cases.

Jenson and colleagues examined the pancreases of 250 children with fatal infections caused by at least fourteen different viruses and found insular pathology in twenty-eight cases. Other surveys have found insular changes in fifteen out of eighty-five cases of neonatal Coxsackie B virus infections, and islet cytopathology has also been reported in cases of disseminated infections due to cytomegalovirus, mumps, varicella–zoster and rubella virus. Therefore, pancreatic islet damage has been found in at least thirteen per cent of fatal viral infections. In these studies, most of the pathological changes were found in neonates and, in most cases, islet cells other than B cells were clearly involved. In cases due to lytic agents, such as Coxsackie B viruses, some islet cells appeared to have undergone lysis and many others had dense pyknotic nuclei; most islets were mildly or moderately insulin-depleted and mononuclear cell infiltrates were present in three to thirty per cent of islets (Fig. 10.16).

Islet cell involvement seems relatively frequent in cases of disseminated varicella–zoster infections. Here, infection of the islets is focal and also involves adjacent acinar cells. Infected cells are detected by the presence of intranuclear inclusion bodies and cells with inclusions are often close to cells that have been lysed. The varicella–zoster virus therefore seems capable of directly destroying islet cells.

Cytomegalovirus is perhaps the agent most frequently responsible for islet cell infection; over thirty cases of islet cell damage due to this agent have been reported. Although most of these cases were congenital or neonatal infections, it appears that cytomegalovirus can also infect islets in adults; such cases are frequent in patients with the acquired immunodeficiency syndrome (AIDS).

Cytomegalovirus-infected cells are easily recognized by typical inclusions which are found not only in B cells but also in other islet cells (Fig. 10.17). Due perhaps to the immunosuppressive activity of this virus, insulitis is a rare finding in these cases. Though the development of diabetes is a frequent sequela of the congenital rubella syndrome, histological evidence for viral cytopathology and insulitis has only rarely been found. Only two cases with islet damage and mild insulitis have been previously described.

In many of these cases, pathological changes in the islets were more prominent than in the surrounding acinar tissue, suggesting that some viral strains may show tropism for islet cells. Thus, these studies provide further *in vivo* support for the observation that, under certain circumstances, viruses can infect and damage human B cells.

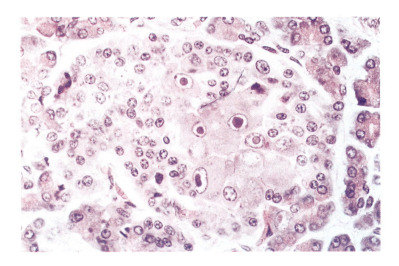

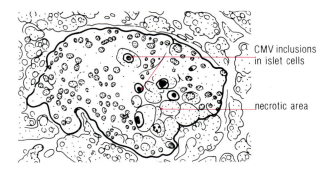

Fig. 10.17 Typical cytomegalovirus (CMV) inclusions ('owl-eye' inclusion bodies) in the islet cells of an eleven-year-old boy who developed a disseminated CMV infection and diabetic ketoacidosis. There is a lack of inflammatory infiltrates (H and E stain). By courtesy of Dr A.B. Jenson.

Clinical Cases

The best way to establish a direct link between viral infections and human diabetes is the recovery of viruses from diabetic patients and the demonstration that the isolated agents are capable of producing diabetes in experimental hosts. So far, this goal has been achieved in only two cases. The first is that of a ten-year-old boy who developed diabetic ketoacidosis three days after the onset of a flu-like illness. Despite intensive therapy, the child's condition deteriorated and he died seven days later. At autopsy, insulitis and B cell necrosis were observed. Yoon, Notkins and colleagues were able to isolate a variant of CBV-4 from his pancreas. He had shown a rise in the titre of neutralizing antibody to this isolate, from less than four on the second hospital day to thirty-two on the day of death. In addition, viral antigens were detected by immunofluorescence in various organs of the child. This provided clear evidence that at the time of death CBV-4 had caused a systemic infection and that the isolated virus was not an inadvertent contaminant from the laboratory.

To prove that this agent was truly related to the child's diabetes, several inbred strains of mice were inoculated with the CBV-4 isolate. Susceptible mice developed acute diabetes, while mice of strains resistant to EMC-induced diabetes did not. As shown in Fig. 10.18, examination of the pancreas from diabetic mice revealed acute insulitis, destruction of B cells and the presence of viral antigens in the islets of Langerhans. All these data led to the conclusion that the diabetes was virus-induced.

The second case is that of a sixteen-month-old girl who was admitted to hospital for thrombocytopenic purpura appearing after one week of fever. Laboratory evidence of diabetes was present from days thirteen to twenty-five, then a remission ensued, but two months later the child developed overt diabetes. On the eighth day after the onset of fever, CBV-5 was isolated from the stools. Antibody titres to this agent rose from less than ten to 640, showing that in the period preceding the onset of diabetes the baby had been infected by CBV-5. When this isolate was inoculated into various strains of inbred mice, glucose intolerance was produced in those strains susceptible to EMC-induced diabetes. Since the common strains of CBV-5 are not diabetogenic in mice, it was concluded that the child had been infected by a pancreatotropic variant of this virus. The child had the high-risk genetic markers, HLA-DR3 and BfF1, and, at the time of admission to hospital, had islet cell antibodies. Thus, it appears that in this case CBV-5 infection combined with genetic and immunological factors to produce diabetes.

In other cases, proof that the isolated agents were diabetogenic in experimental animals has not been provided. However, in these cases a virus has been identified and its relation to the disease has been established by histopathological findings. A five-year-old girl developed myocarditis and acute diabetes seven days after open-heart surgery. She died in diabetic ketoacidosis; at autopsy, there was degeneration and necrosis of the islet cells and an associated insulitis. CBV-4 antigens were found in the islets by immunofluorescence and high levels of antibody to this virus were found in the serum. Thus it appeared that the development of insulin-deficient diabetes in this girl was the direct consequence of acute CBV-4 infection.

One case of diabetes due to CBV-1 infection occurred in a newborn twin who acquired the virus from the mother a few days before birth. Immediately after birth, he deteriorated and developed thrombocytopenia and cardiomyopathy. On the twelfth day, his blood glucose level rose to over 28mmol/l (500mg/dl) and he died four days later. At autopsy, there was insulitis with islet cell degeneration and CBV-1 was recovered from the pancreas. It is of interest that his twin brother, though developing a severe infection due to the same strain of CBV-1, did not become diabetic and was discharged from hospital twenty-five days after birth. Thus it appears that infection with a diabetogenic virus does not always result in the development of diabetes in humans.

Another case concerned a fourteen-month-old boy with well documented congenital rubella syndrome. He died five days after developing diabetes. Insulin-containing B cells could not be detected. A subacute insulitis was observed, but most islets were partially hyalinized indicating prior damage.

Other cases of acute-onset Type I diabetes have been associated with various viral infections with less convincing evidence. So far, over fifteen other cases have been reported: one was attributed to CBV-1, one to CBV-2, two to CBV-5, one to CBV-6, three to mumps virus, five to Epstein–Barr virus (the aetiological agent of infectious mononucleosis) and others to the rubella virus. It is difficult to establish whether, in these cases, the reported viral agents were directly responsible for the development of diabetes or whether they acted as triggering factors superimposed on a progressive diabetogenic process. Those cases which have been reported during the neonatal period, however, undoubtedly represent a direct consequence of viral attack. Although many questions remain, these studies support the contention that at least some cases of Type I diabetes have a viral aetiology.

Diabetes and the Congenital Rubella Syndrome: A Possible Link between Viruses and Genetic Factors in Causing Autoimmunity and Diabetes

The most convincing evidence that a persistent viral infection may cause Type I diabetes comes from studies of patients with the congenital rubella syndrome (CRS). It has been shown that after intra-uterine infection, the rubella virus can be isolated from patients for over twenty years and that, among other organs, it can produce persistent infection of the pancreas. Prospective studies from Australia, the U.S.A. and other countries have established that the prevalence of diabetes among these patients is between five and twenty per cent and that a latent period of many years is required for diabetes to develop. So far, over sixty cases of diabetes have been reported worldwide in such patients and the mean age of onset is approximately thirteen years (range 1–30 years).

The high prevalence and long latent period of diabetes in these subjects makes them an ideal group for the study of the pathogenic events preceding diabetes. Accordingly, Ginsberg–Fellner, Rubinstein and colleagues have found either or both cytoplasmic and surface islet cell antibodies in over twenty per cent of the CRS patients they have studied, and in over seventy per cent of those who developed diabetes. In addition, many of these patients have antithyroid antibodies, showing that persistent infection with this agent can stimulate endocrine autoimmunity against several organs.

It has also been shown that only those CRS patients with the high-risk genetic markers (HLA-DR3 and/or DR4) become diabetic and that it develops in virtually all of these individuals. Even in these patients, the DR2 genotype seems to afford protection. Thus it appears that this severe intra-uterine infection can increase the penetrance of the common susceptibility genotype towards one hundred per cent. How this virus induces diabetes is unknown, but it appears that a persistent viral insult, together with a permissive genotype, can trigger an autoimmune response leading to B cell failure.

Besides rubella virus, a number of other pancreatotropic viruses have the potential to infect the fetus without necessarily causing immediate pathological effects; these include: cytomegalovirus, mumps and BK virus. Therefore the question arises whether exposure to these agents *in utero* predisposes to the later development of diabetes.

From Viral Infection to Diabetes in Humans: Possible Mechanisms

Models requiring viral infection of islet B cells

The experimental models together with the few reported human cases of viral diabetes indicate that certain viruses can damage pancreatic B cells. Based on the current view of viral pathogenesis, it is possible to suggest four major pathways leading from viral infection of islet cells to the development of diabetes (Fig. 10.19).

The first possibility is that of a lytic virus tropic for islet B cells. The intracellular replication of this agent directly kills the cell and

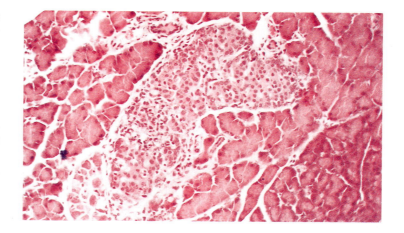

Fig. 10.18 Section of pancreas from SJL mice infected with a diabetogenic strain of CBV-4 isolated from the pancreas of a ten-year-old boy. The boy died of diabetic ketoacidosis a few days after developing an acute infection. Marked degeneration of the islet cells and inflammatory changes can be seen one week after inoculation. H and E stain.

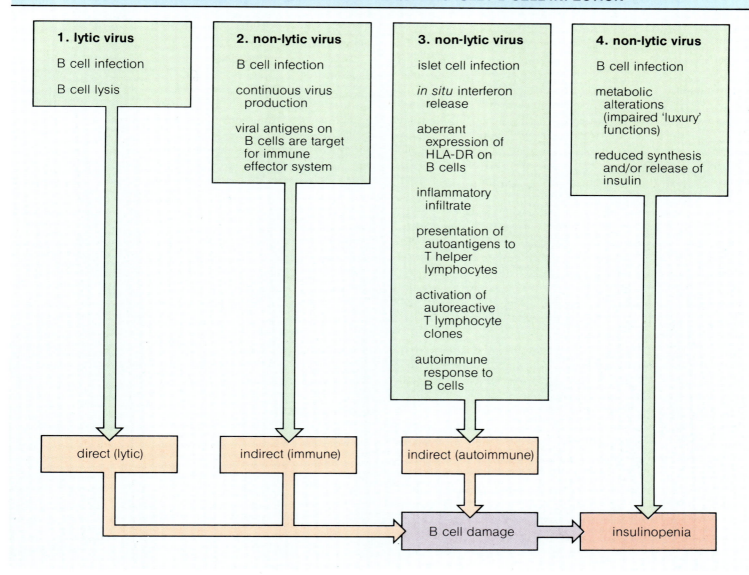

VIRUSES AND DIABETES: MODELS REQUIRING ISLET B CELL INFECTION

1. lytic virus

B cell infection

B cell lysis

2. non-lytic virus

B cell infection

continuous virus production

viral antigens on B cells are target for immune effector system

3. non-lytic virus

islet cell infection

in situ interferon release

aberrant expression of HLA-DR on B cells

inflammatory infiltrate

presentation of autoantigens to T helper lymphocytes

activation of autoreactive T lymphocyte clones

autoimmune response to B cells

4. non-lytic virus

B cell infection

metabolic alterations (impaired 'luxury' functions)

reduced synthesis and/or release of insulin

direct (lytic)   indirect (immune)   indirect (autoimmune)

B cell damage   insulinopenia

Fig. 10.19 Pathogenesis of virus-induced diabetes: (1). Models requiring viral infection of islet B cells. These models are mostly derived from studies on experimental animals.

diabetes ensues within a few days or a few weeks of the onset of systemic infection. In animals, a similar process is caused by EMC, CBV-4 and FMDV. In humans, it may be associated with the few described cases of CBV-induced diabetes which were usually lethal.

The second mechanism may be triggered by a persistent infection of B cells with a non-lytic or mildly-lytic agent. In this situation, B cell failure would be promoted by an immune attack against viral antigens expressed on the surface of B cells. Thus the immune system indirectly kills virus-replicating cells. This process is notably slower than the first since it requires the triggering of an antiviral immune response as well as the penetration of immune effectors into the islets. In addition, the speed of this process is modulated by the rate at which the viral antigens are inserted into the B cell membrane; this, in turn, depends upon the intracellular replication rate of each particular agent. Although this mechanism is activated in the course of most viral infections, it may be of particular relevance to the pathogenesis of those forms of human diabetes due to slowly replicating agents such as rubella or cytomegalovirus.

It is widely accepted that viruses can induce autoimmunity, but the precise mechanisms are unknown. The third model proposes a pathway leading from a local insult to organ-specific auto-immunity. It has been observed that HLA-class II antigens are expressed in certain tissues from patients with a variety of autoimmune endocrine diseases. Since the expression of these molecules is normally restricted to antigen-presenting cells, B lymphocytes, activated T lymphocytes, thymic epithelium and to certain endothelial cells, the finding of these antigens on endocrine cells is considered an aberrant expression of the HLA-D region products. The physiological role of these molecules is to allow the interaction of macrophages with lymphocytes during antigen presentation. If other cells which are neither designed for antigen processing nor presentation express HLA-DR antigens, these cells can then be viewed as antigen-presenting cells if interactions with lymphocytes occur.

The possibility that endocrine DR-positive cells can present autoantigens to autoreactive T cells has been verified *in vitro* and it was observed that treatment of certain endocrine cells with physiological concentrations of either interferon or various lymphokines caused the inappropriate expression of DR by cultured epithelial cells. In the islets of Langerhans *in vivo*, this sequence of events might be triggered by the local production of interferon in response to viral infection. Even if mild, this infection would stimulate lymphocytes and other inflammatory cells to enter the islets. Under these conditions, B cells would have the opportunity of presenting autoantigens to autoreactive T helper lymphocytes. The ensuing autoimmune response would allow the self-perpetuation of this mechanism and its extension to islets which had not been infected (see *Chapter 9*).

Since the interferon response is not virus-specific, any pancreatotropic virus could theoretically initiate this sequence. In addition, this model does not even require that B cells are infected, since damage to any other cell type within the islets would suffice to trigger, via interferon, the aberrant expression of HLA-DR antigens on B cells. Nevertheless, to explain the specific destruction of B cells alone, in theory, only B cells would be capable of presenting autoantigens. Though hypothetical, this mechanism would explain the present inability to associate specific causal viruses with diabetes and would explain the long prediabetic period. The infection might occur months or even years before the onset of overt diabetes and initiate slow autoimmune damage.

The fourth mechanism refers to viruses producing silent persistent infection of B cells. Such agents have never been detected in the human pancreas. Experimental models, however, have shown that LCM and VEE viral infections in mice can cause a long-term reduction of either insulin synthesis or release by subverting insulin biosynthesis. As described above, these infections produce an insulinopenic syndrome reminiscent of some forms of Type II diabetes.

Models not requiring viral infection of B cells
Experimental work in viral immunology suggests that viruses might cause autoimmune diabetes and other endocrine diseases by mechanisms other than islet cell infection (Fig. 10.20). There are three possibilities.

First, the virus could trigger autoimmunity by acting on the immunoregulatory system. One of the best examples comes from studies with Epstein–Barr virus (EBV). *In vitro*, this agent infects and specifically transforms B lymphocytes into lymphoblastoid cell lines that proliferate indefinitely, secreting immunoglobulins of different specificities (polyclonal activation). Some of these antibodies react with antigens of normal cells of endocrine organs such as thyroid, pituitary and pancreatic islets. *In vivo*, EBV is thought similarly to induce lymphoproliferation and autoantibody production, but this phenomenon is usually transient because infected B lymphocytes are killed by cytotoxic T lymphocytes. Thus persistent autoantibody production might occur in individuals with immunoregulatory defects.

A second possibility is that of 'molecular mimicry'. Antibodies raised against certain viral antigens may cross-react with normal host cell antigens. Monoclonal antibodies to viruses are now beginning to substantiate this hypothesis. For instance, cross-reactivity has been observed between certain viral antigens and intermediate filaments, thymic epithelium, pituitary cells and islet cells. Hence infection of any organ with agents having structural similarities with islet cell constituents might trigger an autoimmune process leading to diabetes.

A third mechanism by which a virus could trigger an autoimmune response is by eliciting anti-idiotypic antibodies. Anti-idiotypic antibodies are viewed as regulatory immuno-globulins directed to the idiotype of a particular antibody. As a consequence, these molecules not only react with the variable site of the antiviral antibody, but are also structurally similar to the eliciting antigen. If this antigen is the viral structure which binds to the viral receptor on host cells, the anti-idiotypic antibody also recognizes the viral receptor and binds to the cell membrane. A few examples of this type have been found; it is an appealing mechanism since it would allow the production of potentially hazardous surface autoantibodies.

CONCLUSION
The studies on viral diabetes demonstrate that several different viruses can cause the disease or contribute to its pathogenesis. In humans, however, only a few cases of virus-induced diabetes have been described so far. The fact that autoimmune phenomena together with alterations of lymphocyte subsets precede the clinical onset of the disease by months or years suggests the possibility that a persistent infection with a slow virus may have occurred well before overt diabetes appeared. If this is the case, it is possible that newer virological techniques will allow the isolation of this unknown agent, which could then lead to a means of prevention. Conversely, it appears equally possible that most cases of Type I diabetes are derived primarily from 'spontaneous' autoimmunity and that viruses or other environmental factors act

(a) polyclonal activation of B lymphocytes

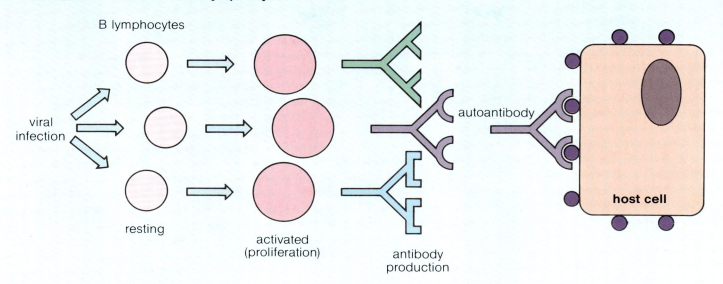

(b) molecular mimicry

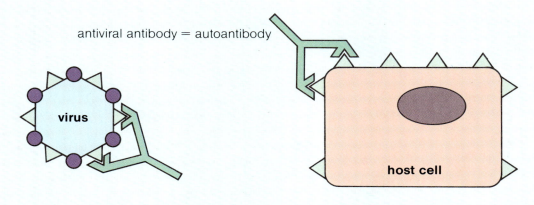

(c) anti-idiotypic antibodies elicited by viral infection

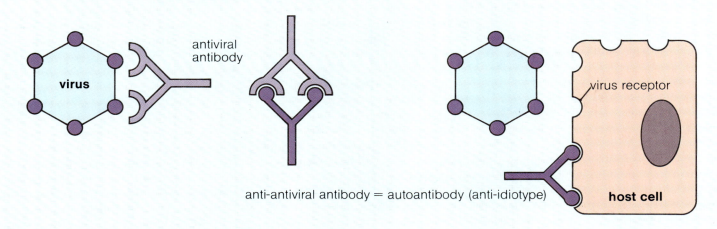

Fig. 10.20 Pathogenesis of virus-induced diabetes: (2). Models not requiring viral infection of islet B cells. These are hypothetical models derived from studies in viral immunology. (a) viral infection causes proliferation of B lymphocytes which secrete antibodies of different specificities. Some may be autoantibodies. (b) antibodies raised against viral antigens may cross-react with normal host antigens. (c) anti-idiotypes to the antiviral antibody may be able to bind to virus receptors on cell membranes. They would thus act as viral antigens and lead to possible immune attack.

merely as triggering agents. In this case, preventative measures would be much more difficult to find.

The solution of this pathogenic puzzle would be facilitated by achieving an understanding of the relationships between HLA type, autoimmunity and viral infections. Nevertheless, even if it is not known why people with certain genetic markers are prone to diabetes or to other autoimmune diseases, an understanding of several chronic idiopathic diseases has rapidly advanced recently.

Various forms of chronic hepatitis, subacute sclerosing panencephalitis, kuru, multiple sclerosis, the acquired immunodeficiency syndrome and some forms of neoplasia have been attributed to conventional or unconventional viruses. To make this issue even more complex, it is clear that some of these diseases represent unusual responses of the host to an infectious agent. If this is also true for diabetes, the identification of the putative aetiological agent, or agents, will require an enormous effort.

REFERENCES

Banatvala JE (1987) Insulin-dependent (juvenile onset, Type I) diabetes mellitus. Coxsackie B viruses revisited. *Progress in Medical Virology*, **34**, 33–54.

Barboni E & Manocchio I (1962) Alterazioni pancreatiche in bovini con diabete mellito post-aftoso. *Archivio Veterinario Italiano*, **13**, 477–489.

Bottazzo GF (1986) Death of a beta cell: homicide or suicide? *Diabetic Medicine*, **3**, 119–130.

Craighead JE (1975) The role of viruses in the pathogenesis of pancreatic disease and diabetes mellitus. *Progress in Medical Virology*, **19**, 161–214.

Craighead JE (1981) Viral diabetes mellitus in man and experimental animals. *American Journal of Medicine*, **70**, 127–135.

Gamble DR (1980) The epidemiology of insulin-dependent diabetes with particular reference to the relationship of virus infection to its etiology. *Epidemiological Reviews*, **2**, 49–70.

Jenson AB & Rosenberg HS (1984) Multiple viruses in diabetes mellitus. *Progress in Medical Virology*, **29**, 197–217.

Notkins AL (1977) Virus-induced diabetes mellitus. Brief review. *Archives of Virology*, **54**, 1–17.

Notkins AL (1979) The causes of diabetes. *Scientific American*, **241**, 62–73.

Notkins AL, Yoon JW, Onodera T, Toniolo A & Jenson AB (1981) Virus induced diabetes mellitus. *Perspectives in Virology*, **11**, 141–162.

Rayfield EJ & Seto Y (1981) Viruses. In *Handbook of Diabetes Mellitus. Volume 1*. Edited by Brownlee M. pp. 95–120. New York: Garland STPM Press.

Toniolo A & Onodera T (1984) Viruses and diabetes. In *Immunology in Diabetes*. Edited by Andreani D, Di Mario U, Federlin FK & Heding LG. pp. 71–93. London: Kimpton Medical Publications.

Type II Diabetes: Epidemiology

Peter H Bennett BSc MB ChB FRCP FFCM

Non insulin-dependent (Type II) diabetes is a clinical designation used to describe those types of diabetes in which spontaneous ketosis does not occur and which are neither malnutrition-related nor secondary to other well-defined causes. The extent to which Type II diabetes represents one or more metabolic disorders is uncertain, but it is a syndrome in which several different pathogenic mechanisms have been implicated. The same clinical syndrome may be associated with a variety of specific abnormalities of insulin or its receptors and also with certain genetic syndromes. At present, however, there is only limited knowledge of the pathogenesis of the more common forms of the disease.

Epidemiology is the study of the occurrence, distribution and determinants of diseases in populations. Knowledge gained through epidemiological studies is important in the identification of the causes of the disease and in describing its natural history and prognosis. Epidemiology also provides information on the scope and impact of the disease in the community and therefore has an important role in the formulation and implementation of strategies to prevent or reduce the impact of the disease. This chapter reviews current knowledge of the epidemiology of Type II diabetes and some of the salient features are shown in Fig. 11.1.

PREVALENCE

Type II constitutes the most frequent form of diabetes. Even in areas where Type I (insulin-dependent) diabetes is common, such as northern Europe, Type II diabetes accounts for at least eighty-five per cent of all patients with diabetes. In other populations, such as Asians, Indians, Japanese, Pacific Islanders (Micronesians, Melanesians and Polynesians) and native Americans (American Indians and Eskimos), Type I diabetes is less common, and Type II constitutes an even greater proportion of the total number of cases. The relative frequencies of Type I and Type II diabetes among black populations of African origin is less certain, but Type I diabetes is less frequent among them than among northern Europeans and hence Type II diabetes predominates. Consequently, in all population groups, Type II diabetes is the predominant form of the disease.

Type II diabetes is a relatively frequent chronic disease in much of the world. In countries such as China, it has been estimated that the prevalence is approximately one per cent of the total population. The prevalence of known diabetes in the U.K. probably lies between one and two per cent, although it is higher in the U.S.A. where it is approximately 3.4% among those aged 20–74 years (Fig. 11.2). In all populations, undiagnosed diabetes constitutes a significant fraction of the total with Type II diabetes. In most western countries, there is usually about one undiagnosed case for each known case. In the U.S.A., for example, it has been shown that 3.2% of those aged 20–74 years have undiagnosed diabetes. This fraction, however, may be very different in other countries or among subgroups of the population where access to health services is more limited. Knowledge of the prevalence of Type II diabetes based only on known cases of the disease is therefore of limited value. Systematic studies of the population are necessary if the true prevalence of the disease is to be

TYPE II (NON INSULIN-DEPENDENT) DIABETES

common chronic disease

most frequent type of diabetes
(especially in non-northern Europeans)

susceptibility genetically determined, but mode of inheritance uncertain

frequency varies in different ethnic groups living in same environment

frequency varies in same ethnic group living in different environments

results from genetic–environmental interaction

Fig. 11.1 Major epidemiological characteristics of Type II diabetes.

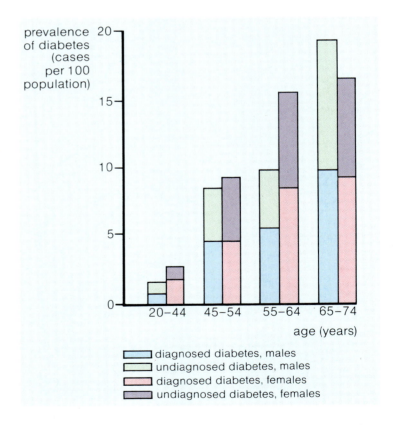

Fig. 11.2 Prevalence of diabetes in a U.S.A. population aged 20–74 years. The data from the U.S. National Health and Nutrition Examination Survey II show the prevalence in 1976–80 according to WHO criteria. The prevalence of Type II diabetes increases with advancing age, is relatively similar in males and females and shows that about equal proportions of previously diagnosed and newly diagnosed disease were found in each age and sex group. From Harris *et al.* (1986), by courtesy of the American Diabetes Association.

determined and require that the population, or a representative sample of those not already known to have diabetes, be tested using an oral glucose tolerance test (OGTT).

Effect of Environment and Ethnic Origin

There are large variations in the prevalence of Type II diabetes in different ethnic groups and in different countries (Fig. 11.3). Until recently the true magnitude of these differences was unclear as different criteria had been used in many of the studies. The adoption of the internationally agreed World Health Organization (WHO) criteria for diabetes in 1980 (revised in 1985, see *Chapter 6*) has led to a much greater standardization which greatly facilitates comparisons of the prevalence of the disease.

Even within countries, there may be large variations in the frequency of Type II diabetes among different ethnic groups (Fig. 11.4). There are also substantial differences in prevalence in populations of the same ethnic origin living in different countries. For example, expatriate Asian Indians in many parts of the world have much higher frequencies than their populations of origin in India (Fig. 11.5). Subgroups of the population of similar ethnic origin, even within the same country, may also show variations in frequency. These differences may relate to socioeconomic status, lifestyle or relative degree of obesity (Fig. 11.6).

In some countries, the frequency of Type II diabetes has increased during the last forty years, but the extent to which this represents a real increase is uncertain (Fig. 11.7). The apparent increase in the prevalence in some countries, such as the U.S.A., may be due to increased use of diagnostic screening during the past forty years. There is, however, evidence from population surveys in which most members of the community have been tested that some of this increase is indeed real. For example, before 1940, Type II diabetes was no more common in American Indian populations than in the general U.S.A. population, yet a clear-cut increase in the true prevalence of the disease in the Pima Indians, as well as much higher rates in other tribes than in the general population have been documented during the past twenty years by systematic epidemiological studies.

Some populations now have extraordinarily high frequencies of diabetes; for example, the Pima Indians and many other American Indian tribes living in the U.S.A., the Nauruans, inhabitants of a small island in the central Pacific (see Fig. 11.3) and retired Japanese Sumo wrestlers all have high prevalence rates. In these groups, the prevalence of Type II diabetes among those aged thirty-five years and over approaches fifty per cent. Increased prevalence rates have been found among groups who have moved from a traditional environment into a more

PREVALENCE OF TYPE II DIABETES IN VARIOUS POPULATIONS

country	ethnic group	age (years)	prevalence (%)
Australia	Caucasian	25+	3.4
U.S.A.	general population	20–74	6.8
	Caucasian	20–74	6.4
	Negroid	20–74	9.9
	Mexican American	25–64	10.6
	Pima Indians	20+	34.1
Nauru	Micronesian	20+	30.3
Fiji	Melanesian	20+	6.9
	Indian	20+	14.8
Western Samoa	Polynesian	20+	4.9
Papua New Guinea	Melanesian	20+	0.0

Fig. 11.3 Prevalence of Type II diabetes in various populations. The results of systematic population surveys that have used the same standardized methods (and criteria) to determine the prevalence of Type II diabetes are shown for individuals aged twenty years and over. The prevalence varies considerably, with that in Australians being only one-tenth that of the Pima Indians or Nauruans; among 308 Melanesians in the highlands of Papua New Guinea, none were found with diabetes. All prevalence results correspond to a two-hour plasma glucose level greater than or equal to 11.1 mmol/l (200 mg/dl) after a 75g glucose load (i.e. 1985 WHO criteria).

EFFECT OF ETHNIC ORIGIN ON PREVALENCE OF TYPE II DIABETES

country	age (years)	ethnic group	subjects tested (n)	prevalence (%)
Singapore	15+	Indians	1169	6.1
		Malaysians	2268	2.4
		Chinese	12,812	1.6
Fiji (Suva)	20+	Indians	836	14.1
		Melanesians	853	6.6

Fig. 11.4 Prevalence of Type II diabetes in different ethnic groups living in a similar environment. These two studies illustrate large differences in prevalence in communities where groups of different ethnic origin live in the same geographical environment. While differences in socioeconomic status and lifestyle may contribute to some of these differences, it appears that the inherent (genetic) susceptibility to Type II diabetes differs considerably among different ethnic groups. The criteria for the prevalence of diabetes differed between the two areas.

DIABETES PREVALENCE IN ASIAN INDIANS

region	age (years)	prevalence (%)
Indian sub-continent:		
rural	≥15	1.3
urban	≥15	3.0
expatriate Indians:		
Singapore	≥15	6.1
Malaysia	≥30	4.2
South Africa	≥20	5.0
South Africa	≥10	6.0 (11.1)*
South Africa	≥15	4.0 (10.4)*
Trinidad	≥20	4.5
Fiji	≥20	14.1
*age adjusted to the European or U.S.A. population		

Fig. 11.5 Prevalence of diabetes in Asian Indians. The prevalence is higher in expatriate Asian Indians than it is in India. Some of the differences in rates may be attributable to differences in diagnostic techniques used in different studies, but the rates in the expatriates are uniformly higher. When rates are adjusted to the age distribution of populations in Europe or the U.S.A., rates become much higher than that seen in Caucasians. This is the result of the relatively younger age distribution of the Indian population in many parts of the world.

EFFECT OF ENVIRONMENT ON PREVALENCE OF TYPE II DIABETES

ethnic group	age (years)	region	prevalence (%)
Japanese	40+	Hiroshima (urban)	6.9
		Hawaii (semi-rural)	12.3
Wallis islanders (Polynesian)	20+	traditional island (rural)	2.4
		Noumea (urban)	14.0
Western Samoans (Polynesian)	20+	Savaii (rural)	2.7
		Apia (urban)	7.0
Kiribatians (Micro-nesian)	20+	Tabiteuea (rural)	3.4
		Betio (urban)	9.7

Fig. 11.6 Prevalence of Type II diabetes in subjects of the same ethnic origin living in different environments. The prevalence of Type II diabetes in many populations is greater in individuals of the same ethnic origin living in an urban than in a rural environment. This difference may be related to changes in socioeconomic status, differences in lifestyle, nutritional habits and physical activity that occur either with migration to an urban area (e.g. Wallis Islanders) or with exposure to a more western environment when compared with others of similar origin who reside in a rural environment (e.g. Samoans and Kiribatians). This view is strengthened by the Japanese study, where despite migration to a more rural environment (Hawaii), the prevalence of diabetes is greater in the more westernized location. These differences provide evidence that environmental factors play a major role in determining the frequency of Type II diabetes in populations with the same genetic background. 1985 WHO criteria for diabetes were used in these studies except for the Japanese one where the criterion for diabetes was a two-hour plasma glucose level $\geq$ 11.1mmol/l (200mg/dl) after a 50g glucose load.

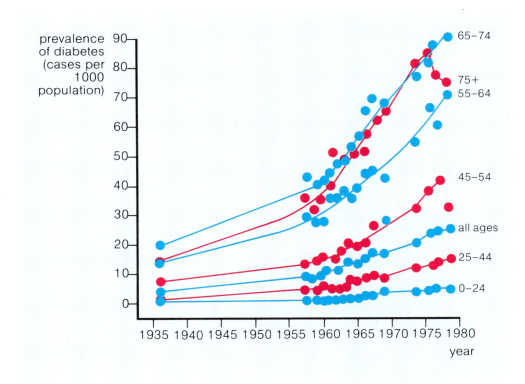

Fig. 11.7 Trends in the prevalence of known diabetes in the U.S.A., 1935–78. The prevalence of diagnosed diabetes determined in the U.S. National Health Interview Surveys has increased considerably in the past forty years. Some of this increase is the result of increased diagnostic screening, especially in the 1960's, but the continued rise, particularly in those aged forty-five years and over, suggests that the more recent increases represent a true increase in the prevalence of Type II diabetes. From NIH Publication No. 85–1468 (1985), by courtesy of the U.S. Department of Health and Human Sciences.

westernized one; for example, Polynesians who have migrated from Pacific islands to New Zealand and New Caledonia, and Japanese who migrated to Hawaii (see Fig. 11.6). These observations indicate the importance of environmental factors in the aetiology of Type II diabetes.

Effect of Age and Sex

Both sexes are affected, but in some communities the disease shows a male preponderance, for example, in India and in Asian Indians in the U.K., whereas in others the majority with the disease are female. The prevalence of Type II diabetes rises with increasing age (see Fig. 11.2) and in many populations the majority of those with diabetes are either middle-aged or elderly. Like Type I diabetes, however, Type II may occur at any age. The incidence (rate of development of new cases) also rises with increasing age in Caucasian populations (Fig. 11.8), but in at least one population, the Pima Indians, the incidence falls after fifty-five years of age, suggesting that the majority of susceptible individuals develop the disease at an earlier age. In populations where Type II diabetes is very frequent, it is not uncommonly encountered in adolescence and among young adults. This form of diabetes, which has a familial distribution compatible with a dominant mode of inheritance, is sometimes referred to as 'maturity onset diabetes of the young' (MODY). Whether or not the pathogenesis of this form differs from that occurring in older people is unknown.

Conclusion

Taken as a whole, this complex pattern of the distribution of Type II diabetes is best explained on the basis that the disease is the result of interaction between environmental influences and genetic susceptibility. Although specific genetic determinants of Type II diabetes have not yet been identified, the very high frequencies among some ethnic groups compared to others living in a similar environment strongly suggest that genetic factors determine the susceptibility to the disease. The inheritance of susceptibility is also suggested by the extent of familial aggregation and by higher concordance for the disease among pairs of identical twins than among non-identical twins.

Evidence that environmental factors are extremely important in the manifestation of the disease is evident from the facts that, at least in some populations, the frequency has increased over a very short time period and that some migrant populations show much higher frequencies of Type II diabetes than those who have remained in a more traditional environment. The specific environmental factors which lead to the expression of the disease, however, are only partially understood.

PUBLIC HEALTH IMPORTANCE OF TYPE II DIABETES

The major public health importance of Type II diabetes (Fig. 11.9) is that it is a chronic disorder which is associated with the development of specific microvascular complications, such as retinopathy, nephropathy and neuropathy, as well as higher frequencies of macrovascular disease, including coronary heart disease, peripheral vascular disease and cerebrovascular disease. These complications give rise to morbidity to a much greater degree than found in persons of similar age and sex without the

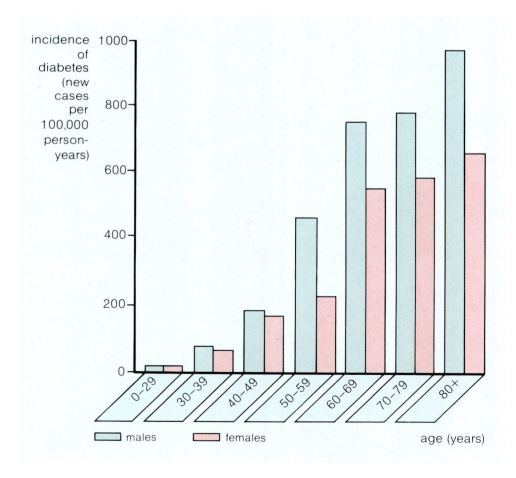

Fig. 11.8 Incidence of Type II diabetes in Minnesota, U.S.A., 1960–69. The proportion of the population developing the condition rises considerably with increasing age, so that the elderly have the highest risk of developing the disease. This example is probably representative of Caucasian populations, but is not seen in all groups. From Palumbo *et al.* (1976), by courtesy of the American Diabetes Association.

disease. Excessive mortality rates are also found. Age-specific mortality rates among those with Type II diabetes are about twice as high as in non-diabetic subjects.

The occurrence of the vascular complications leads to increased loss of work and disability, as well as increased health care costs. In the U.S.A. in 1984, for example, it was estimated that the economic impact of diabetes was at least $14 billion per year and that the per capita cost of health care of diabetic patients was two to three times that of non-diabetic subjects. Diabetes is among the ten leading causes of death in Europe and the U.S.A. despite the fact that the impact of diabetes is underestimated from analysis of death certificates. This is because of the coding rules that result in diabetes only infrequently being designated as the underlying cause when death occurs as a result of its complications.

NATURAL HISTORY

The development of Type II diabetes can be divided into four stages: (i) genetic susceptibility; (ii) insulin resistance; (iii) impaired glucose tolerance; and (iv) diabetes.

Genetic Susceptibility

Type II diabetes shows considerable familial aggregation which may result from either the inheritance of disease susceptibility or the sharing of a common environment by members of the same family. As there is considerable evidence of environmental determinants in Type II diabetes and as there is no method for recognizing the specific gene or genes predisposing to this condition at present, evidence for the occurrence of genetic susceptibility is somewhat indirect. There are, however, several lines of evidence that strongly support the concept of inherited susceptibility to Type II diabetes.

Evidence from twin studies, reviewed in *Chapter 12*, indicates that the degree of concordance for diabetes of monozygotic (identical) twins is high and much greater than in dizygotic twins. While all twin studies point to a greater degree of concordance in monozygotic twins, the degree of concordance varies from approximately fifty per cent to over ninety per cent depending upon the age at which the twins were studied and the ways in which the affected twins were identified or ascertained. Ascertainment because one or other of the twins had diabetes is almost certain to lead to an overestimate of the degree of concordance, as the likelihood of recognizing a pair in which both twins are affected is greater than when only one is afflicted. Two other lines of evidence, however, also provide evidence for a genetic component.

In populations where there is genetic admixture, the frequency of Type II diabetes in those of mixed blood is intermediate between that of the parent populations. Evidence that such genetic admixture plays an important role has been obtained in several closed communities with a high prevalence of diabetes, such as among the Nauruans, inhabitants of a small central Pacific island, and among several tribal groups of American Indians (Fig. 11.10). In these communities, the rates of diabetes correlate strongly with the degree of admixture. Assuming that all individuals in these populations are exposed to a similar environment, the only explanation for these differences is that they have inherited different degrees of genetic susceptibility to Type II diabetes. These data also complement the inferences

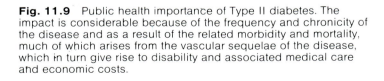

PUBLIC HEALTH IMPORTANCE OF TYPE II DIABETES

common chronic disease

associated vascular complications lead to increased morbidity and mortality

common cause of:
  blindness
  amputation
  renal failure

excessive frequencies of coronary heart disease, stroke and peripheral vascular disease

among the top ten causes of mortality in most countries, yet impact underestimated from death certificates

age-sex specific mortality approximately twice that of non-diabetic subjects

leads to:
  reduced life expectancy
  excess medical care expenditure
  disability and economic burden for society

Fig. 11.9 Public health importance of Type II diabetes. The impact is considerable because of the frequency and chronicity of the disease and as a result of the related morbidity and mortality, much of which arises from the vascular sequelae of the disease, which in turn give rise to disability and associated medical care and economic costs.

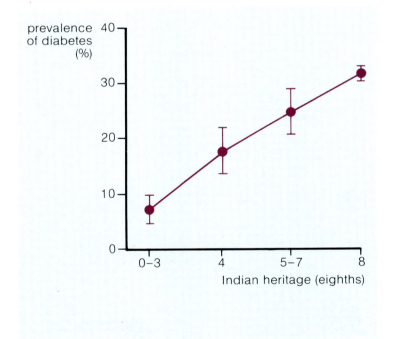

Fig. 11.10 Age-sex adjusted prevalence of Type II diabetes according to the degree of genetic admixture among the Pima Indian population. The proportion of the population with Type II diabetes is directly related to the extent of genetic admixture. In full-blood (8/8) Pima Indians, the prevalence is over 30%, whereas among those of less than half-Pima heritage (0–3/8), living on the same Indian reservation, the prevalence of Type II diabetes is less than 10% (mean ± 95% confidence intervals).

made from studies of different racial groups living in the same community where, as shown earlier, large differences in the prevalence of diabetes may be found.

For MODY, there is a pattern consistent with inheritance as a dominant trait. Pedigrees of such families, in which the disease occurs in three generations, show that about half of the offspring of an affected parent have diabetes. This pattern is compatible with a dominant mode of inheritance. In addition, in some populations where the disease is common, mathematical (segregation) analyses of pedigrees also indicate, as the most plausible explanation for the distribution of the disease within families, a pattern of inheritance most compatible with that of a single major gene expressed in a dominant manner (Fig. 11.11).

Until specific evidence for a diabetes susceptibility gene, or genes, can be found, it cannot be determined whether a specific individual without the disease is likely to carry the gene, unless they happen to be the identical co-twin of a diabetic subject.

Thrifty gene hypothesis
While the specific mode of the inheritance of Type II diabetes is presently unknown, there has been speculation about the nature of the diabetes genotype. Such hypotheses may help to explain why diabetes is so common and why the frequency of Type II diabetes among populations with the same genetic background living in different environments may vary.

It has been postulated that the diabetes gene may confer a selective advantage in some circumstances. In populations who now have very high frequencies of diabetes, such as the Pima Indians, in whom there is strong evidence that the frequency of the disease has increased recently, many individuals must carry the genetic susceptibility to diabetes. If diabetes had been as frequent in the past as it is now, there would almost certainly have been negative selection for the gene and, over the course of many generations, its frequency would have diminished. It is therefore necessary to postulate that the gene must have had a positive selective value in the past and that those who carried it were those who were most likely to survive and procreate. The gene may either allow for or promote the storage of excessive calories when food is abundant so that when food supplies were erratic, as they often were, those with this characteristic would have been the best prepared to survive a famine and procreate. If so, the gene would gradually increase in frequency when there were alternating periods of feast and famine as there have been in many populations throughout human history.

In more recent times, however, food shortages have been largely eliminated and at the same time the caloric requirements for day-to-day living and, in particular the gathering of food, have become vastly reduced. Carriage of the gene could then lead to deleterious effects in terms of excessive degrees of obesity and the appearance of high frequencies of Type II diabetes with all of its associated complications. This hypothesis, the 'thrifty gene hypothesis', could account for the extraordinary frequencies of

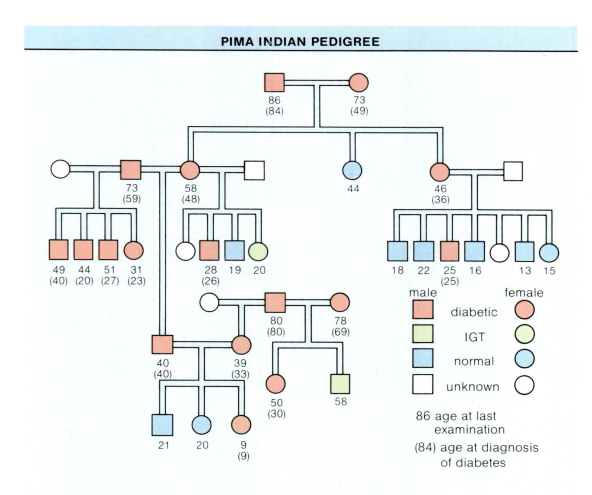

PIMA INDIAN PEDIGREE

Fig. 11.11 Pedigree of a Pima Indian kindred showing the presence of Type II diabetes in four generations. The diagnoses were made according to WHO criteria. While this pedigree is compatible with the inheritance of the disease as a dominant trait, caution must be exercised because of the high frequency of the disease in this population and because many of the unaffected members are young and may develop the disease as they become older. From Köbberling & Tattersall (1982), by courtesy of Academic Press.

diabetes now seen in some populations, such as the Pima Indians and the Nauruans, and explain why migrants to affluent parts of the world, from such countries as India, have much higher frequencies of diabetes than the indigenous populations.

Insulin Resistance

There is an increasing body of evidence which suggests that insulin resistance, or reduced insulin-mediated glucose uptake, is characteristic of those either developing or susceptible to Type II diabetes. The epidemiological evidence for this relationship is twofold: first, among individuals with normal glucose tolerance, those with relatively higher insulin levels are more likely to develop diabetes (Fig. 11.12); secondly, among populations with a high risk of developing diabetes, insulin levels in individuals with normal glucose tolerance are higher than in those of similar age, sex and degree of obesity from populations with lower frequencies of Type II diabetes (Fig. 11.13).

Higher insulin levels in the presence of normal glucose tolerance imply the presence of abnormal insulin action, that is, insulin resistance. Insulin resistance may be due to several factors. In a few families, high insulin levels have been shown to be due to the presence of structurally abnormal insulins caused by genetic mutations. While study of these families is important to attempt to understand further the mechanisms of insulin action, they are extremely rare. Insulin gene mutations cannot account for the hyperinsulinaemia found in most populations with a high frequency of diabetes.

Hyperinsulinaemia also occurs when insulin binding is abnormal. This can result from the presence of anti-insulin receptor antibodies, which block the binding sites for insulin. In a few rare syndromes of insulin resistance there is an abnormality of receptor number or affinity that results in impaired insulin action and compensatory hyperinsulinaemia. These abnormalities are very rare and do not account for the great majority of cases of Type II diabetes. The insulin resistance seen prior to development of Type II diabetes in the majority of cases probably results from a post-binding intracellular defect in insulin action, the nature of which has yet to be elucidated.

Impaired Glucose Tolerance

Impaired glucose tolerance (IGT) is a category designated by the WHO classification of diabetes to describe individuals who lie between the categories of 'diabetic' and 'normal'. They show evidence of impairment of glucose utilization as manifested by abnormalities of post-load glucose levels in the presence of fasting glucose levels which are not abnormally high. According to the WHO (1985) criteria, individuals with venous plasma levels from 7.8mmol/l to less than 11.1mmol/l (140–199mg/dl), two hours after a 75g oral glucose load, and with a fasting venous plasma glucose level of less than 7.8mmol/l (140mg/dl) fall into this group (see also *Chapter 6*).

The main interest from an epidemiological and clinical viewpoint is that individuals with IGT have a high risk of

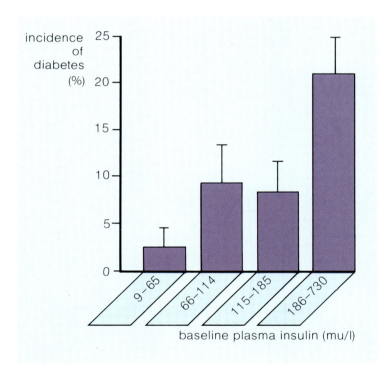

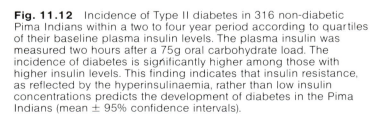

Fig. 11.12 Incidence of Type II diabetes in 316 non-diabetic Pima Indians within a two to four year period according to quartiles of their baseline plasma insulin levels. The plasma insulin was measured two hours after a 75g oral carbohydrate load. The incidence of diabetes is significantly higher among those with higher insulin levels. This finding indicates that insulin resistance, as reflected by the hyperinsulinaemia, rather than low insulin concentrations predicts the development of diabetes in the Pima Indians (mean ± 95% confidence intervals).

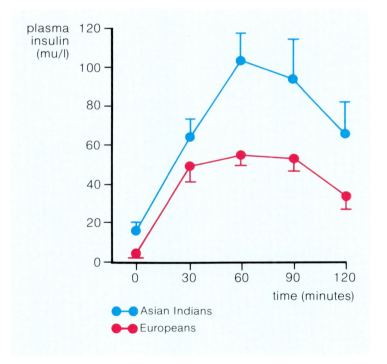

Fig. 11.13 Plasma insulin concentrations during a 75g OGTT in non-diabetic Asian Indians and Europeans of similar age, sex, obesity and glucose tolerance. The Indians, who have a higher prevalence of Type II diabetes, show significantly higher concentrations of insulin, both fasting and throughout the test, compared to the Europeans. Similar findings, first reported among the Pima Indians, have also been made among Mexican Americans and Australian Aborigines. In each of these populations, the likelihood of developing the condition is greater than among Europeans (mean ± 2 SEM). From Mohan *et al.* (1986), by courtesy of Springer Verlag.

11.7

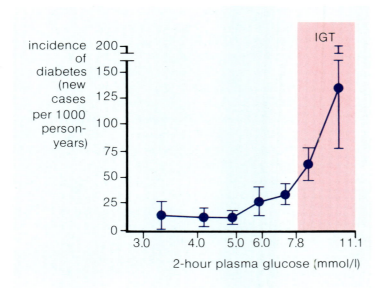

developing Type II diabetes in the future (Fig. 11.14). IGT, however, is a stage at which progression to diabetes is not inevitable and indeed an appreciable proportion of those with IGT will subsequently return to normal glucose tolerance, while others will remain impaired for many years. IGT therefore represents a stage at which progression to diabetes is not inevitable and theoretically is a point where it appears possible to reverse its development.

The frequency of IGT varies considerably from population to population. In general, those with IGT are more obese than those with normal glucose tolerance and IGT is associated with high fasting and post-glucose load insulin levels (Fig. 11.15).

Subjects with IGT have lower rates of insulin-mediated glucose disposal than subjects with normal glucose tolerance. As a group, their degree of insulin resistance is intermediate between those with normal glucose tolerance and those with Type II diabetes (Fig. 11.16). Recent evidence also indicates that those with IGT

Fig. 11.14 Incidence of Type II diabetes in Pima Indians according to baseline plasma glucose levels measured two hours after a 75g oral carbohydrate load. The risk of developing diabetes (by WHO criteria) is appreciably higher among those with IGT (2 hour plasma glucose levels 140–199mg/dl or 7.8–<11.1mmol/l) than in those without IGT. Similar results were found in the Bedford and Whitehall, U.K., studies, and the Nauruans. These studies indicate that 20–30% of subjects with IGT will develop Type II diabetes within five years, whereas up to one-half will return to normal glucose tolerance (mean ± 95% confidence intervals; 1mmol/l ≡ 18mg/dl). From Bennett *et al.* (1982), by courtesy of Elsevier Science Publishers B.V.

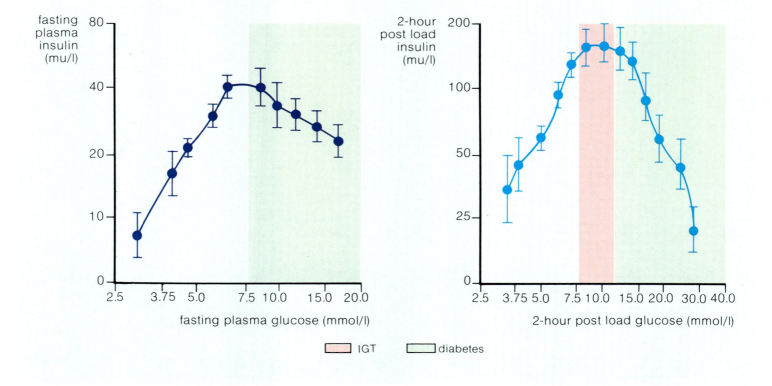

Fig. 11.15 Fasting and two-hour post-glucose plasma insulin concentrations in Pima Indians and the corresponding plasma glucose levels. Fasting insulin levels increase with glucose up to the level at which glucose levels are diagnostic of diabetes. The two-hour post-glucose insulin levels in relation to the corresponding glucose levels form an inverted U, with the highest insulin levels occurring in individuals with IGT. With Type II diabetes, mean fasting insulin levels remain high regardless of the degree of hyperglycaemia. Conversely, the post-load levels fall and the insulin increment (2-hours post-load, minus fasting) decreases with increasing degrees of hyperglycaemia (mean ± 95% confidence intervals). From Bennett *et al.* (1982), by courtesy of Elsevier Science Publishers B.V.

often also have increased systolic and diastolic blood pressures, higher very low density lipoprotein (VLDL) levels and lower high density lipoprotein (HDL) cholesterol levels than those with normal glucose tolerance, as well as hyperinsulinaemia. There is also an association between IGT and the presence of central obesity, as measured by having either greater waist-to-hip or waist-to-thigh measurements or larger central skinfold measurements, such as the subscapular skinfold thickness.

Type II (Non Insulin-dependent) Diabetes

Type II diabetes is present when the WHO criteria for its diagnosis are met (see *Chapter 6*). Subjects with Type II diabetes also have very low rates of insulin-mediated glucose disposal, but variable plasma insulin levels. The fasting insulin levels are often quite high, but these may fall with increasing duration of the disease. Insulin responses following a glucose load, however, are much lower than in subjects with IGT which, while very variable,

may be as high or higher than in individuals with normal glucose tolerance. Despite reduced insulin responses, spontaneous ketosis does not occur as basal insulin levels remain sufficient to prevent uncontrolled ketogenesis.

DETERMINANTS AND RISK FACTORS
Genetics

Evidence that there are genetic determinants for Type II diabetes has been reviewed earlier. Despite many studies, however, the mode of its inheritance has remained elusive. There are a number of reasons for this. In most populations, the age of onset is in the later adult years making it difficult to find pedigrees where two or three generations are affected. Furthermore, there is always uncertainty over whether the younger members of such families, who have not yet developed the disease, will do so in later life. As the disease may remain asymptomatic for many years, it is necessary to test members of the pedigree not already known to have diabetes, to determine whether or not they are affected. In addition, there is doubt about the extent to which Type II diabetes in its more common forms represents a single disease, or whether there might be several common types of the disease, possibly with different modes of inheritance.

Recently, detailed genetic studies of some of the populations who show an unusual frequency of Type II diabetes, such as the Nauruans and Pima Indians of Arizona where the onset of the disease is frequently at an early age, appear to show a dominant mode of inheritance most compatible with the inheritance of a single major gene. Whether or not a single dominant gene is responsible for the susceptibility to the disease in populations where the age of onset is much older remains to be determined.

If indeed Type II diabetes is the result of a single major gene, it should now be possible to identify the chromosomal location of such a gene, in pedigrees in which there is more than one generation affected, by use of DNA probes for restriction fragment length polymorphisms (RFLP). RFLP's that are on the same chromosome and close to the diabetes gene should be inherited in a pattern concordant with that of the disease itself. If this is true, it should be possible within pedigrees to identify subjects who carry the disease susceptibility gene and, ultimately, to identify the specific gene or genes responsible for the disease.

Whatever the reason, Type II diabetes shows a strong degree of familial aggregation. The presence of a family history in parents or siblings is a risk factor for the disease and is a factor which enhances the prediction of the development of the disease over and above that which can be inferred from the degree of glucose intolerance or the degree of obesity (see below).

Obesity

The relationship between Type II diabetes and obesity is relatively complicated and somewhat controversial. In part, the controversy has arisen from the difficulty of interpreting data on obesity gathered when the patient was already known to be diabetic. As mentioned earlier, Type II diabetes is often asymptomatic and the likelihood of diagnosis increases with the appearance of symptoms. However, by the time symptoms have appeared, the patients have often experienced some degree of weight loss making measured weights unreliable as an estimate of the weight at the time the disease actually appeared, or prior to it.

Nevertheless, the majority of comparisons of newly diagnosed Type II diabetic patients indicate an excessive degree of obesity compared with control subjects of similar age and sex. Studies of the incidence of diabetes uniformly indicate that obesity increases

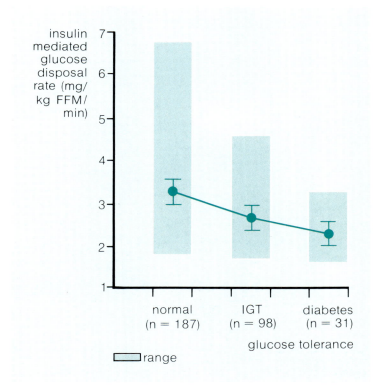

Fig. 11.16 Insulin-mediated glucose disposal rates (M) measured using the euglycaemic clamp technique in Pima Indians with normal, impaired and diabetic glucose tolerance. The results show that insulin resistance (low M values) is characteristic of those with Type II diabetes. Those with IGT also have low M values compared to those with normal glucose tolerance. Prospective studies carried out among normal subjects have shown that low M values predict the development of IGT and progression of IGT to Type II diabetes (mean ± 95% confidence intervals). FFM = free fat mass.

the risk of developing the disease (Fig. 11.17). Thus there is no doubt that obesity is a risk factor for the disease, especially when there is a positive family history. Obesity aggravates insulin resistance and is therefore likely to precipitate diabetes in those otherwise predisposed.

Type II diabetes, however, does occur in individuals who are not obese by conventional criteria and many such patients have a family history of diabetes. It has been postulated therefore that diabetes not associated with obesity may have a different aetiology and pathogenesis from the more typical form that is obesity-related. The relative frequency of obesity in patients with Type II diabetes varies markedly from population to population, such that about half of new cases in Caucasians in the U.K. occur among those who are not obese.

Whether the pathogenesis of the non-obese and obese forms of Type II diabetes is different, however, is unknown. While it is generally believed that insulin resistance plays an important role in the pathogenesis of the obese type, it has been postulated that the non-obese type may result more frequently from a defect in pancreatic B cell function and may thus perhaps be primarily the consequence of insulin deficiency rather than of insulin resistance. The interpretation of the available data, however, is complicated by the fact that hyperglycaemia itself may result in either the worsening or development of insulin resistance and lead to desensitization of the normal B cell responsiveness to a glucose challenge.

On the basis of the available evidence, it is impossible to determine whether the non-obese type and the obese type of Type II diabetes share a common aetiology and pathogenesis. Unless similar or different specific genetic mechanisms for these two sub-types are identified, it seems likely that only long-term prospective studies of the development of Type II diabetes among both obese and non-obese individuals, with measurement of insulin resistance and islet cell function at various stages during the development of the disease, will resolve this issue. Such a prospective study among obese Pima Indians who have a family history of diabetes is being carried out. In this study, the results indicate that those who develop diabetes have a greater degree of insulin resistance than those who do not. Conversely, no evidence of a deficiency in

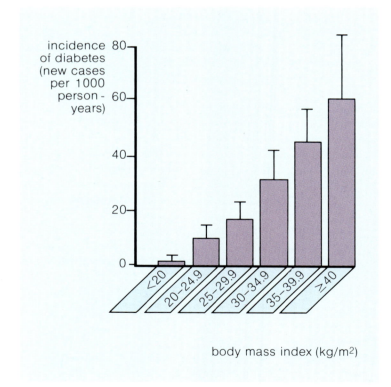

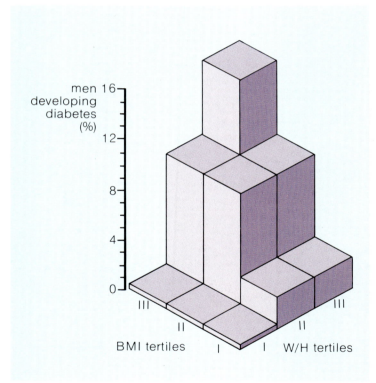

Fig. 11.17 Incidence of Type II diabetes according to body mass index among Pima Indians. The development of diabetes is directly related to the degree of obesity, as measured by the body mass index. Studies of the prevalence of Type II diabetes and obesity do not always show a clear-cut relationship, presumably because the presence of diabetes may lead to weight loss. Studies in the Pima Indians and in a population from Israel both indicate that the duration of obesity is a further factor in predicting the development of Type II diabetes (mean ± 95% confidence intervals). From Knowler *et al.* (1981), by courtesy of the *American Journal of Epidemiology*.

Fig. 11.18 Percentage of Swedish men, initially aged fifty-four years, who developed Type II diabetes over the subsequent 13.5 years according to tertiles of body mass index (BMI) and waist/hip (W/H) circumference. The measurement of W/H circumference adds appreciably to the prediction for the development of diabetes from that obtained from the measurement of BMI alone. The ability to predict the development of diabetes is greatest in men whose BMI is in the upper one-third of the distribution for the population. From Ohlson *et al.* (1985), by courtesy of the American Diabetes Association.

islet cell function has been demonstrated prior to the development of IGT suggesting the primacy of a defect in insulin-mediated glucose disposal in the pathogenesis of this type of diabetes.

While most studies relating obesity to Type II diabetes have relied on measures of height and weight to estimate obesity, there is now convincing evidence that the form of obesity plays a major role in determining the risk of development of diabetes. The distribution of fat among those with Type II diabetes more frequently has a central, truncal pattern than in individuals without diabetes. This pattern of obesity is reflected in greater waist-to-hip or waist-to-thigh ratios and in greater subscapular or abdominal skinfolds than in non-diabetic subjects of similar height and weight. The importance of central obesity as a risk factor for Type II diabetes has been convincingly demonstrated among a cohort of Swedish men in whom the risk of developing this condition varies directly with the waist-to-hip ratios within strata of body mass index (Fig. 11.18).

A family history of diabetes, the degree of obesity (especially of the central type), the existing degree of glucose intolerance and age are all risk factors for the development of Type II diabetes. Furthermore, the more of these factors that are present in a given individual, the greater the risk (Fig. 11.19). Recognition of the presence of these factors facilitates the assessment of the likelihood that a patient currently has or will develop Type II diabetes.

Physical Activity
It has long been believed that physical inactivity has a role in the development of Type II diabetes; historically it has been associated with sloth and indolence. In some countries, those with sedentary occupations have been reported to have higher frequencies of diabetes than manual workers. Only recently, however, has more direct evidence concerning the role of physical activity been forthcoming. Fig. 11.20 shows the frequency of diabetes among women who were active in college athletics compared to those who were not. Women who had been active during their college years as a group tended to maintain such activity in later years compared to those who were less active;

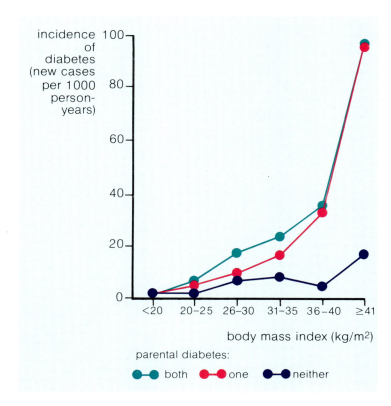

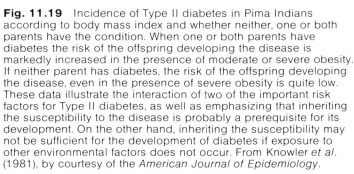

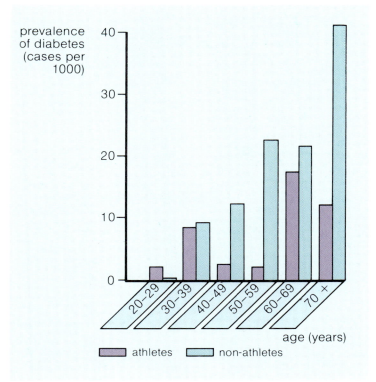

Fig. 11.19 Incidence of Type II diabetes in Pima Indians according to body mass index and whether neither, one or both parents have the condition. When one or both parents have diabetes the risk of the offspring developing the disease is markedly increased in the presence of moderate or severe obesity. If neither parent has diabetes, the risk of the offspring developing the disease, even in the presence of severe obesity is quite low. These data illustrate the interaction of two of the important risk factors for Type II diabetes, as well as emphasizing that inheriting the susceptibility to the disease is probably a prerequisite for its development. On the other hand, inheriting the susceptibility may not be sufficient for the development of diabetes if exposure to other environmental factors does not occur. From Knowler et al. (1981), by courtesy of the American Journal of Epidemiology.

Fig. 11.20 Prevalence of Type II diabetes in women who either had or had not participated in athletics in college. The prevalence of diabetes is lower in those who had been active in athletics and who in general had remained more active in later years. Overall, the frequency of Type II diabetes is more than twice as high in the non-athletes than in the athletes. From Frisch et al. (1986), by courtesy of the American Diabetes Association.

among the latter, the prevalence of self-reported diabetes was significantly higher. These data, although of an observational nature, lend support to the hypothesis that physical activity may help to prevent the development of Type II diabetes.

Nutrition

As with physical inactivity, there is a strong belief that Type II diabetes is related to overeating. Through the years a number of specific dietary components have been implicated in the development of the condition. For example, fat consumption on a national basis appears to be related to mortality from diabetes and similarly there is a correlation between national sugar consumption and mortality attributed to diabetes. However, the intake of each

of these foodstuffs is highly correlated with the other. High calorie diets almost always contain a relatively high proportion of fat and a high proportion of sugar and, inversely, a lower proportion of dietary fibre.

No studies to date have provided convincing evidence that any specific nutrients lead to increased risk of developing non insulin-dependent diabetes. However, decreases in diabetes-related mortality were demonstrated in a number of countries during and after World Wars I and II (Fig. 11.21). Countries which experienced extreme food deprivation or were subject to strict food rationing showed decreased diabetes-related mortality, which persisted for some time after the wars.

While these data cannot be used to implicate specific types of

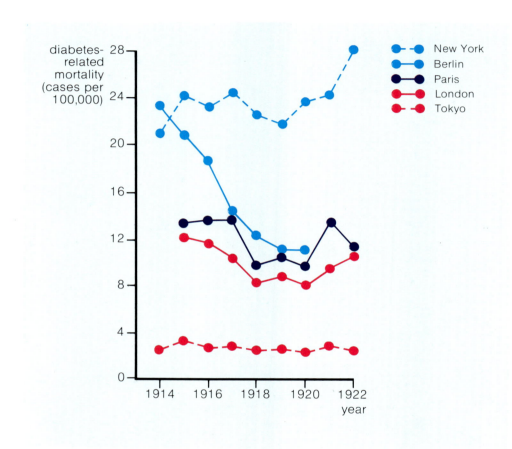

Fig. 11.21 Mortality attributed to diabetes in several cities during World War I. Cities which experienced food shortages and rationing, such as Berlin, Paris and London, showed marked falls in diabetes-related mortality, whereas those where the food supply was not affected, such as New York and Tokyo, showed no consistent changes. Similar trends were seen in World War II. From West (1978), by courtesy of Elsevier North-Holland Inc.

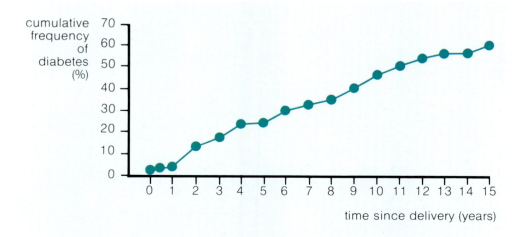

Fig. 11.22 Development of diabetes in women who had experienced gestational diabetes (O'Sullivan criteria). Women who have gestational diabetes have a high risk of developing Type II diabetes in subsequent years, despite the fact that glucose tolerance almost always returns to normal shortly after delivery. From O'Sullivan (1975), by courtesy of Academic Press.

food as being aetiologically related to the development of diabetes, they do suggest that calorific restriction, either on a national or individual basis, may partly prevent Type II diabetes. It seems reasonable to conclude that moderate calorie restriction, which would result in a lower prevalence of obesity in most western countries, can either reduce the incidence of Type II diabetes or prolong the longevity of those who already have the disease.

Pregnancy and Gestational Diabetes

Several investigations have suggested that parity is related to the risk of developing Type II diabetes. These studies, however, also show that parity is related to obesity and that, when the frequency of diabetes according to completed family size in women aged forty-five years and over is examined according to the degree of obesity, no excessive frequency of diabetes is seen in multiparous women. It now seems unlikely that the number of pregnancies is related to the prevalence of Type II diabetes despite the fact that pregnancy is often associated with some deterioration in glucose tolerance in the third trimester and, in some women, the appearance of gestational diabetes.

The occurrence of gestational diabetes, that is, diabetes which either first appears or is first recognized during pregnancy and which often resolves in the immediate post-partum period, is associated with increased risk for the development of diabetes in

subsequent years (Fig. 11.22). Thus, women who experience gestational diabetes should be considered a high risk group for the development of Type II diabetes.

Recently, an intriguing relationship has been found between pregnancy and diabetes in Pima Indians. It has been shown that the risk of development of Type II diabetes in the offspring of women who were diabetic at the time of pregnancy is much greater than in the offspring of women who were not diabetic during pregnancy, but who subsequently developed the disease (Fig. 11.23). If it is assumed that women who were diabetic during pregnancy and those who subsequently developed the disease both carry the genetic susceptibility to diabetes and pass this to their offspring to a similar extent, these data implicate the abnormal intra-uterine environment of the diabetic pregnancy as playing an important role in precipitating Type II diabetes in the offspring. Such offspring also develop obesity more frequently, which presumably plays a role in precipitating their diabetes.

The effect of the diabetic pregnancy on the expression of diabetes in the offspring further emphasizes the crucial role of environmental factors in the manifestation of Type II diabetes in those genetically predisposed to the disease.

MORTALITY AND LIFE EXPECTANCY

Many studies of mortality in diabetes have made no distinction between the major forms of the disease. Some have classified patients according to the age of onset of the disease assuming that the majority of those with an onset beyond thirty or forty years of age had Type II diabetes. A further problem in assessing the impact of Type II diabetes on mortality has been the notorious lack of reliability and validity of death certificate information. Death certificates in those with this condition frequently do not mention diabetes, either as the underlying or contributory cause of death. Diabetes may not be mentioned on the death certificate in 25–75% of those with the disease. This under-reporting influences calculations of life expectancy and makes it very difficult to obtain an unbiased description of the frequency and causes of death that are associated with diabetes in representative populations.

Other factors also influence the representativeness of the available data. Bias is inherent in analyses of life insurance data and in series which emanate from diabetes centres due to the inevitable referral bias. The most reliable data would be expected from prospective surveys of defined cohorts recruited from general population surveys. On the other hand, reports from such surveys often include data from only a relatively small number of diabetic subjects. Furthermore, changes in criteria for the diagnosis of diabetes and appreciable changes in the treatment of diabetes during the past twenty years further compound the difficulties in interpreting much of the available data.

The results of all cause-specific mortality analyses among subjects with Type II diabetes performed prospectively indicate that overall mortality rates of patients with Type II diabetes are approximately twice those of non-diabetic subjects of similar age and sex. The overall mortality rates in Type II diabetic females are equal to or exceed those of males, contrasting with findings in the population at large where females characteristically have lower age-specific mortality rates and greater life expectancy. Thus, Type II diabetes has a relatively greater impact on overall mortality in females than in males.

As many of the complications of diabetes are more frequent with increasing duration of the disease, it might be expected that the excess mortality would be greater in those with longer duration than in those of the same age with shorter duration.

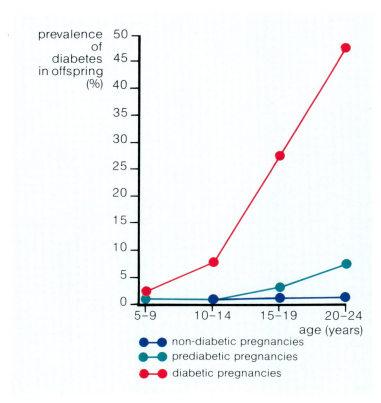

Fig. 11.23 Prevalence of Type II diabetes in offspring of Pima Indians according to whether the mother was non-diabetic or diabetic during the pregnancy. The 'prediabetic' group are the offspring of women who had normal glucose tolerance during pregnancy, but who subsequently developed diabetes. The offspring of the diabetic pregnancies develop a high prevalence of Type II diabetes at an early age. The differences in the rates between the offspring of the diabetic and prediabetic pregnancies suggest that the intra-uterine environment of the diabetic pregnancy plays an important role in determining the age at which Type II diabetes occurs in the offspring.

Cause of Death

Many investigations have shown that cardiovascular disease and cerebrovascular disease are the leading causes of mortality in patients with Type II diabetes. Age-adjusted cause-specific mortality rates for coronary heart disease are two to four times higher than in comparable non-diabetic subjects (Fig. 11.24). Furthermore, females have a relatively greater excess risk of coronary heart disease than males. The excess coronary heart disease mortality is attributable to a higher incidence of myocardial infarction as well as an increased case fatality rate. There is also strong evidence that congestive heart failure, without significant atherosclerosis, occurs more frequently in diabetic patients than in the general population.

Cerebrovascular disease probably constitutes the second most frequent cause of death among diabetic patients and accounts for about fifteen per cent of deaths. About seventy-five per cent of all deaths in Type II diabetes are due to vascular disease and there is a two- to fourfold higher risk of cardiovascular disease in patients with the disease than in non-diabetic subjects of similar age.

In contrast to Type I diabetes, where it has been estimated that about forty per cent of deaths are attributable to diabetic nephropathy, end-stage renal disease is the underlying cause in only 2–6% of the total deaths among Type II diabetic patients in most western countries.

These generalizations may not be true in all parts of the world, or in all racial groups. Among Japanese diabetic patients, cerebrovascular disease and coronary heart disease have been reported to be equally frequent as underlying causes of death and together account for about thirty per cent of deaths; renal disease accounts for about twelve per cent of deaths. Among the Pima Indians, twenty per cent of deaths in diabetic patients were attributed to renal disease.

To some extent, the frequency of cardiovascular diseases among diabetic patients appears to mirror that of the general population from which they are drawn. This appears to be particularly true of coronary heart disease, which is known to be much less frequent in the Japanese and Pima Indians than in the Caucasoid population. Nevertheless, all studies to date reflect an excessive risk of coronary heart disease among diabetic patients compared to their respective general populations. Furthermore, in the U.S.A., where there has been an appreciable fall in coronary heart disease mortality during the last fifteen years, mortality attributed to diabetes has fallen in parallel.

Variations in mortality rates in Type II diabetic patients and differences in the cause-specific rates in various parts of the world and different ethnic groups have been confirmed in a recent follow-up study performed as part of the 'WHO Multinational Study of Vascular Disease among Diabetics'.

In less developed areas of the world, it seems likely that other causes of death, rather than vascular disease, may predominate. In areas where infectious diseases, such as tuberculosis, are still major causes of death, those with Type II diabetes are likely to have even higher rates of infectious disease as the underlying cause of death.

MORTALITY RISK RATIOS FOR CORONARY HEART DISEASE IN TYPE II DIABETES

study location	year	age (years)	follow-up (years)	mortality risk ratio males	females
Dupont Company U.S.A.	1970	< 20–64	10	2.87	
Israel	1977	≥ 40	5	3.4	
Massachusetts, U.S.A.	1979	45–74	20	1.7	3.3
Georgia, U.S.A.	1980		4.5	1.0	2.8
California, U.S.A.	1983	40–79	7	2.4	3.5
Warsaw, Poland	1984	18–68	9.5	1.33	1.65
Whitehall, U.K.	1985	40–64	10	3.45	
Illinois, U.S.A.	1986	35–64	9	3.8	4.7
Finland	1986	40–69	11	2.0	4.1

Fig. 11.24 Mortality risk ratios for coronary heart disease in Type II diabetes compared to the general population in prospective population based studies. From Panzram (1987), by courtesy of Springer Verlag.

There is also a small proportion of diabetes mortality which is directly attributable to the acute metabolic derangements of the disease. Hyperosmolar coma and, in some instances, diabetic ketoacidosis or lactic acidosis, occurring in conjunction with other fulminating illnesses, do occur in Type II diabetes but the overall frequency as a cause of death in patients is quite small (see also *Chapter 21*).

The reasons for excessive cardiovascular and renal mortality in Type II diabetic patients are not certain. Hypertension may contribute to the risk and it has been known for many years that the presence of proteinuria is associated with a marked increase in risk of death. Recently, the presence of albuminuria in the subclinical range has also been shown to predict mortality. While it is known that microalbuminuria is predictive of the development of renal disease, it is also apparent that the extent of the deaths that are predicted by its presence can only partly be attributed to renal failure. Thus it appears that the presence of albuminuria of any degree is an indicator of susceptibility to vascular disease, not only in the kidney, but in other arterial beds, which, in many instances, results in death from coronary artery or cerebrovascular disease.

Life Expectancy

For patients with Type II diabetes, there is a reduction in life expectancy (Fig. 11.25). The extent of this reduction declines continuously with increasing age at diagnosis. There are three studies, each with rather similar results, which indicate that life expectancy in patients aged 40–59 years at the time of diagnosis is shortened on average by 5–10 years. There is no clear evidence that life expectancy is reduced, however, when diabetes is diagnosed after the age of seventy years.

CONCLUSION

Type II (non insulin-dependent) diabetes varies in frequency from population to population. While it is a common disease in western Europeans, it is even more frequent in certain groups, such as in expatriate Asian Indians, some tribes of American Indians and some Pacific islanders. While there is certainly more than one type, the pathogenesis of the more common forms of the disease is only partially understood. There is strong evidence that genetic susceptibility plays an important role, but the specific nature of the gene, or genes, concerned is unknown.

Environmental factors play an important role in the expression of the disease. While in many populations the onset of Type II diabetes is in middle-aged or elderly individuals, in some populations it occurs with high frequency at younger ages. Factors such as obesity and physical inactivity are risk factors for the disease. Other factors of a metabolic nature also play an important role. In particular, reduced insulin-mediated glucose disposal (insulin resistance), impaired glucose tolerance and higher than normal insulin levels are associated with the development of the disease. Furthermore, exposure of the fetus to a diabetic intra-uterine environment leads to the development of the disease at an early age.

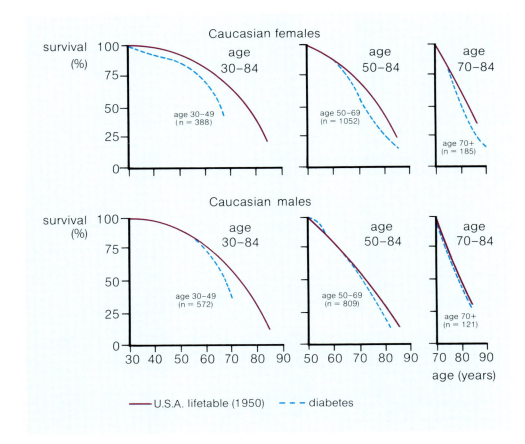

Fig. 11.25 Survival among diabetic patients according to age at diagnosis and compared with U.S.A. lifetable data. Survival is reduced among the diabetic patients, especially in females, and the survival rates in those diagnosed at an earlier age are reduced to a relatively greater degree than those diagnosed aged seventy years and over, when diabetes appears to have little effect on life expectancy. From Królewski *et al.* (1985), by courtesy of Lea and Febiger.

The aetiology of Type II diabetes is multifactorial and the effects of metabolic and lifestyle risk factors, and genetic susceptibility combine to determine if and at what age the disease becomes apparent. It may remain asymptomatic for many years, but both the asymptomatic and symptomatic stages of the disease are associated with the development of both specific and non-specific vascular complications. These vascular complications are responsible for the majority of the excess morbidity and mortality which are associated with the disease. Because of its frequency and the related medical care costs, disability, excessive mortality and shortened life expectancy, Type II diabetes constitutes an important public health problem in many countries.

For the clinician, knowledge of the epidemiology of the disease, its risk factors, precipitants and prognosis are important for the proper clinical management of patients. For the clinical investigator, knowledge of the epidemiology of the disease provides an understanding of the time sequence in which the various metabolic and other abnormalities occur, both before and after the disease becomes established, so that these events may be related to each other. Furthermore, good epidemiological data on Type II diabetes are essential for health planning purposes to determine the type and amount of preventative and curative services that are required for specific population groups.

REFERENCES

Bennett PH, Knowler WC, Pettit DJ, Carraher MJ & Vasquez B (1982) Longitudinal studies of the development of diabetes in Pima Indians. In *Advances in Diabetes Epidemiology*. Edited by Eschwege E. pp. 65–74. Amsterdam: Elsevier Science Publishers B.V.

Bennett PH, LeCompte PM, Miller M & Rushforth NB (1976) Epidemiological Studies of Diabetes in the Pima Indians. *Recent Progress in Hormone Research*, **32**, 333–376.

Bennett PH & Miller M (Eds) (1978) International studies in the epidemiology of diabetes. *Advances in Metabolic Disorders*, **9**, 1–281.

Frisch RE, Wyshak G, Albright TE, Albright NL & Schiff I (1986) Lower prevalence of diabetes in female former college athletes compared with nonathletes. *Diabetes*, **35**, 1101–1105.

Harris MI, Hadden WC, Knowler WC & Bennett PH (1986) Prevalence of diabetes and impaired glucose tolerance and plasma glucose levels in U.S. population aged 20–74 Yr. *Diabetes*, **36**, 523–534.

Knowler WC, Pettit DJ, Savage PJ & Bennett PH (1981) Diabetes incidence in Pima Indians: contributions of obesity and parental diabetes. *American Journal of Epidemiology*, **113**, 144–156.

Köbberling J & Tattersall R (Eds) (1982) *The Genetics of Diabetes Mellitus*. London: Academic Press.

Królewski AS & Warram JH (1985) Epidemiology of Diabetes Mellitus. In *Joslin's Diabetes Mellitus*. 12th edition. Edited by Marble A, Krall LP, Bradley RF, Christlieb AR & Soeldner JS. pp. 12–42. Philadelphia: Lea & Febiger.

Królewski AS, Warram JH & Christlieb AR (1985) Onset, course, complications, and prognosis of diabetes mellitus. In *Joslin's Diabetes Mellitus*. 12th edition. Edited by Marble A, Krall LP, Bradley RF, Christlieb AR & Soeldner JS. pp. 251–277. Philadelphia: Lea & Febiger.

Mann JI, Pyörälä K & Teuscher A (Eds) (1983) *Diabetes in Epidemiological Perspective*. Edinburgh: Churchill Livingstone.

Mohan V, Sharp PS, Cloke HR, Burrin JM, Schumer B & Kohner EM (1986) Serum immunoreactive insulin responses to a glucose load in Asian Indian and European type 2 (non-insulin-dependent) diabetic patients and control subjects. *Diabetologia*, **29**, 235–237.

National Diabetes Data Group (1985) *Diabetes in America: Diabetes Data Compiled 1984*. U.S. Department of Health and Human Services. NIH Publication No. 85–1468.

Ohlson L-O, Larsson B, Svärdsudd K, Welin L, Eriksson H, Wilhelmsen L, Björntorp P & Tibblin G (1985) The influence of body fat distribution on the incidence of diabetes mellitus. 13.5 years of follow-up of the participants in the study of men born in 1913. *Diabetes*, **34**, 1055–1058.

O'Sullivan JB (1975) Long term follow-up of gestational diabetes. In *Early Diabetes in Early Life*. Edited by Camerini-Davalos RA & Cole HS. pp. 503–510. New York: Academic Press.

Palumbo PJ, Elveback LR, Chu C-P, Connolly DC & Kurland LT (1976) Diabetes mellitus: incidence, prevalence, survivorship, and causes of death in Rochester, Minnesota, 1945–1970. *Diabetes*, **25**, 566–573.

Panzram G (1987) Mortality and survival in Type 2 (non-insulin-dependent) diabetes mellitus. *Diabetologia*, **30**, 123–131.

West KM (1978) *Epidemiology of Diabetes and its Vascular Lesions*. New York: Elsevier North-Holland Inc.

Zimmet P (1982) Type 2 (non-insulin-dependent) diabetes—an epidemiological overview. *Diabetologia*, **22**, 399–411.

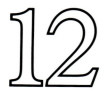

12 Type II diabetes: genetic implications from studies in identical twins

David A Pyke MD FRCP ● **R David G Leslie** MD MRCP

Non insulin-dependent (Type II) diabetes and insulin-dependent (Type I) diabetes are two separate entities. This was suggested by twin studies and further evidence has been provided by the association of certain HLA types with Type I but not with Type II diabetes.

In identical twin pairs, the concordance rate for Type II diabetes is very high. Thus, if one twin has diabetes, the other is also highly likely to have the condition. The second twin may not know that he or she too has the disease, but in such cases glucose tolerance testing nearly always demonstrates the presence of diabetes.

Among fifty-three pairs in which one twin had diabetes, the identical co-twin was also diabetic in fifty-one (Fig. 12.1). This high rate of concordance was found even when both pairs were middle-aged or elderly and the twins lived apart. If non-genetic factors are the cause of this type of diabetes, it would be expected that many pairs would be discordant, that is, only one twin is diabetic in each pair, yet this is not so.

Obesity is often considered to be a strong contributor to Type II diabetes. If this were the case, it would be expected that, in twin pairs with one twin obese and the other non-obese, the obese one would be diabetic and the non-obese co-twin not diabetic. However, current evidence shows that such twin pairs tend to be concordant even when they differ in weight (Fig. 12.2). This raises questions about the aetiological significance of obesity in Type II diabetes.

Not only do both twins develop diabetes, but they do so at about the same time. The period between the first and second twin becoming diabetic is usually less than five years and nearly always less than ten (Fig. 12.3). Indeed, these figures may be an exaggeration, as the second twin, in many cases, is not tested at the time the first twin is discovered to be diabetic. If the second

OCCURRENCE OF DIABETES IN 200 PAIRS OF IDENTICAL TWINS

	number of pairs		
	concordant	discordant	total
Type I diabetes	80	67	147
Type II diabetes	51	2	53
	131	69	200

Fig. 12.1 Concordance and discordance for diabetes in 200 pairs of identical twins.

BODY WEIGHT DIFFERENCES BETWEEN TWIN PAIRS CONCORDANT FOR TYPE II DIABETES

weight difference (kg)	n	weight difference (percentage of average body weight)	n
0–4	5	0–9	6
5–9	8	10–19	5
10–14	1	20–29	6
15–19	5	30+	1
20+	2		
	21		18

Fig. 12.2 Differences in body weight between twin pairs concordant for Type II diabetes. Twins are concordant even when their body weights differ.

PERIOD OF DISCORDANCE IN TYPE II DIABETIC TWINS

	number of pairs	
years	concordant	discordant
0–5	35	1
6–10	14	1
11–15	2	

Fig. 12.3 Period of discordance in twins with Type II diabetes. The number of years is for the time between diagnosis of diabetes in the first and second twin in concordant pairs, and between the diagnosis of diabetes in the affected twin and the most recent test for diabetes in the unaffected twin in discordant pairs.

twin had been tested, diabetes might have been discovered earlier. Therefore, the real discordance interval may be even shorter than is shown in Fig. 12.3.

Even in those few co-twins of diabetic patients who are not overtly diabetic, there is some evidence of impairment of carbohydrate tolerance. Compared to control subjects, they show higher glucose values and lower serum insulin levels (Fig. 12.4). Therefore it seems likely that all pairs will be concordant in time, suggesting that Type II diabetes is predominantly, or perhaps even entirely, due to genetic factors.

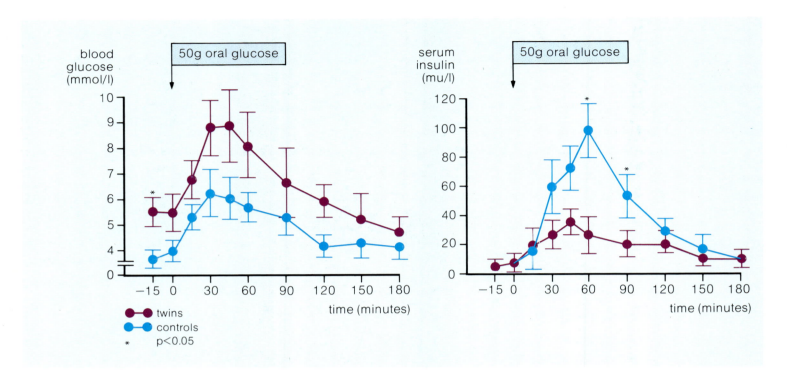

Fig. 12.4 Blood glucose and serum insulin concentrations in the fasting state and after a 50g oral glucose challenge in discordant co-twins of probands with Type II diabetes and control subjects (mean ± SEM). From Barnett *et al.* (1981), by courtesy of the British Medical Journal.

REFERENCES

Barnett AH, Eff C, Leslie RDG & Pyke DA (1981) Diabetes in identical twins. A study of 200 pairs. *Diabetologia*, **20**, 87–93.
Barnett AH, Spiliopoulos AJ, Pyke DA, Stubbs WA, Burrin J & Alberti KGMM (1981) Metabolic studies in unaffected co-twins of non-insulin-dependent diabetics. *British Medical Journal*, **282**, 1656–1658.
Harvald B, Hauge M (1963) Selection in diabetes in modern society. *Acta Medica Scandinavica*, **173**, 459–465.
Stunkard AJ, Sørensen TIA, Hanis C, Teasdale TW, Chakraborty R, Schull WJ & Schulsinger F (1986) An adoption study of human obesity. *New England Journal of Medicine*, **314**, 193–198.

13 Type II Diabetes: Pathophysiology

Richard H Jones MA MB BChir FRCP ● **Jonathan J Benn** MA MB BChir MRCP

Unlike Type I (insulin-dependent) diabetes mellitus, which usually presents with a dramatically apparent metabolic abnormality resulting from severe insulin deficiency, Type II (non insulin-dependent) diabetes forms a continuum from normal, both in cross-sectional population studies and with the passage of time in the individual. Diagnosis therefore requires the arbitrary definition of a dividing line from normal.

The World Health Organisation (WHO) Expert Committee on Diabetes Mellitus (1985) proposed that diabetes should be defined by a fasting venous whole blood glucose concentration of 6.7mmol/l (120mg/dl) or greater (7.8mmol/l, 140mg/dl, for venous plasma) and/or a value of 10mmol/l (180mg/dl) or greater (11.1mmol/l, 200mg/dl, for venous plasma) two hours after a 75g oral glucose load, if symptoms of diabetes are present. In the absence of symptoms, a second abnormal glucose value is required to confirm the diagnosis. A 'grey area' between normal glucose tolerance and diabetes was also defined, in which fasting venous whole blood glucose is less than 6.7mmol/l, but a value two hours after oral glucose falls between 6.7 and 10mmol/l. This 'grey area' is termed 'impaired glucose tolerance' (see also *Chapter 6*).

It is of interest that the definitions allow the diagnoses to be made when the fasting glucose concentration is normal but the response to glucose loading is inadequate. This inclusion is significant as changes in insulin dynamics may be more important than changes in total secretion in the pathogenesis of Type II diabetes.

Mechanisms of causation of Type II diabetes must incorporate both inherited and environmental factors. Attempts to unravel the genetics of this group of patients have yet to reveal defects that can be linked biochemically to the physiological disturbance. More progress has been made in the examination of environmental, or more specifically behavioural, associations with the disease. Lack of exercise, dietary indiscretion and particularly the consequent obesity, dramatically increase the quantity of insulin required to maintain euglycaemia. However, it is known that if sufficient exogenous insulin is administered, blood glucose concentration can be reduced to normal in such patients and it therefore follows that they have inadequate amounts of insulin for their needs, that is, they are relatively insulin-deficient. It is still an area of active debate and, indeed, of disagreement whether either insulin resistance or B cell insufficiency can be regarded as a primary causative abnormality in this disease. There is now a wealth of data relating to both of these variables such that, in the light of recent observations, the conflict can be regarded as largely semantic.

INSULIN RESISTANCE IN TYPE II DIABETES

Insulin reduces hepatic glucose production and stimulates peripheral glucose disposal predominantly in muscle. Quantitative information about these activities has come primarily from the use of techniques which 'clamp' plasma glucose concentration either at euglycaemic or hyperglycaemic levels. The principle of this method is illustrated in Fig. 13.1. Over a range of insulin concentrations achieved by exogenous insulin infusion, the quantity of glucose required to maintain or clamp the plasma glucose concentration is recorded.

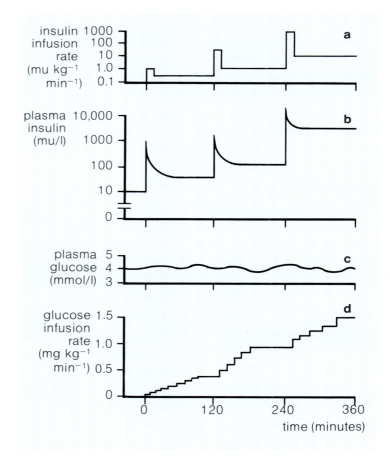

Fig. 13.1 Example of a glucose clamp experiment. Insulin infusion (a) raises plasma insulin concentration to three different steady state concentrations which are determined by radioimmunoassay (b). Repeated measurements of plasma glucose allow its value to be clamped at euglycaemic values (c) by adjustment of a peripheral glucose infusion (d). The three steady-state values of insulin concentration and glucose infusion rate allow construction of an insulin dose-response curve for glucose disposal.

Insulin and Glucose Disposal Rates

The insulin dose-response relationships for glucose disposal in groups of non-diabetic subjects and Type II diabetic patients is shown in Fig. 13.2. The curve for the diabetic subjects is abnormal in two respects. It is shifted to the right of the normal curve such that a higher concentration of insulin is required to achieve half maximal glucose disposal. This phenomenon is described as reduced insulin sensitivity. In addition, the diabetic subjects display a reduced maximal capacity for glucose disposal, or impaired responsiveness. This distinction is of interest because, as explained in *Chapter 5*, a reduction in the number and affinity of insulin receptors can impair sensitivity, but only in extreme cases influence the maximal response. Only the rate-limiting step in the process of glucose disposal, which must occur at some stage later than the initial binding of insulin to its receptor, is capable of reducing responsiveness. These data then demonstrate unequivocally the existence of a post insulin-receptor or, at least, post-binding defect in glucose disposal in the diabetic subjects.

In attempts to explain the loss of sensitivity, many efforts have been made to observe abnormalities of insulin receptor number or affinity in Type II diabetes. Although in some studies differences from normal have been reported, it is now clear that except in a few rare specific syndromes such abnormalities cannot be implicated in the insulin resistance of Type II diabetes. Insulin clearance is largely receptor mediated and the normal metabolic clearance rates for insulin almost uniformly reported in Type II diabetes, strongly support this conclusion.

In retrospect, it can be argued that attempts to implicate abnormalities of insulin receptor interaction in the aetiology of Type II diabetes were misguided. It is easy to assume that insulin resistance, as defined by the dose-response curve, inevitably implies an increased demand for insulin secretion. This would not

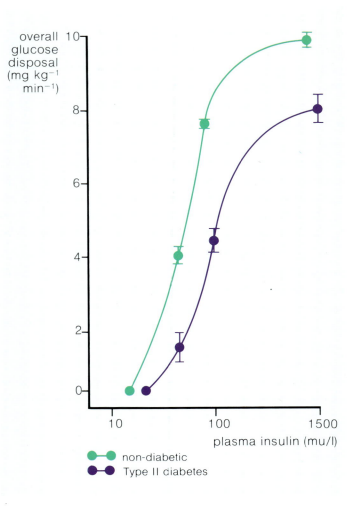

Fig. 13.2 Dose-response curves for overall glucose disposal derived from glucose clamp experiments in non-diabetic subjects and patients with Type II diabetes. In the patients, insulin resistance is apparent in terms of both sensitivity and responsiveness (mean ±SEM). From Gerich (1984), by courtesy of C.V. Mosby Company.

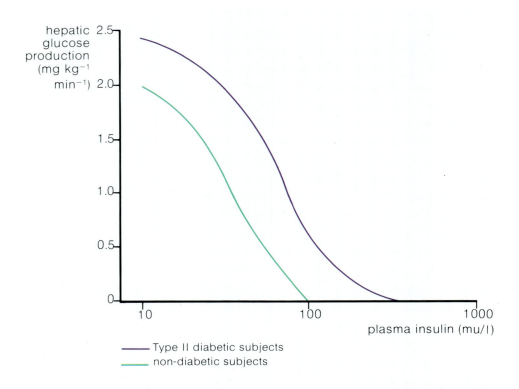

Fig. 13.3 Insulin dose-response curves for hepatic glucose production. Higher insulin levels are required at all rates of glucose output in Type II diabetes, although complete suppression can still be achieved.

be the case if the resistance were due to a reduced receptor number or affinity. In these circumstances, as described in *Chapter 5*, reduced insulin clearance would compensate for the abnormality and result in higher insulin concentrations at a particular secretion rate.

Post-receptor abnormalities can themselves impair sensitivity rather than responsiveness if they occur at steps in the pathway which are not rate-limiting. It would appear that in Type II diabetes major peripheral defects in insulin action exist, but not at the level of insulin binding. The site or sites of these defects remain to be established, although, in two recent studies, reduced tyrosine kinase activity of the receptor per unit of insulin binding has been reported. In addition, the problem may relate specifically to glucose metabolism rather than to all aspects of insulin action, as it appears that in Type II diabetes the ability of insulin to inhibit lipolysis is unimpaired.

Hepatic Contribution to Insulin Resistance

The euglycaemic clamp technique as described allows measurement of glucose disposal rate only at insulin concentrations which completely inhibit hepatic glucose production. If clamp experiments are combined with an infusion of tracer quantities of radioactive glucose, the degree to which the tracer is diluted by endogenously released unlabelled glucose allows calculation of absolute rates of glucose appearance from the liver as well as of overall utilization. The result of such an experiment is shown in Fig. 13.3. It is clear that in this sense too, Type II diabetic subjects are insulin resistant. Their dose-response curve is shifted to the right of that of non-diabetic subjects. Insulin is capable, however, even in Type II diabetes, of completely inhibiting hepatic glucose output. In this case too, it is now apparent that the major defect is at a post-binding step rather than directly the result of any defect in insulin binding.

A further aspect of hepatic function deserves more consideration. In normal individuals, elevated glucose concentrations in the portal vein result in net hepatic glucose uptake rather than output. This glucose-mediated glucose disposal is largely independent of insulin concentration and would be dominant in a normal liver exposed to the glucose and insulin concentrations found in Type II diabetes. It follows that in such patients the liver can be regarded as 'glucose resistant' in a sense that is distinct from abnormalities of insulin action. It is now clear that this failure of the liver to respond by itself to high blood glucose concentrations in Type II diabetes contributes considerably to the observed hyperglycaemia.

Conclusion

Given these observations, can it be concluded that defects in insulin action and the response to hyperglycaemia exert such undue demands on normal pancreatic function so as to cause Type II diabetes? The answer is no, for two reasons. First, many individuals, particularly the obese, are profoundly insulin resistant and yet the majority are not diabetic. At least in these people, the B cell reserve is sufficient to maintain normoglycaemia. Perhaps this potential for reserve capacity should be regarded as a criterion of normality in pancreatic function. Secondly, it has been repeatedly observed that diabetes itself, however caused, induces insulin resistance. In insulin-dependent diabetes, in which the established primary lesion is destruction of the B cells, insulin resistance can be profound and is inversely related to the quality of metabolic control achieved by treatment. Fig. 13.4 illustrates one of the many observations relevant to this point. Furthermore, in many animal models in which diabetes is induced by surgical pancreatectomy or chemical B cell destruction, the same phenomenon has been observed. It is against this background that B cell function in Type II diabetes has been extensively studied.

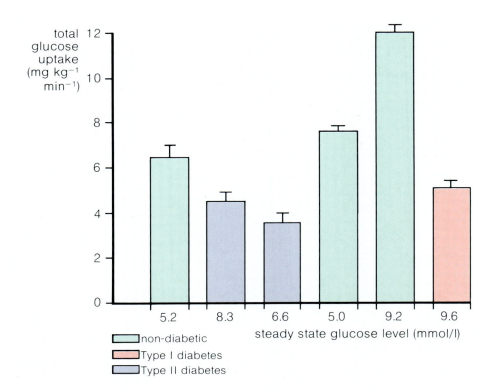

Fig. 13.4 Rate of steady-state glucose uptake in non-diabetic subjects and patients with Type I or II diabetes during an infusion of insulin at $1\,mu\,kg^{-1}min^{-1}$. A glucose clamp was used to maintain the glucose concentrations at the levels indicated below the columns. Even in Type I diabetes where B cell destruction is the primary lesion, considerable insulin resistance is apparent (mean ±SEM). From DeFronzo *et al.* (1982), by courtesy of Springer Verlag.

13.3

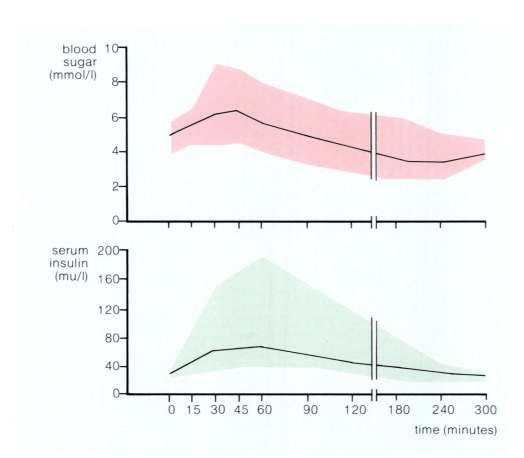

Fig. 13.5 Blood sugar and serum insulin concentrations before and after 100g oral glucose in a group of non-diabetic men aged 15–45 years. A wide range of insulin responses is a striking feature in this non-diabetic population (log mean ±2SD).

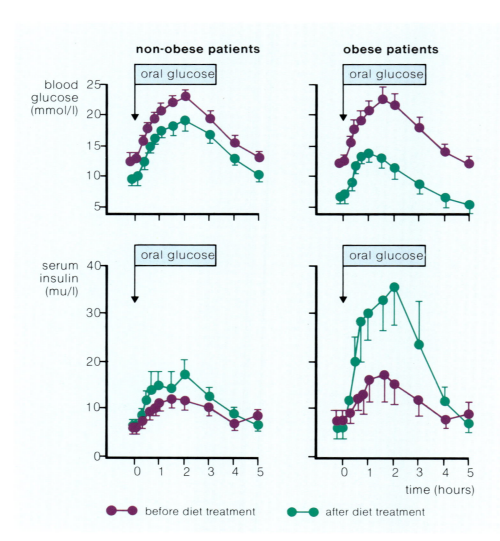

Fig. 13.6 Blood glucose and insulin concentrations before and after diet treatment in non-obese and obese subjects with Type II diabetes. In all four studies, the B cell mass demonstrates some ability to respond to oral glucose and in some cases this response could be regarded as normal. In the obese group, the improved carbohydrate tolerance following diet therapy results in a significantly greater insulin response to glucose. From Perkins *et al.* (1977), by courtesy of Springer Verlag.

INSULIN SECRETION IN TYPE II DIABETES

In the post-absorptive state, fasting plasma insulin and C peptide concentrations are not below the normal range, particularly in early stages of the disease. Even when a control group is matched for weight in addition to age and sex, in many cases the fasting insulin concentrations are still above the normal range. It cannot be concluded from this that these individuals have normal B cell function. It is known that the arterial plasma glucose concentration is a major determinant of insulin secretion and, by definition, the normal and diabetic groups are not matched for arterial plasma glucose concentration. Elevation of this variable in normal subjects, by glucose infusion, to levels which reflect those found in Type II diabetes results in considerably higher insulin concentrations than observed in the diabetic group. The B cell response to glucose is unequivocally blunted in Type II diabetes.

Insulin Response to an Oral Glucose Load

Comparisons are even more difficult after an oral glucose load. As shown in Fig. 13.5, the range of insulin responses in normal subjects is broad indicating a wide natural variation. More importantly, after oral glucose, diabetic subjects will, by definition, experience higher arterial plasma glucose levels which persist for a longer time than those in the non-diabetic group (Fig. 13.6). The equivalence of the oral dose does not equate to an equivalence of the stimulus to the B cell. The observation that in some diabetic subjects the area under the insulin curve is equal to or greater than that seen in non-diabetic subjects cannot be interpreted as an indication of normal B cell function.

First Phase Insulin Release

Intravenous glucose causes an acute rise in plasma glucose in all individuals to levels that can be expected to provoke a maximal insulin response. With this stimulus, major defects in insulin secretion in Type II diabetes become apparent. Fig. 13.7 shows this abnormality clearly. The B cell responds to glucose with a biphasic release of insulin. Fig. 13.7a demonstrates that in the group with Type II diabetes, the rapid first phase response is severely blunted, whereas the later, second phase is relatively preserved. That this deficiency is not due to a lack of insulin within the B cells is shown in Fig. 13.7b which reveals that the ability to respond to the non-glucose stimulant arginine is completely preserved.

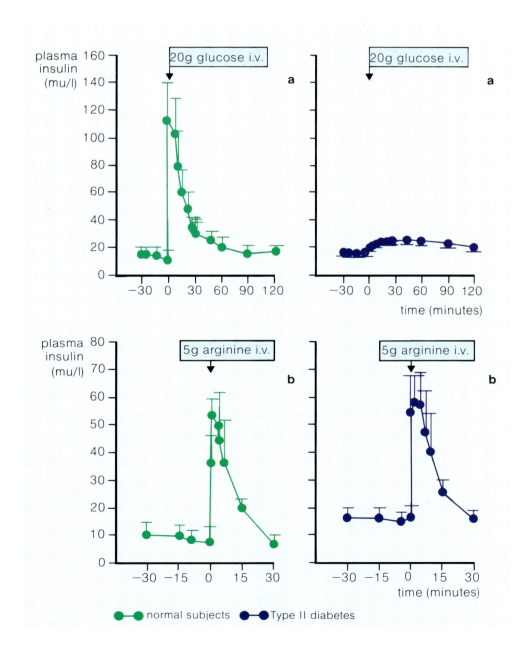

Fig. 13.7 Insulin concentrations in response to intravenous glucose or arginine in normal and diabetic subjects. (a) in the group with Type II diabetes, first phase insulin release is absent after intravenous glucose. However, the pancreatic response to intravenous arginine (b) is maintained (mean ±SEM). From Pfeifer *et al.* (1981), by courtesy of Yorke Medical Group.

Interaction between Insulin Resistance and Secretion

In one of few studies which have attempted to quantify the effects of impaired B cell function, it was concluded that even severe insulin resistance will exert little influence on plasma glucose concentration unless insulin secretion is abnormal (Fig. 13.8). The possibility that this functional defect may be of primary aetiological importance is enhanced by investigation of first degree relatives of subjects with Type II diabetes. These studies have shown that subjects with glucose intolerance who progress to diabetes are those who have deficient insulin secretion.

Reduced B cell function was demonstrable in all degrees of glucose intolerance, whereas only the more severely hyperglycaemic relatives had impaired insulin sensitivity. Even this is not conclusive evidence as it could be argued that the mild hyperglycaemia of impaired glucose tolerance could itself impair the B cell responsiveness to glucose.

The balance of these and many other observations can be stated as follows: the process of ageing reduces the capacity of the B cell mass to maintain normoglycaemia and reduces the sensitivity and responsiveness of target tissues to insulin. These changes are partly genetically programmed and partly induced by behavioural or other environmental factors. In those individuals in whom the insulin requirement comes to exceed insulin secretory capacity before the end of their lives, Type II diabetes develops.

Implicit in this is an acceptance of the validity of 'insulin requirement' and 'insulin secretory capacity' as single variables. In practice this is hard to justify. In both cases, complex dynamic factors operate and the values derived depend upon the nature of the experimental observation. However, they are conceptually useful, and accepted on that basis, they allow a degree of understanding of this complex disease.

In Fig. 13.9, the simplest application of this idea is illustrated. Both insulin requirement (IR) and insulin secretory capacity (ISC) are conceived empirically as approximately normally distributed in the population. At birth, there is no overlap but the

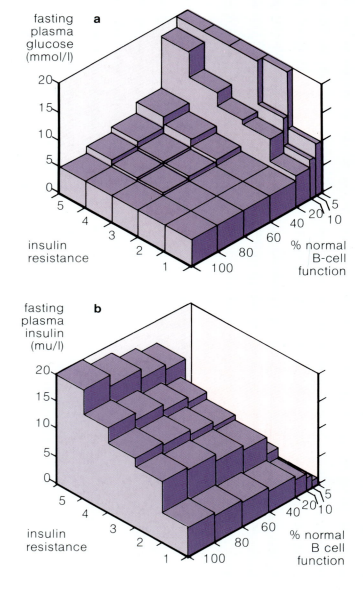

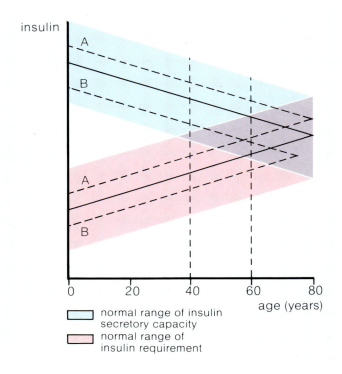

Fig. 13.8 Three-dimensional representation of the effect on (a) fasting plasma glucose concentration and (b) fasting plasma insulin concentration of increasing insulin resistance or falling insulin secretory capacity, or both. The findings are the predictions of a mathematical model which incorporates many of the known features of insulin and glucose physiology and suggest that a normal pancreas can accommodate the demands of even severe insulin resistance. Fasting insulin concentration is predicted to increase with increased insulin resistance even when B cell function is considerably impaired. From Turner *et al.* (1982), by courtesy of *Lancet*.

Fig. 13.9 Representation of the natural ranges of two global variables: insulin secretory capacity (ISC) and insulin requirement (IR) during the course of the human lifespan. It is proposed that, with the passage of time, ISC naturally declines and IR increases. From the age of approximately thirty-five years the population can be expected to include individuals whose IR exceeds their ISC and who therefore have Type II diabetes. As examples, two individuals are depicted. Subject A, although more insulin resistant than the population mean, never achieves an IR greater than his own innate ISC and never becomes diabetic. In contrast, subject B is less insulin resistant than A, but nevertheless, becomes diabetic at age seventy-five when his normal, albeit below average, B cell capacity fails to match his IR.

process of ageing approximates IR and ISC such that, by the age of thirty-five years, the variables are no longer entirely separated. In a few individuals, IR can now outstrip ISC and they can be defined as diabetic. This proportion increases with the further passage of time.

In this model, the choice of the statistically normal distribution of both IR and ISC implies natural biological variation. The semantic implication of this is that Type II diabetes, like baldness in men, could be considered as one manifestation of the natural ageing process and may not require a cause in any other sense. Also apparent is that, by this analysis, it is inappropriate to regard an abnormality of either IR or ISC as an initial causative event upon which the other is consequent. Further, it serves to explain why metabolic studies have led to confusion. For example, suppose that a group of subjects with Type II diabetes between the ages of forty and sixty years are selected for investigation. In Fig. 13.9, these individuals will comprise those from within the shaded area whose IR exceeds ISC. It is obvious that for both of these variables the group will be 'abnormal'. That is, their IR will be greater than an age-matched non-diabetic control group and their ISC will be less. However, the conclusions reached will be influenced by the nature of the experimental observations. A euglycaemic clamp study would reveal insulin resistance and, as judged by fasting insulin concentration or overall insulin response during an oral glucose tolerance test, possibly no defect in B cell

function. In contrast, an intravenous glucose tolerance test would throw emphasis on the loss of first phase insulin release as a defect in ISC with the insulin resistance regarded as secondary to the consequent hyperglycaemia. In the circumstances described, neither conclusion would be correct.

CONCLUSION

In an attempt to resolve these difficulties, it is often argued that Type II diabetes is a heterogeneous disease; the implication being that we may in time identify distinct sub-groups within this diagnosis. In some individuals, a primary defect of IR is predicted; in others, an abnormal ISC. The approach depicted in Fig. 13.9 suggests that even this suggestion may be unproductive. The expectation that both ISC and IR exist as continuous variables within the population reduces the concept of heterogeneity to the truism that each individual is unique.

Figs 13.10 and 13.11 are two examples of life histories which are shown to lead to Type II diabetes in middle age and illustrate the course of subsequent events. From the above discussion, it will be appreciated that within the current framework of understanding, an infinite variety of such time courses can be constructed.

In therapeutic terms, it can be expected that whereas there may be many potential new forms of treatment for Type II diabetes, the prospect of prevention depends upon advances in gerontology.

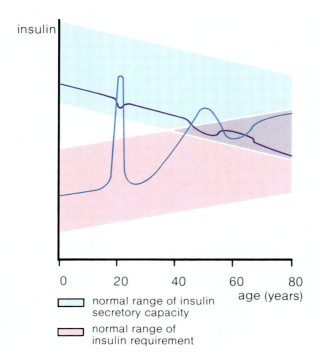

normal range of insulin secretory capacity

normal range of insulin requirement

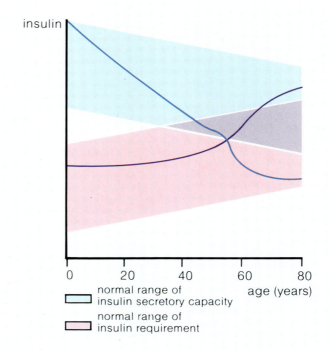

normal range of insulin secretory capacity

normal range of insulin requirement

Fig. 13.10 Theoretical time course of insulin secretory capacity and insulin requirement in a woman who develops Type II diabetes in middle age. She displays an average IR and somewhat below average ISC due to inherited factors. A pregnancy at the age of twenty years acutely increases her insulin requirement to a level above the ability of her B cell mass to respond and she presents with gestational diabetes. In the fourth and fifth decades, increasing obesity again induces resistance, until Type II diabetes is apparent. A brief respite is achieved by dietary weight loss at approximately the age of sixty years, but shortly after, the inexorable effects of declining function with increasing age render diabetes inescapable

Fig. 13.11 Example of a boy with a high innate IR in whom an above average ISC at birth nevertheless declines more rapidly than average with the passage of time. He remains at ideal weight but diabetes occurs at about the age of fifty years. In this case, the diabetes itself further impairs both IR and ISC to beyond their normal ranges. It is clear that in the last twenty years of this man's life, B cell function will fall far short of what is required. It is likely that he would be an example, common in practice, of a patient with Type II diabetes who nevertheless requires insulin treatment.

REFERENCES

DeFronzo RA, Simonson D & Ferrannini E (1982) Hepatic and peripheral insulin resistance: a common feature of Type 2 (non-insulin-dependent) and Type 1 (insulin-dependent) diabetes mellitus. *Diabetologia*, **23**, 313–319.

Horton ES (1983) Role of environmental factors in the development of non-insulin-dependent diabetes. *American Journal of Medicine*, **30**, 32–40.

Perkins JR, West TET, Sönksen PH, Lowy C & Iles C (1977) The effects of energy and carbohydrate restriction in patients with chronic diabetes mellitus. *Diabetologia*, **13**, 607–614.

Pfeifer MA, Halter JB & Porte D Jr. (1981) Insulin secretion in diabetes mellitus. *American Journal of Medicine*, **70**, 579–588.

Turner RC, Matthews DR, Holman RR & Peto J (1982) Relative contributions of insulin deficiency and insulin resistance in maturity-onset diabetes. *Lancet*, **1**, 596–598.

Ward WK, Beard JC, Halter JB, Pfeifer MA & Porte D Jr. (1984) Pathophysiology of insulin secretion in non-insulin-dependent diabetes mellitus. *Diabetes Care*, **7**, 491–502.

Weir GC (1982) Non-insulin-dependent diabetes mellitus: interplay between B cell inadequacy and insulin resistance. *American Journal of Medicine*, **73**, 461–464.

Weir GC, Leahy JL & Bonner-Weir S (1986) Experimental reduction of B cell mass: implications for the pathogenesis of diabetes. *Diabetes/Metabolism Reviews*, **2**, 125–161.

14 Insulin Treatment

Robert B Tattersall MD FRCP

The introduction of insulin treatment in 1923 proved life-saving for many diabetic patients. Since then, a profusion of insulin preparations and proposed insulin regimens has confused many physicians who do not regularly deal with diabetes. Familiarity with these preparations and regimens is usually confined to specialists in diabetic clinics. However, most clinicians can become adept at insulin treatment by familiarizing themselves with a small representative range of insulins and a few standard regimens. Many clinicians are wary of insulin treatment as there is no standard dose. However, insulin is given largely on an empirical basis and most cases of insulin-requiring diabetes can be treated by individual adjustment.

INDICATIONS FOR INSULIN TREATMENT

The first thing that all newly diagnosed diabetic patients want to know is whether they will need injections. Sometimes the decision is easy; when insulin was first introduced it proved life-saving for the ketosis-prone diabetic patient and one episode of ketoacidosis remains an absolute indication for permanent insulin therapy, whatever the age of the patient.

A commoner clinical problem is deciding if the symptomatic outpatient is ketosis-prone and whether they ought to be either given a trial of tablets or put straight on to insulin. In this context, it is important to have a clear idea of what constitutes 'typical' Type I or insulin-dependent diabetes (IDDM; Fig. 14.1). Most patients will be under forty years of age, of normal or subnormal body weight and will present with a short (<6 weeks) history of thirst, polyuria and weight loss. The severity of the onset is best assessed from the degree of weight loss and nocturia. The typical patient will have heavy glycosuria and moderate to heavy ketonuria. In practice, the commonest error is failure to recognize this clinical picture in a middle-aged patient because of a fixed idea that older people always have Type II or non-insulin dependent diabetes (NIDDM).

Fig. 14.1 Typical presenting features of Type I diabetes. Tests for islet cell antibodies, HLA antigens and C peptide are not routinely available.

FEATURES OF TYPE I DIABETES AT PRESENTATION

onset <40 year of age in 75% of cases

<6 weeks of symptoms

severe symptoms, especially nocturia

marked weight loss

may have family history of Type I diabetes or other autoimmune endocrine diseases

heavy glycosuria with moderate to heavy ketonuria

islet cell antibodies (ICA) in 80–90% of young patients at diagnosis

HLA-DR3 or DR4 positive in 70–80% of cases and HLA-DR3/DR4 heterozygosity in 40–50%

C peptide concentration in fasting state is normal or low and there is reduced or absent response after stimulation by food or i.v. glucagon

Three laboratory tests can be used to confirm the diagnosis of Type I diabetes for research or epidemiological purposes. They are: (i) islet cell antibodies (eighty to ninety per cent of Type I diabetic patients under forty years will have autoantibodies to the islets of Langerhans at diagnosis); (ii) HLA antigens (more than a third of patients with Type I diabetes will be heterozygous for the histocompatibility antigens, DR3 and DR4, and most will have either DR3 or DR4); and (iii) C peptide (it is a convenient marker of endogenous insulin secretion and a random level below 0.2nmol/l indicates insulin deficiency). It should be stressed that these laboratory tests are not widely available and are mainly of use for retrospective categorization. The decision to start a patient on insulin injections is a clinical one. A useful algorithm is shown in Fig. 14.2.

A difficult problem is posed by the young person with a subacute onset of symptoms who does not have any of the indications for immediate insulin treatment (steps 5, 6 and 7, Fig. 14.2). This type of patient is probably better on insulin for several reasons. First, virtually all normal weight diabetic patients under the age of forty years at diagnosis will need insulin within eighteen months and tablets merely postpone the inevitable and encourage false optimism. Secondly, there is some evidence that early insulin

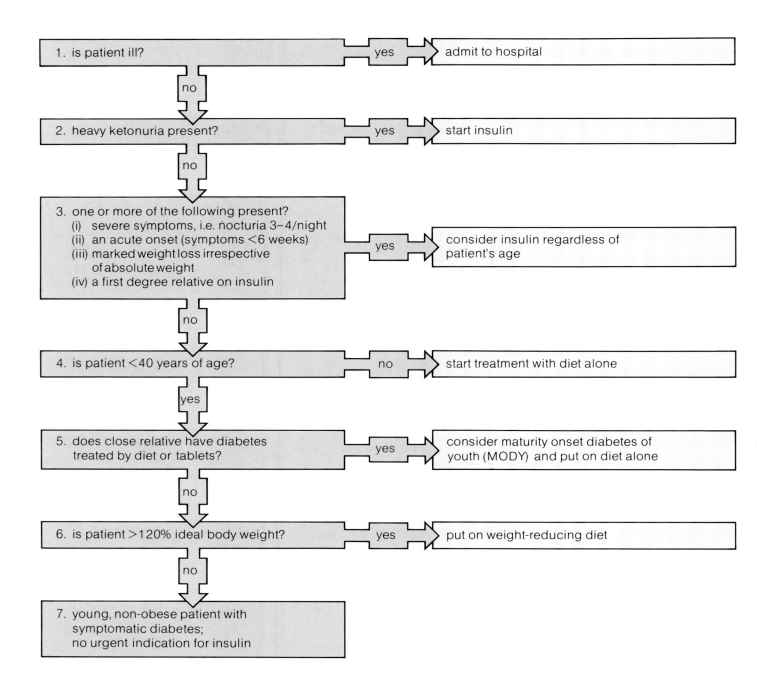

Fig. 14.2 Algorithm for a therapeutic decision in a newly diagnosed diabetic patient. If any of the features 3(i) to 3(iv) are present, serious consideration should be given to starting insulin immediately. This is not an irreversible decision, it can be reviewed, whereas the penalty for not starting insulin injections may be an admission with ketoacidosis.

treatment preserves B cell function and makes control easier in the years to come and thirdly, it is easier to educate people in the routine of insulin injection when they feel well rather than after the drama of an admission with ketoacidosis.

Many middle-aged or elderly patients are not insulin-dependent in the sense that they need the hormone to prevent ketoacidosis. Nevertheless, on maximal doses of tablets they have high blood glucose levels and feel chronically unwell with symptoms such as tiredness, nocturia and pruritus vulvae. Such people are often reluctant to start insulin, although at least half will feel better with it, even if glycaemic control is not improved. A trial of insulin is always worthwhile in these cases, with the clear understanding that it can be stopped if the patient wishes.

The following points about the decision to start insulin should be stressed: (i) blood glucose concentration is a poor guide as to its need; (ii) typical Type I diabetes does occur in the elderly and overweight and can be identified on clinical grounds (Fig. 14.2); and (iii) any outpatient with newly diagnosed diabetes and moderate or heavy ketonuria should be started on insulin.

PRINCIPLES OF INSULIN TREATMENT

The first use of replacement therapy for a hormone deficiency disorder was that of thyroid extract for myxoedema. This was introduced in 1896 and by the time insulin came into use in 1923 thyroid hormone was known to be simple, effective and free from short- or long-term complications; at first it was hoped that insulin would cure diabetes in the same way. However, diabetes has turned out to be a special case for several reasons. First, insulin is not protein-bound and plasma levels in healthy people fluctuate from minute-to-minute depending on, for example, food and exercise. Hence, hormone replacement in diabetes is a dynamic process; a single daily injection cannot mimic normal physiological insulin secretion.

Secondly, insulin is a polypeptide which has to be given parenterally. The only convenient route is subcutaneously which leads to higher peripheral than portal levels, the opposite to that in normal physiology and an undesirable situation since the liver is the main target of insulin action (see *Chapter 5*). Finally, insulin prevents death from ketoacidosis but its use over the past sixty years has not prevented long-term microvascular complications affecting the eyes, kidneys and nervous system.

It now seems certain that either hyperglycaemia or a closely-related abnormality is the main cause of long-term complications. The aim of insulin treatment should therefore be to achieve continuous normoglycaemia, provided the patient's life expectancy is sufficient for the prevention of complications to outweigh the side-effects and arduous nature of the treatment. Such a rigorous objective may not always be appropriate and it is useful with each newly diagnosed patient with Type I diabetes to draw up a theoretical cost/benefit analysis and on this basis to set realistic aims and objectives. As Dr R.D. Lawrence put it, we should 'use insulin as physiologically as possible to suit the life of the diabetic man'.

Designing an Insulin Regimen: Theoretical Considerations

The normal daily patterns of blood glucose concentrations and insulin secretion are shown in Fig. 14.3. Blood glucose is tightly controlled in the healthy subject between a minimum of 3.5–4mmol/l in the fasting state and 5–8mmol/l post-prandially. Any schedule of insulin administration which fails to mimic the normal pattern of plasma insulin secretion is unlikely to produce normoglycaemia in the totally insulin-deficient patient. Nearly perfect control can be achieved in such patients by means of a glucose-controlled insulin infusion system, the so-called artificial endocrine pancreas (AEP), the principle of which is discussed in detail in *Chapter 15*. It operates by continuously monitoring blood glucose concentration so that a computer can instruct two pumps to infuse either insulin or glucose as appropriate and thus maintain near-normoglycaemia.

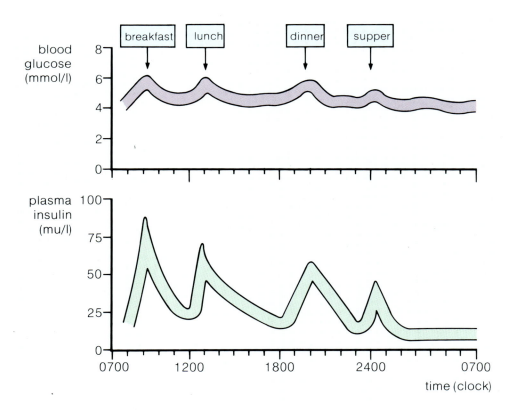

Fig. 14.3 Daily blood glucose and plasma insulin ranges in normal subjects.

Studies of normal physiology and the insulin delivery patterns of the AEP have shown that an ideal insulin regimen should: produce prompt short-lived peaks of plasma insulin to coincide with meals; produce a low but constant basal insulin concentration between meals and more especially at night with, if possible, a slight rise between 0500h and 0800h when insulin sensitivity is at the lowest point of its circadian rhythm; and deliver more insulin at breakfast to overcome the reduced sensitivity at this time even though other meals have a higher carbohydrate content.

This physiological pattern cannot be achieved with a daily dose of intermediate-acting insulin which produces a parabolic curve (Fig. 14.4) with a peak of free insulin concentration four to eight hours after injection followed by a gradual fall to pre-injection levels after fifteen to twenty-four hours. With this regimen, if the plasma insulin concentration is high enough to prevent hyperglycaemia with a meal, it will be too high between meals and will cause hypoglycaemia unless counterbalanced by snacks. Conversely, if the dose is low enough to prevent hypoglycaemia between meals it will not prevent hyperglycaemia after them. However, a single injection of intermediate- or long-acting insulin may be successful if all that is required is to boost basal insulin levels in patients whose pancreas still functions sufficiently to produce some endogenous insulin with meals. This is true, for example, in some Type II diabetic patients or in some Type I patients in the first year or two after diagnosis.

Apart from being closer to real physiological patterns, regimens of two or more insulin injections per day have two other advantages: they offer the patient more flexibility compared with one injection of long-acting insulin per day, in that the size of each injection can be individually adjusted to cope with changing circumstances; and there is less risk of severe and prolonged hypoglycaemia.

The most common multiple injection schedule is a twice-daily combination of short-acting or soluble and intermediate-acting insulins, either lente or isophane type, shown schematically in Fig. 14.5b. In theory, the two injections of intermediate-acting insulin cover basal insulin requirements and the short-acting insulin covers meals. As a general rule, two-thirds of the daily insulin requirement is given in the morning and one-third at night. In practice, this type of regimen, often called twice-daily soluble and isophane, is often unsatisfactory. This is because it both fails to produce adequate peaks of free insulin with meals and leads to hyperinsulinaemia in the middle of the night with inadequate insulin levels in the dawn hours from 0500h onwards. The free insulin profile and the blood glucose curve associated with this regimen are shown in Fig. 14.6.

Two alternative regimens which conform more closely to physiological principles are: (i) thrice-daily soluble insulin given fifteen to thirty minutes before meals with a small injection of isophane last thing at night (Fig. 14.5c) and (ii) twice-daily slow-acting insulin (ultralente) to provide basal insulin requirements with thrice-daily soluble insulin before meals (Fig. 14.5d).

Use of Insulin in Practice

Insulin treatment is a dynamic and rapidly changing process and it follows that patients must be actively involved so they become their own doctor, dietician and laboratory technician. The success of the AEP results from it being a closed-loop system in which constant feedback is translated into action. The same process should underlie self-treatment by the insulin-dependent patient,

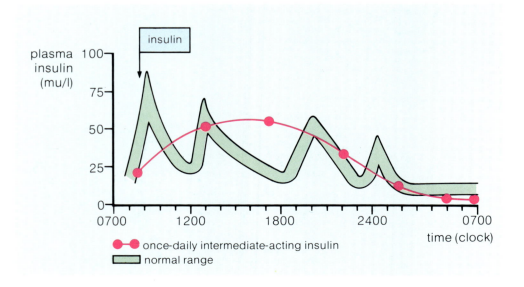

Fig. 14.4 Effect of a single daily dose of an intermediate-acting insulin on plasma insulin levels through the day. The single dose produces a parabolic curve. The normal daily range of insulin concentration is also shown.

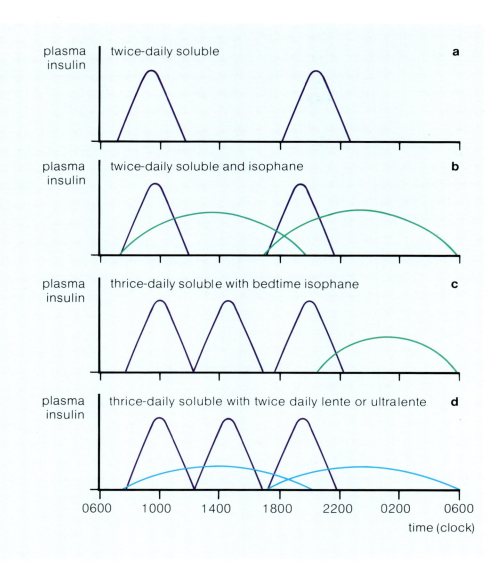

plasma insulin — twice-daily soluble — **a**

plasma insulin — twice-daily soluble and isophane — **b**

plasma insulin — thrice-daily soluble with bedtime isophane — **c**

plasma insulin — thrice-daily soluble with twice daily lente or ultralente — **d**

0600   1000   1400   1800   2200   0200   0600

time (clock)

Fig. 14.5 Effect on plasma insulin concentration of various insulin regimens.

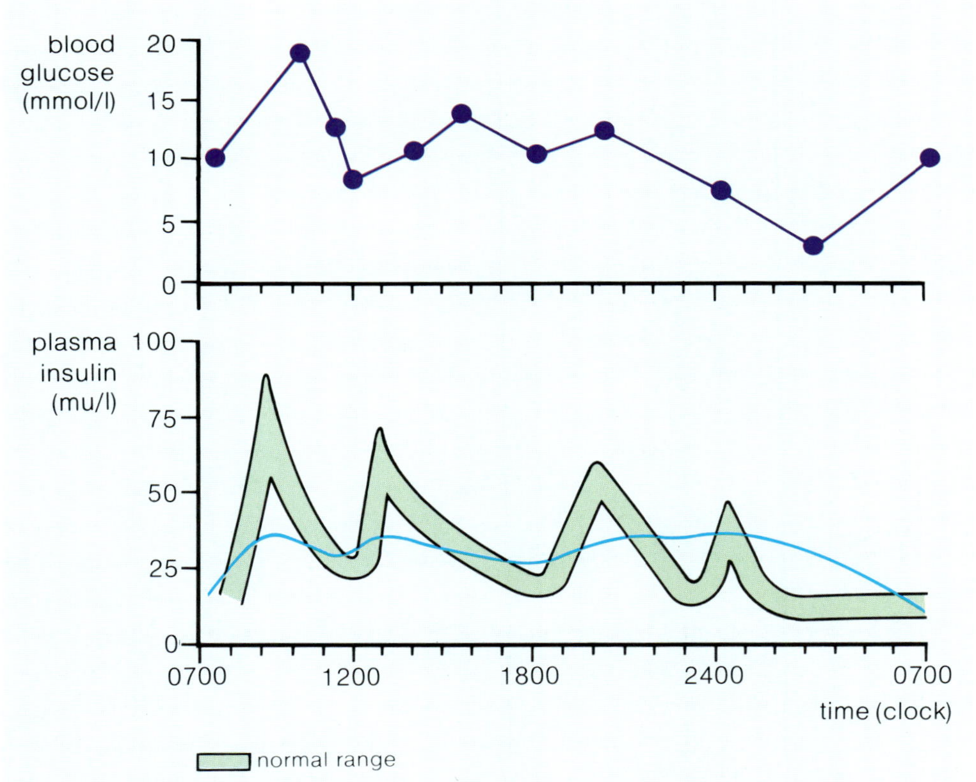

blood glucose (mmol/l)

20
15
10
5
0

plasma insulin (mu/l)

100
75
50
25
0

0700   1200   1800   2400   0700

time (clock)

normal range

Fig. 14.6 Plasma insulin and blood glucose concentrations which result from an insulin regimen of twice-daily injections of a short-acting and intermediate-acting insulin. This regimen does not produce adequate peaks of insulin after meals and leads to hyperinsulinaemia in the middle of the night as can be seen by comparison with the normal range.

with the patient's brain taking the place of the computer and feedback being produced by frequent self-monitoring of either blood or urine glucose. This process is depicted schematically in Fig. 14.7.

Education

To achieve good metabolic control, the patient must have received comprehensive education about his condition and have understood and retained that information. If control is poor, the physician may presume that the patient is 'non-compliant' with the treatment, although the patient may have had inadequate education to cope with diabetes. Therefore, before judging someone as 'non-compliant', the level of diabetic education should be considered.

Failure of diabetic education may stem from low intelligence in the patient, lack of appreciation of the patient's misconceptions about insulin, education when the patient is unwell and thus unable to understand and retain information, poor teaching and trying to give too much information at once. Each department should regularly review the efficiency of its own teaching programme, paying attention to the ability of the teachers, their level of knowledge, the uniformity of the teaching programme throughout the hospital, adaptation of the programme according to the patient's ability, assessment of retained information and the provision of refresher courses.

A checklist is useful to ensure that no aspects of the educational programme are omitted in each case (Fig. 14.8).

Diet

If one searches for the ideal dietary structure for a patient with Type I diabetes it is possible to find articles advocating almost every conceivable permutation of carbohydrate, fat, protein and fibre. Over the past decade there has been a swing away from traditional low carbohydrate, high fat diets to high carbohydrate,

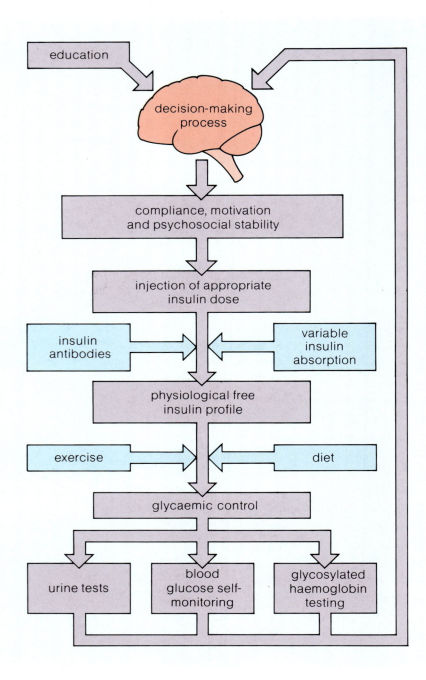

Fig. 14.7 Closed-loop control of diabetes by self-monitoring by the patient.

14.6

EDUCATIONAL CHECKLIST FOR PATIENTS STARTING INSULIN THERAPY

- injection technique
- diet
- self-monitoring
- hypoglycaemia
- exercise
- intercurrent illness
- inheritance and aetiology
- driving
- identification bracelet

Fig. 14.8 Checklist of points in which each patient starting insulin therapy should be educated. A note should be made of when and by whom each stage of the educational process was carried out.

high fibre and low fat diets. This should not obscure the fact that the most important principle of diet for the patient with Type I diabetes is consistency of carbohydrate intake with the same amount of carbohydrate being eaten at the same time each day (see *Chapter 18*).

Insulin absorption

Most patient handbooks give tables of the duration and peak action of the various types of insulin and, as a result, most patients and many physicians believe that absorption of insulin by the subcutaneous route is relatively constant and predictable. This is unfortunately not the case and variation in absorption is one of the main problems in conventional insulin treatment. Some factors have a predictable effect on the speed of insulin absorption (Fig. 14.9). However, even when insulin is injected in a standardized fashion into the same anatomical site, there is considerable day-to-day variation in absorption within and between patients.

Absorption of unmodified (soluble) insulin is less variable than that of modified preparations. For example, with monocomponent lente insulin there is an individual daily range of absorption of 19–104% of the injected insulin. A further example of the between-patient variation of absorption of highly purified porcine isophane insulin is shown in Fig. 14.10.

The effect of insulin antibodies on the absorption process has not been well studied but, in general, it is thought that antibodies retard absorption and also prolong the action of a given insulin. For example, where a patient has a moderate level of insulin antibodies, the duration of action of an injection of soluble insulin is more like that of isophane in a patient without antibodies.

FACTORS AFFECTING THE ABSORPTION OF SUBCUTANEOUS INSULIN

lipohypertrophy
slow from these areas

anatomical area
fastest from abdominal wall and slowest from thigh

exercise
increased when injected limb is exercised

subcutaneous blood flow
rise increases absorption, e.g. hot bath or sauna

size of dose
slower with larger injection volumes

Fig. 14.9 Various factors affecting the absorption of insulin which has been injected subcutaneously.

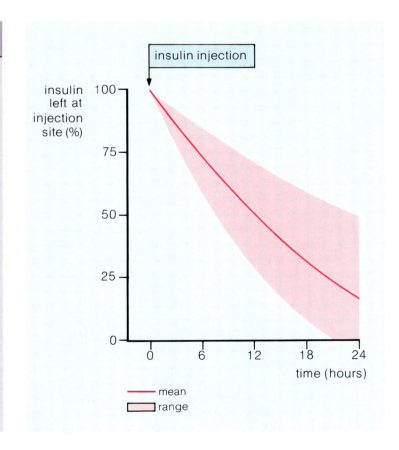

Fig. 14.10 Variation between patients of the absorption of highly purified porcine isophane insulin.

SELF-MONITORING

Some form of self-monitoring is necessary to close the feedback loop (see Fig. 14.7). Urine testing (Fig. 14.11) is convenient and cheap but too insensitive and inaccurate for patients making a serious attempt to obtain near-normoglycaemia. Fig. 14.12 shows how very marked fluctuations in blood glucose levels in an individual patient are completely missed by four-times-daily urine testing. A further example of the ineffectiveness of urine tests for estimating real time blood glucose concentrations is shown in Fig. 14.13. It will be seen that a negative urine test for reducing sugars could be associated with a blood glucose concentration anywhere from 3–16mmol/l while a two per cent test covered a range from 3–20mmol/l.

Given the inaccuracy of urine tests, it is logical that patients should measure their own blood glucose directly and this was first done on a widespread scale in the U.K. in 1978. There are now a variety of systems and accessories available; Fig. 14.14 shows a strip with a double reagent pad which can be read either by eye or a meter. Other strips with a single reagent pad can only be read accurately in a meter of which a variety are shown in Fig. 14.15.

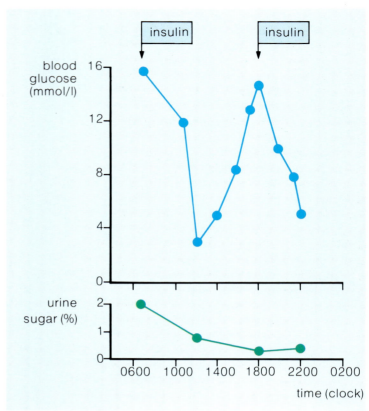

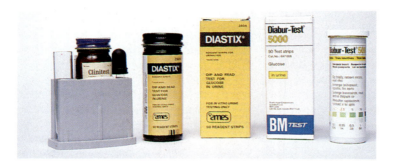

Fig. 14.11   Range of urine testing kits.

Fig. 14.12   Actual blood glucose levels and results of urine testing in a diabetic patient. The urine tests fail to show the pronounced variation in blood glucose levels through the day.

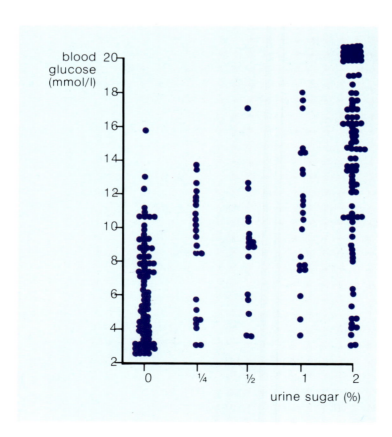

Fig. 14.13   Ineffectiveness of urine tests for estimating blood glucose concentrations. The results are of 250 simultaneous blood glucose and urine tests in forty-five diabetic children.

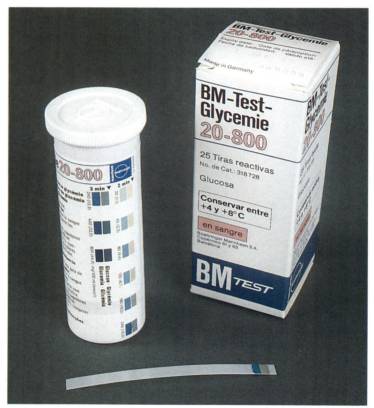

Fig. 14.14   Strip with double reagent pad for testing blood glucose.

Several semi-automatic, spring-loaded, finger-pricking devices are shown in Fig. 14.16. All these systems are capable of measuring blood glucose to within plus or minus ten per cent of a reference value provided they are used properly by patients who have been carefully instructed. Fig. 14.17 shows the very good correlation between laboratory blood glucose estimations and those obtained by trained patients using a typical testing stick.

Similar figures have been published for all available sticks and meters with correlation coefficients usually over 0.85.

Home blood glucose monitoring is not always used appropriately and will probably only lead to improved control if done several times every day. However, it still has advantages over urine testing which are summarized in Fig. 14.18. It should be

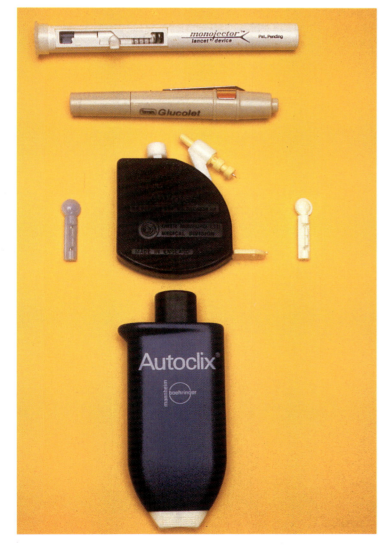

Fig. 14.15 Variety of meters for reading blood glucose testing strips.

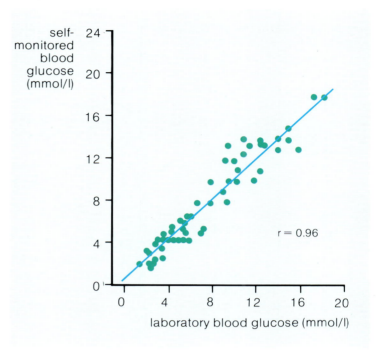

Fig. 14.17 Correlation between blood glucose concentrations obtained by self-monitoring and in the laboratory. All patients were experienced at self-monitoring (n = 57).

Fig. 14.16 Variety of semi-automatic, spring-loaded, finger-pricking devices.

ADVANTAGES OF BLOOD GLUCOSE MONITORING OVER URINE TESTING

only method for self-monitoring normoglycaemia accurately

enables goals to be clearly defined

improvement of diabetic control and outpatient stabilization

indicates which symptoms are due to hypoglycaemia

detects nocturnal hypoglycaemia

makes patients feel secure when accompanying negative urine tests

allows an estimation of renal threshold

often preferred by patients

Fig. 14.18 Advantages of blood glucose self-monitoring over urine testing.

emphasized that for patients being treated either with a pump or intensive conventional therapy who maintain their blood glucose concentration within the normal range, blood glucose monitoring is the only technique which gives useful information, since urine tests will always be negative and will give no warning of abnormally low blood glucose levels.

Glycosylation and the Assessment of Glycaemic Control

Glucose becomes non-enzymatically attached to many body proteins, a process termed 'glycosylation'; the higher the blood glucose level, the more glucose is attached. Haemoglobin is glycosylated and by measuring the proportion of total haemoglobin with glucose attached, an indication is provided of the average blood glucose values over the previous two to three months, which is the lifespan of the red cell. Glycosylated haemoglobin (HbA$_1$ or HbA$_{1c}$) may be estimated by a variety of methods including column chromatography, isoelectric focusing and colorimetry. In non-diabetic subjects, approximately 4–8% of total haemoglobin is glycosylated, the precise normal range depending upon method, whereas in diabetic subjects higher values reflect recent elevated blood glucose levels.

INSULIN INJECTIONS AND ACUTE COMPLICATIONS OF INSULIN TREATMENT

Most patients have a fear of injections, usually based on the misconception that they are performed with as large a needle as is used for venepuncture and that they will be as complicated. This fear can be easily allayed by showing them a 27 gauge needle and making them give a 'dummy' injection.

Provided that patients are not acutely ill, they can be started on insulin as outpatients with twice-daily injections of 6–10u intermediate-acting insulin given thirty minutes before both breakfast and the evening meal. These small doses were originally chosen as being unlikely to lead to hypoglycaemia in the first week but in fact almost invariably abolish acute diabetic symptoms within four or five days even though they do not produce perfect control. The insulin dose can then be raised at weekly intervals and fast-acting insulin added as necessary to control post-prandial hyperglycaemia.

Whatever time of day the patient arrives, the first injection should be performed as soon as possible. Teaching is done by a full-time diabetes nurse as follows: (i) the nurse shows how to draw up the correct dose of insulin; (ii) she demonstrates the injection technique on herself with an empty syringe and needle; (iii) the patient injects themself with the full syringe; and (iv) the patient now learns how to draw up.

This sequence was devised to get the first injection over as quickly as possible since it is only after having done it that patients relax and concentrate on other instructions. In the first session, no attempt should be made to educate the patient. All that is necessary is survival information to enable the patient to get through the first week. The choice of injection equipment is shown in Fig. 14.19. Plastic syringes are preferred by most patients and can be safely reused for at least a week. They do not become infected because traces of insulin, which contains phenol or orthocresol as a preservative, remain in the syringe between injections and act as a disinfectant.

Injection abscesses with conventional insulin delivery are very uncommon, but more common with continuous subcutaneous insulin infusion. When injection abscesses do occur they are usually caused by staphylococci. Fig. 14.20 shows a rare type of

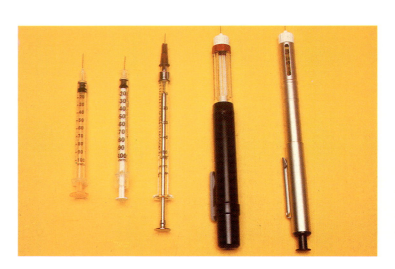

Fig. 14.19   Insulin injection equipment. Left to right: two plastic syringes with integral needles, glass syringe with detachable needle, Accupen and Novopen. Both the latter use pre-cartridged insulin and are much more convenient than any other means of injection.

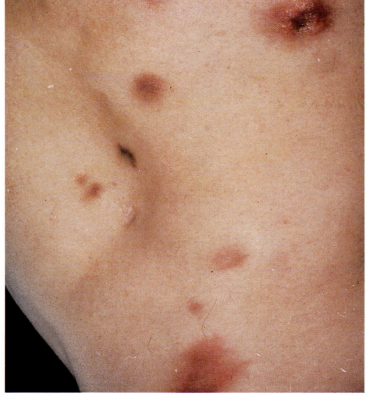

Fig. 14.20   Injection abscess caused by *Mycobacterium chelonei*.

injection abscess caused by *Mycobacterium chelonei* which tends to be indolent and spread. Injections must be given subcutaneously rather than intradermally. Intradermal injections are painful and produce pock marks (Fig. 14.21). Allergic reactions to insulin are rare, especially with the increasing use of highly purified insulin. The most common form of allergic reaction is either urticaria or red, itchy lumps which occur during the first two or three weeks after starting insulin. These usually resolve spontaneously. If a patient complains of pain or swelling at injection sites, these should be inspected and the injection technique thoroughly checked.

During the first three weeks on insulin there may be marked refractive changes leading to blurred vision. These are thought to be due to rehydration of the lens and resolve spontaneously within three weeks. However, patients should be warned of their possible occurrence to prevent them getting their eyes tested unnecessarily. Very rarely, patients started on insulin will develop ankle oedema within the first week ('insulin oedema'). This is most usual if the original presentation has been in ketoacidosis. Again, it resolves spontaneously within a couple of weeks.

Lipoatrophy at injection sites (Fig. 14.22) is thought to be a consequence of high circulating levels of insulin antibody and is most common with impure bovine insulins. It can be cured by changing to highly purified porcine or human insulin. Lipohypertrophy or fatty tumours at injection sites (Fig. 14.23) is a consequence of the lipogenic effect of insulin and results from repeated injections into the same site. It is most common in children and patients on highly purified insulins.

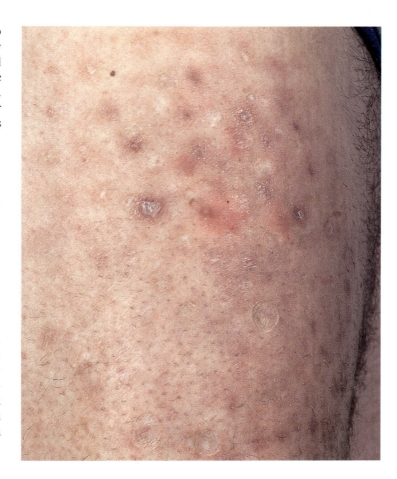

Fig. 14.21 Pock marks in the thigh caused by intradermal injection of insulin.

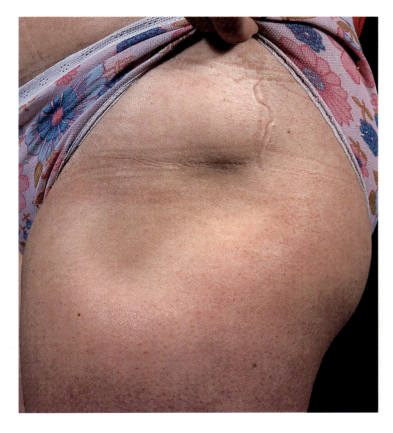

Fig. 14.22 Lipoatrophy at insulin injection sites. This is caused by high circulating levels of insulin antibody.

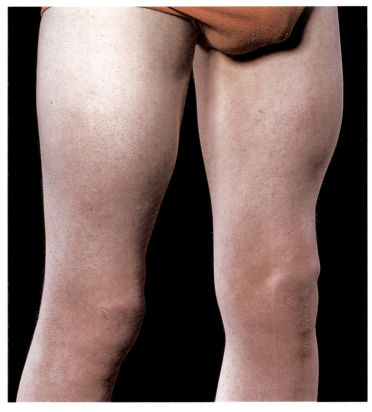

Fig. 14.23 Lipohypertrophy at insulin injection sites. This is a consequence of the lipogenic effect of insulin.

CONCLUSIONS

Conventional insulin treatment as described here has been used for over sixty years, mainly with impure bovine insulins. During these sixty years fashions have changed from four-times daily unmodified insulin with a strict diet, to once-daily insulin with a free diet, back to twice-daily mixtures of short- and intermediate-acting insulins and finally, in the 1980's, to more sophisticated regimens involving two or more daily injections of different insulin types.

It is undeniable that most patients do not achieve normoglycaemia on subcutaneous insulin injections and it is understandable that many physicians seek new approaches to the problems of poor glycaemic control. It is unlikely that this can ever be achieved by some technological miracle alone, such as supplying every patient in the clinic with a pump and a box of blood glucose testing strips. Instead, the solution to the problem lies much more in the area of improving education and motivation of patients with insulin-dependent diabetes.

REFERENCES

Ireland JT, Thomson WST & Williamson J (1980) *Diabetes Today: A Handbook for the Clinical Team*. Aylesbury: H.M. & M Publishers.

Keen H & Ng Tang Fui S (1982) The definition and classification of diabetes mellitus. *Clinics in Endocrinology and Metabolism*, **11**, 279–305.

Sonksen P, Fox C & Judd S (1985) *The Diabetes Reference Book*. Philadelphia: Harper and Row Publishers.

Tattersall RB (1986) *Diabetes: A Practical Guide for Patients on Insulin*. 2nd edition. Edinburgh: Churchill Livingstone.

Tattersall RB & McCulloch DK (1984) Modern aspects of insulin therapy. *Annals of Clinical Research*, **16**, 107–117.

15 Insulin Infusion Systems

John C Pickup MA BM BCh DPhil MRCPath

Electromechanical devices for administration of insulin to the diabetic patient aim to improve metabolic control by simulating patterns of insulin secretion in non-diabetic subjects; essentially a slow delivery throughout the twenty-four hours with superimposed boosts at meal-times (Fig. 15.1). There are two infusion strategies (Fig. 15.2): closed-loop systems, where there is automatic sensing of blood glucose and feedback control of the insulin delivery rate, and open-loop systems, where there is no glucose sensing or feedback, although the patient may be said to complete the loop by blood glucose self-monitoring and by altering the insulin infusion rates accordingly.

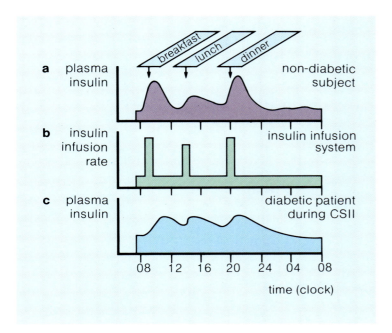

Fig. 15.1 Aim and result of insulin infusion. Graph (a) shows plasma insulin concentrations throughout the day in non-diabetic subjects, where there is a clear separation between slow basal delivery throughout the night and between meals (restraining glucose output from the liver) and boosts at meal-times (stimulating glucose uptake into the liver and periphery and inhibiting glucose output from the liver).
  Graph (b) delineates insulin infusion rates from an electromechanical divice; basal rate (approximately 1u/h for continuous subcutaneous insulin infusion (CSII)) and prandial boosts.
  Graph (c) shows plasma free insulin concentrations in diabetic patients being treated by an infusion system (levels illustrated are those occurring during CSII). Note the 'best fit' of insulin peak and meal-times and the simulation of non-diabetic basal insulin levels.

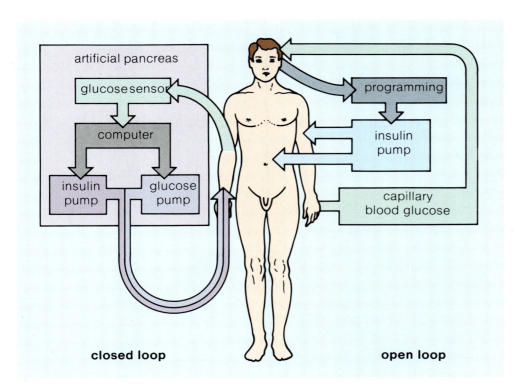

Fig. 15.2 Principle of closed- and open-loop insulin infusion devices. With a closed-loop system, commonly called an artificial pancreas, venous blood is pumped from the patient to the glucose analyser in the machine. The computer calculates the amount of insulin or glucose which has to be infused back into the patient's circulation to maintain a given glycaemic level.
  With open-loop devices there is no blood glucose sensing by the machine and consequently no feedback control. Insulin is infused from a portable pump at a variety of rates (basically prandial and basal rates) and can be delivered to a number of sites (subcutaneous, intravenous or even intraperitoneal). Self-monitoring of capillary blood glucose by the patient may be said to close the loop.

THE ARTIFICIAL ENDOCRINE PANCREAS

The artificial endocrine pancreas, or AEP, which is a closed-loop insulin infusion device, is commercially available (Fig. 15.3). The principle is that blood is pumped from a peripheral vein of the patient to the machine, where the glucose concentration is continuously and automatically measured, the results fed to the 'on-board' computer and the amount of insulin or glucose required to either maintain or restore a desired blood glucose concentration (usually euglycaemia) is calculated. The required insulin or glucose is then infused into a peripheral vein. The computer of the AEP uses pre-set algorithms or rules to translate blood glucose information into appropriate insulin or glucose delivery rates (Fig. 15.4).

The AEP takes into account not only the absolute glucose level but also the rate of change of blood glucose. This ensures a rapid initial insulin delivery at meal-times (imitating the first phase of non-diabetic insulin secretion) and attenuation of the insulin infusion rate when the blood glucose concentration is falling (thus preventing hypoglycaemia); it also corrects for the delay between blood withdrawal and glucose measurement.

The AEP very successfully returns blood glucose levels in the diabetic patient to normal throughout the entire twenty-four hours (Fig. 15.5). It has been used clinically in a number of circumstances as an alternative treatment strategy where short-term glycaemic control is difficult, for example, during surgery, parturition, ketoacidosis and for the management of insulinoma patients at operation. It has been a most valuable research tool in such studies as the comparison of glucose normalization with changes in other metabolites and hormones known to be disordered in conventionally-treated diabetic patients; for measuring the change in insulin requirements during adminis-

Fig. 15.3 An example of a closed-loop system, or artificial endocrine pancreas, in use at a patient's bedside. This machine is the 'Biostator[R]', made by Life Science Instruments. Photograph by courtesy of Professor K.G.M.M. Alberti.

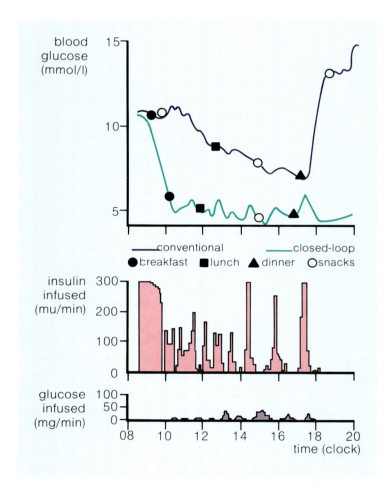

Fig. 15.4 An algorithm for calculating the rate of glucose or insulin infused by a closed-loop device according to the prevalent blood glucose. In this case, the desired blood glucose level has been set at a euglycaemic concentration. The artificial endocrine pancreas also takes into account the rate of change of blood glucose over the previous few minutes (sometimes called the difference factor) in its calculation of the necessary rate of either insulin or glucose delivery to the patient.

Fig. 15.5 Illustration of short-term blood glucose control in one insulin-dependent diabetic patient treated by a closed-loop device. The upper graph shows the patient's blood glucose concentration during conventional injection treatment (55u lente insulin before breakfast) and the same patient's blood glucose levels in response to infusion of insulin and glucose by an artificial pancreas.

tration of an antidiabetic drug such as somatostatin; for maintaining the blood glucose at a desired level whilst other substances like insulin are varied; and for titrating absorbed insulin with glucose in studies of the pharmacokinetics of insulin absorption.

The present AEP is unsuitable for prolonged use for the following reasons: its intravenous insulin infusion route would present problems of infection and thrombosis if used on a long-term basis; it is not portable; it is complex, requiring several operators; and it is expensive.

CONTINUOUS SUBCUTANEOUS INSULIN INFUSION

In the early 1970's several investigators showed that glycaemic control almost as efficient as with closed-loop systems could be achieved in diabetic patients by open-loop intravenous insulin infusion from a portable, battery-operated pump (Fig. 15.6). A number of groups have now shown strict control for many months using continuous ambulatory infusion systems, usually with the delivery cannula in a central vein. However, the intravenous route of administration has again restricted its widespread application.

Our own group conceived and developed the open-loop technique of continuous subcutaneous insulin infusion (CSII) specifically to overcome the problems of long-term intravenous infusion and thus allow periods of near-normoglycaemia sufficient to test the links between diabetic control and complications. Insulin is infused from a portable pump into the subcutaneous tissue of the anterior abdominal wall. Boosts are given about half an hour before main meals to allow for the delay in absorption from the subcutaneous site (Figs 15.7 and 15.8).

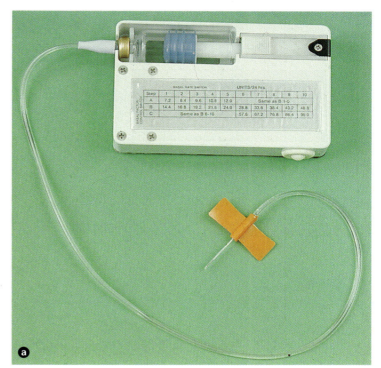

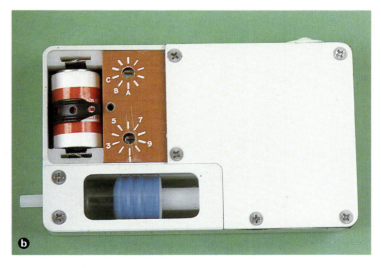

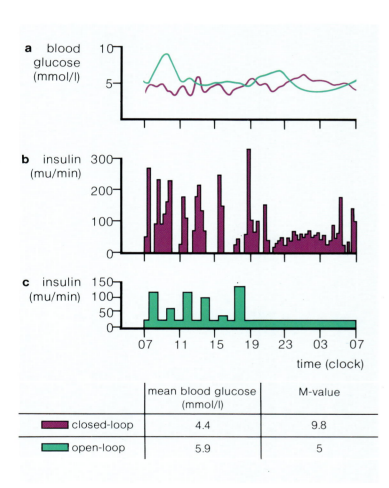

	mean blood glucose (mmol/l)	M-value
closed-loop	4.4	9.8
open-loop	5.9	5

Fig. 15.6 Illustration of the comparable results obtained with closed-loop and open-loop systems. Graph (a) shows blood glucose control throughout the day in a diabetic patient treated by either a closed-loop device or a portable open-loop intravenous infusion system. Note the equivalent degree of near-normoglycaemia.

Graphs (b) and (c) show the insulin infusion profile during closed-loop or open-loop treatment. The box insert shows the mean daily blood glucose and M-value on both regimes. The M-value is a mathematical derivation of the blood glucose and an index of control which gives extra weighting for hypoglycaemia; the normal range is 0–4.

Fig. 15.7 Portable syringe pump used for CSII. The Nordisk Infuser is an example of a syringe pump used for open-loop insulin delivery. The delivery cannula incorporates a 25G winged needle (a). The basal rate can be altered by rotary switches inside the pump (b). The pre-prandial insulin boost is activated by pressing a button on the side of the infuser.

Diabetic patients can achieve and maintain near-normoglycaemia and lowered glycosylated haemoglobin concentrations for periods of years using CSII (Figs 15.9–15.11). Infection and severe lipodystrophy at the infusion site occur only occasionally, particularly if the site is regularly changed. Accompanying the strict glycaemic control there is a return towards normal of other metabolites such as lactate, ketone bodies and lipids, and hormones such as glucagon (Fig. 15.12). There is also evidence that exercise-induced hypoglycaemia is less manifest during CSII than during conventional injection treatment.

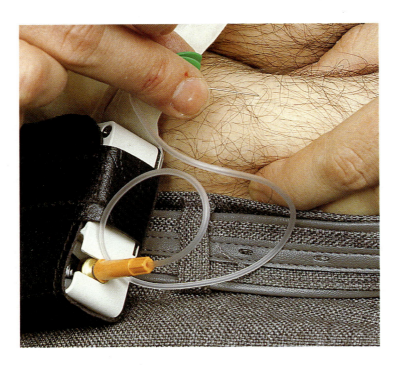

Fig. 15.8 Patient wearing an infusion pump attached to a belt. The delivery cannula is inserted in the subcutaneous tissue of the anterior abdominal wall.

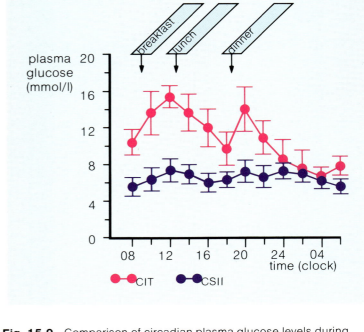

Fig. 15.9 Comparison of circadian plasma glucose levels during treatment with conventional insulin treatment (CIT) and CSII. Circadian plasma glucose concentrations were measured in nine insulin-dependent diabetic patients who were treated in random order by either CIT or CSII. The period of CSII therapy was three weeks. Values represent mean and SEM calculated from a day profile performed in hospital on each regimen.

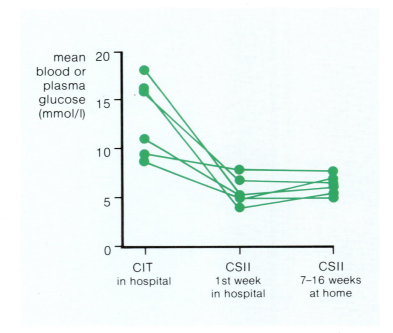

Fig. 15.10 Illustration of the effectiveness of CSII in long-term therapy. Blood or plasma glucose concentrations in six insulin-dependent diabetic patients during CIT, after stabilization in hospital on CSII and during long-term CSII at home. Results for hospital samples were for plasma and home values were calculated as the mean of all self-monitored capillary blood samples using Dextrostix.

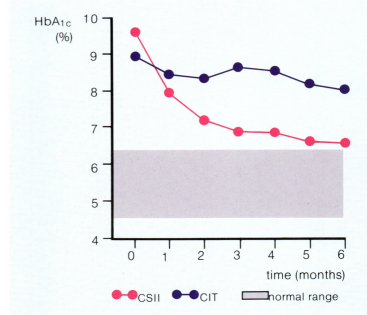

Fig. 15.11 Comparison of glycosylated haemoglobin levels during long-term treatment with CIT and CSII. The percentage of glycosylated haemoglobin (HbA1c) in diabetic patients, randomly assigned to either unchanged conventional treatment or CSII, was measured over a period of six months.

Consequences of CSII

Research into the effect of CSII on diabetic complications is very active. Just a few days of CSII-induced strict control reduces the elevated microalbuminuria present in some conventionally treated patients (Fig. 15.13), arguing against structural causes such as basement membrane thickening for the increased glomerular capillary permeability. Unfortunately, in most diabetic patients with severe nephropathy and persistent proteinuria, up to two years of CSII does not alter indices of renal function such as macroalbuminuria, or the decline of glomerular filtration rate.

Short-term CSII reverses various indices reflecting retinal capillary permeability such as vitreous fluorescence. Several major clinical trials are in progress which randomly assign diabetic patients with early background retinopathy either to their unchanged injection treatment or to CSII. Retinopathy is assessed by fundus photographs and serial fluorescein angiograms.

First results show that after an initial slight deterioration, the progress of retinopathy is slower in CSII-treated patients than in those on conventional injection therapy. With diabetic peripheral neuropathy, CSII has been shown to increase motor nerve conduction velocities and to give symptomatic improvement to some patients with painful neuropathy.

Future Developments in CSII

The clinical role of CSII in the routine treatment of diabetic patients is as yet uncertain and will partly depend on technological developments. Infusers are being developed which are not only smaller and lighter and have alarm systems for events such as malfunction and low battery state, but have more flexible rate adjustments such as the facility for automatic basal rate changes at pre-set times during the day or night (Fig. 15.14).

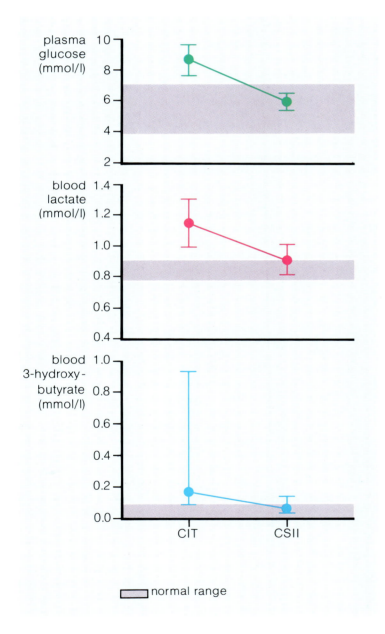

normal range

Fig. 15.12 Blood or plasma metabolite levels during CIT and CSII in seven insulin-dependent diabetic patients. Values represent the mean ± SEM (glucose and lactate) or the mean ± range (3-hydroxybutyrate) of the daily levels for each patient. The normal range for non-diabetic patients (mean ± 2 SD) is shown.

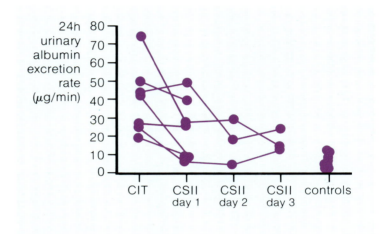

Fig. 15.13 Illustration of the reduction of urinary albumin excretion rate achieved by CSII therapy. Twenty-four-hour urinary albumin excretion was measured by radioimmunoassay in seven insulin-dependent diabetic patients treated by either CIT or 1–3 days of strict glycaemic control achieved by CSII. Non-diabetic control values are also shown.

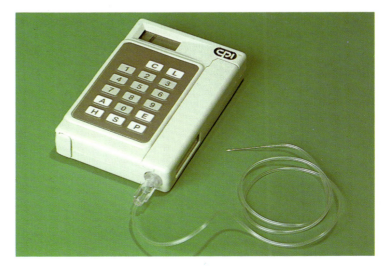

Fig. 15.14 Infusion pump for CSII with facility for sophisticated rate changes (CPI Betatron II, CPI Inc.).

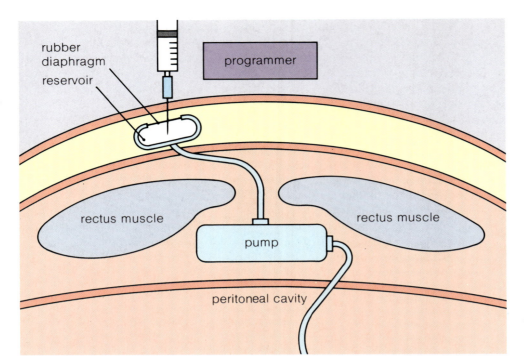

Fig. 15.15 Implanted open-loop insulin infusion device with intraperitoneal delivery of insulin. Pump rates are controlled from an external programmer. An insulin reservoir is sited just below the skin; refill is by injection through the skin and puncture of a resealable rubber diaphragm. The peristaltic pump is located below the rectus muscles, with an output cannula inserted into the peritoneal cavity.

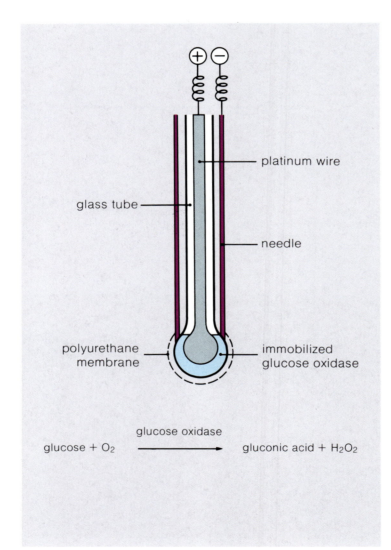

Fig. 15.16 Diagram of a needle-type implantable glucose sensor based on electrochemical detection of hydrogen peroxide.

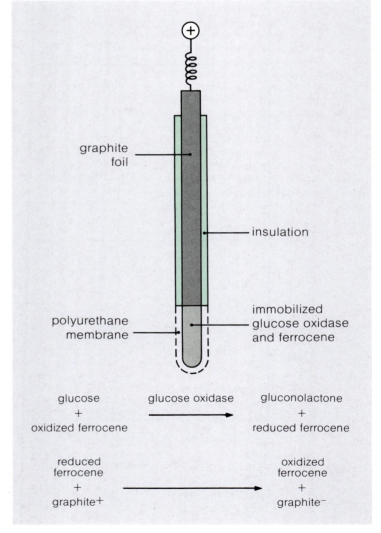

Fig. 15.17 Diagram of an implantable glucose sensor based on ferrocene-mediated electron transfer. In this type of sensor, molecular oxygen is not the final electron acceptor and the device is relatively insensitive to changes in oxygen tension at the site of implantation.

Alternative delivery routes for insulin infusion are being explored and one of the most promising is intraperitoneal (Fig. 15.15). Both extracorporeal and totally implanted open-loop intraperitoneal pumps are undergoing trial. Enthusiasts are encouraged by the possibility of slightly more rapid absorption of insulin delivered to the peritoneum compared to subcutaneous sites and the theoretical advantages of presumed absorption into the hepatic portal circulation.

This last point may account for the lower peripheral plasma free-insulin levels which have been reported for intraperitoneal delivery compared to continuous intravenous, subcutaneous and AEP treatments. Implanted pumps may also be less prone to mechanical damage and they reduce infection from outside sources. Disadvantages include the danger of reservoir leakage, the need for multiple refill through the skin, the need for operative procedures for implantation and the risk of aggregation and precipitation of insulin when kept in a reservoir for more than a few days at body temperature. The solutions to these problems are being actively pursued.

DEVELOPMENTS IN GLUCOSE SENSORS

Implantable electrodes are now being developed for continuous glucose sensing and for eventual closed-loop operation of portable insulin delivery systems. Although many sensing strategies have been proposed, they mainly fall into the categories of amperometric (current-measuring) and potentiometric (voltage-measuring) enzyme electrodes, electrocatalytic sensors, which use a noble metal as a catalyst, and optical devices. With the enzyme electrode which has been investigated the most, immobilized glucose oxidase catalyses the oxidation of glucose and the hydrogen peroxide which is produced is detected electrochemically at a positively charged platinum wire (Fig. 15.16).

An alternative amperometric enzyme electrode (Fig. 15.17) uses an organic mediator such as ferrocene, an iron-containing compound, to shuttle electrons from glucose to a graphite base electrode, without the intervention of molecular oxygen. These sensors have the advantage of being insensitive to changes in the partial pressure of oxygen at the implantation site.

Both types of sensor have been successfully tested *in vivo*, using the subcutaneous tissue as an implantation site, and the hydrogen peroxide-detecting electrode has been coupled to an infusion pump in a prototype artificial pancreas that can be worn.

REFERENCES

Albisser AM, Leibel BS, Ewart TG, Davidovac Z, Botz CK, Zingg W, Schipper H & Gander R (1974) Clinical control of diabetes by the artificial pancreas. *Diabetes*, **23**, 397–404.

Claremont DJ, Sambrook IE, Penton C & Pickup JC (1986) Subcutaneous implantation of a ferrocene-mediated glucose sensor in pigs. *Diabetologia*, **29**, 817–821.

Irsigler K & Kritz H (1979) Long-term continuous intravenous insulin therapy with a portable insulin dosage-regulating apparatus. *Diabetes*, **28**, 196–203.

Pickup JC & Keen H (1979) The value of good control. *Irish Journal of Medical Science*, **148** (suppl. 2), 54–62.

Pickup JC, Keen H, Parsons JA, Alberti KGMM & Rowe AS (1979) Continuous subcutaneous insulin infusion: improved blood glucose and intermediary metabolite control in diabetics. *Lancet*, **1**, 1255–1258.

Pickup JC & Rothwell D (1984) Technology and the diabetic patient. *Medical and Biological Engineering and Computing*, **22**, 385–400.

Pickup JC, White MC, Keen H, Kohner EM, Parsons JA & Alberti KGMM (1979) Long-term continuous subcutaneous insulin infusion in diabetics at home. *Lancet*, **2**, 870–873.

Schade DS, Eaton RP, Edwards WS, Doberneck RC, Spencer WJ, Carlson GA, Bair RE, Love JT, Urenda RS & Gaona JI Jr (1982) A remotely programmable insulin delivery system. Successful short-term implantation in man. *Journal of the American Medical Association*, **247**, 1848–1853.

Schlichtkrull J, Munck O & Jersild M (1965) The M-value, an index of blood sugar control in diabetics. *Acta Medica Scandinavica*, **177**, 95–102.

Service FJ, Molnar GD, Rosevear JW, Ackerman E, Gatewood LC & Taylor WF (1970) Mean amplitude of glycemic excursions, a measure of diabetic instability. *Diabetes*, **19**, 644–655.

Steno Study Group (1982) Effect of 6 months of strict metabolic control on eye and kidney function in insulin-dependent diabetics with background retinopathy. *Lancet*, **1**, 121–124.

Viberti GC, Pickup JC, Bilous RW, Keen H & Mackintosh D (1981) Correction of exercise-induced microalbuminuria in insulin-dependent diabetics after 3 weeks of subcutaneous insulin infusion. *Diabetes*, **30**, 818–823.

Viberti GC, Pickup JC, Jarrett RJ & Keen H (1979) Effect of control of blood glucose on urinary excretion of albumin and β_2-microglobulin in insulin-dependent diabetics. *New England Journal of Medicine*, **300**, 638–641.

16 Antibodies to Insulin

Antony B Kurtz PhD FRCP

Insulin is immunogenic because it is a protein. In the 1920's insulin preparations were associated with skin reactions which were probably caused by contaminants. In the 1930's insulin resistance, caused by antibodies capable of neutralizing insulin, was documented in a patient undergoing insulin shock therapy. During the 1950's it was realized that nearly all insulin-treated diabetic patients had circulating antibodies to insulin.

Immunogenicity can be related to the presence of proinsulin and polymerized insulin in insulin preparations. In addition, bovine insulin appears to be more immunogenic than porcine or human insulin. In insulin formulations, the absorption of insulin can be retarded by precipitating the insulin either with protamine (a basic polypeptide; Fig. 16.1) or a high zinc concentration (Fig. 16.2).

Insulin administration can cause Type I urticarial skin reactions, delayed skin reactions and occasionally anaphylaxis. Type I reactions can occur to protamine and delayed skin sensitivity can be caused by zinc. A common side-effect of insulin is lipohypertrophy at injection sites (Fig. 16.3). This is a direct local effect of

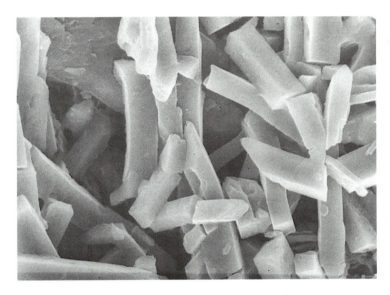

Fig. 16.1 Isophane or neutral protamine Hagedorn (NPH) insulin. An insulin preparation at neutral pH without excess protamine or zinc (magnification × 10,000).

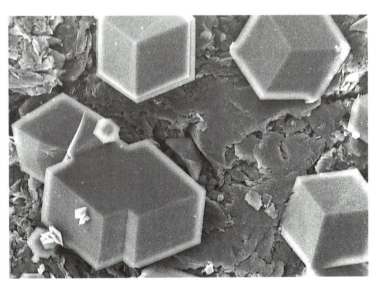

Fig. 16.2 Lente insulin. This is a mixture of 70% crystalline insulin and 30% amorphous insulin (magnification × 10,000).

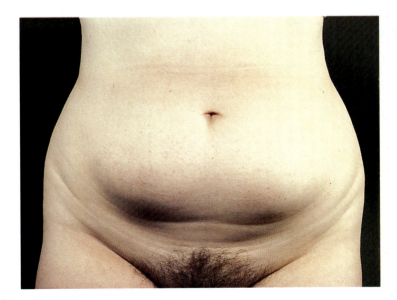
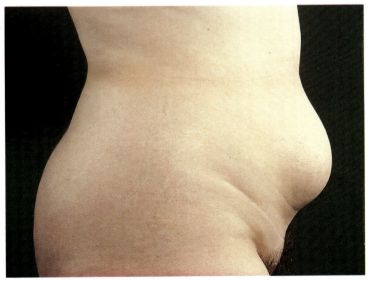

Fig. 16.3 Lipohypertrophy at injection sites on the abdomen. This localized hypertrophy of adipose tissue is a direct result of insulin action on fat cells.

insulin rather than an immunological problem. Lipoatrophy, on the other hand (Fig. 16.4), is caused by an immunological process in which immunoglobulins react with insulin and are deposited in the affected areas. With the increasing use of insulins of high purity all of these local reactions, apart from lipohypertrophy, are rarely seen.

INSULIN-TO-ANTIBODY BINDING

Insulin can be bound to antibody in the circulation. The possible presence of antibodies can be assessed by incubating serum with labelled insulin and determining the percentage of labelled insulin bound to antibody. An alternative method is measurement of the concentration of antibody-bound insulin in the circulation. The size of the antibody-bound pool of insulin varies widely from patient to patient and can be considerable. This insulin pool is biologically available as, by dissociation, it is in equilibrium with free insulin (Fig. 16.5).

In insulin-treated diabetic patients, insulin is available from several sources: subcutaneous injection sites, residual secretion from pancreatic islet B cells and from the bound pool (Fig. 16.6).

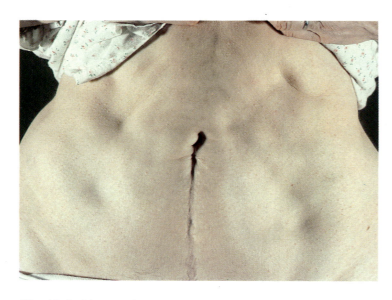

Fig. 16.4 Lipoatrophy at multiple injection sites on the abdomen. Localized disappearance of subcutaneous fat is the result of an immunological process in which immunoglobulins react with insulin and are deposited in the affected area. It is sometimes also seen at non-injection sites. With the increasingly widespread use of highly purified insulins, it is seen rarely now.

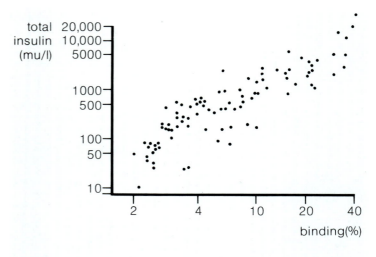

Fig. 16.5 Relationship between the binding of labelled insulin by serum and the total concentration of insulin. The size of the antibody-bound insulin pool can be considerable and varies widely between patients.

Fig. 16.6 The various sources of insulin in the insulin-treated diabetic patient. Insulin may come from the subcutaneous injection site, the pancreatic islet B cells, if there is residual secretion, and from the antibody-bound pool.

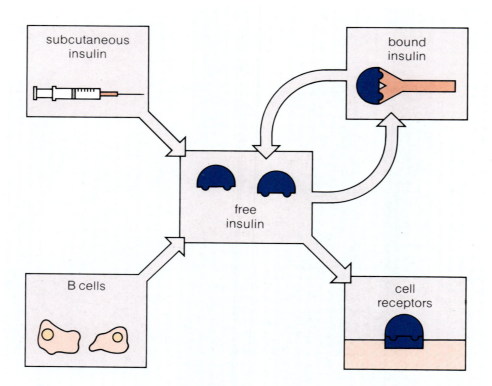

The effect of an antibody-bound pool of insulin can be seen when insulin treatment is stopped; patients, selected because of absent endogenous insulin secretion, were treated with intravenous insulin in order to deplete their subcutaneous insulin depots; the infusion was then stopped. The results from two subjects, one with and one without antibodies to insulin, are shown in Fig. 16.7. Insulin supplied from the bound insulin pool maintained an effective free insulin concentration for twelve hours in the patient with antibodies. In the patient without antibodies there was a rapid fall in free insulin and a rise in blood glucose concentration after insulin withdrawal.

CONCLUSION

Over recent years there has been a shift towards treatment with insulins of increasing purity as well as a tendency towards the use of human insulin rather than either porcine or bovine. With the use of less immunogenic insulins, insulin antibody levels in patients are falling. High levels were found in a clinic population treated with conventional bovine insulin (Fig. 16.8) while in a group treated with highly purified porcine insulin much lower

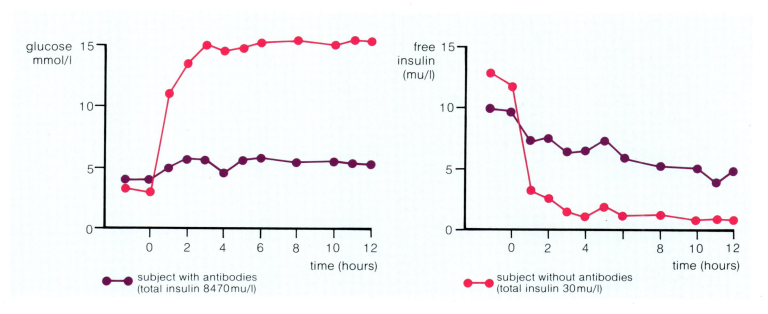

Fig. 16.7   Results of insulin withdrawal in one subject with and one without insulin antibodies. Both had their subcutaneous insulin reserves entirely depleted during a prolonged intravenous insulin infusion. When the infusion was stopped, insulin released from the bound pool maintained near-normoglycaemia in the subject with antibodies for nearly twelve hours. The antibody-free subject showed a rapid rise in blood glucose and a fall in free insulin.

Fig. 16.8   Frequency distribution of insulin binding in patients treated with conventional bovine insulin. Out of 210 patients, only four (1.9%) had 2% or less bound insulin. The median value was 18.5% bound insulin.

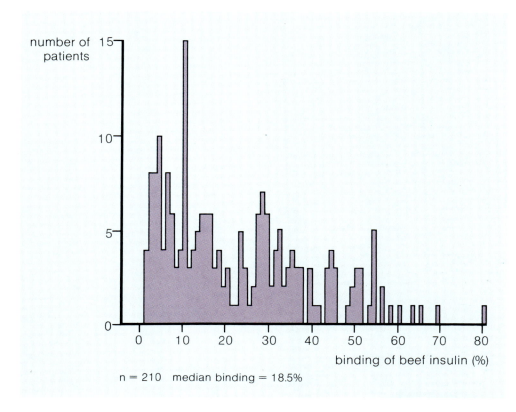

levels occurred (Fig. 16.9). Similarly, low antibody levels have been reported in patients treated with human insulin. Such low antibody levels are without clinical effects; there is insufficient bound insulin to act as a buffer and there is therefore no inter-ference with the duration of action of injected insulin. The prolongation of insulin action, delayed hypoglycaemia and insulin resistance, all of which are effects of very high antibody levels, are now very rare.

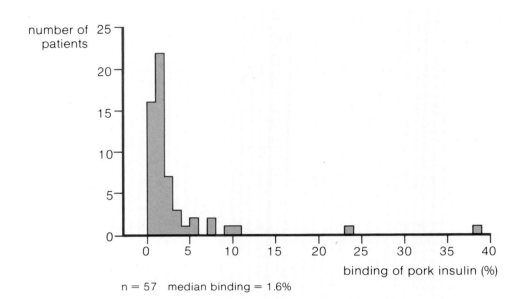

Fig. 16.9 Frequency distribution of insulin binding in patients treated with highly purified porcine insulin. Out of fifty-seven patients, thirty-eight (67%) had 2% or less bound insulin. The median value was only 1.6% bound insulin.

REFERENCES

Kurtz AB & Nabarro JDN (1980) Circulating insulin-binding antibodies. *Diabetologia*, **19**, 329–334.
Vaughan NJA, Matthews JA, Kurtz AB & Nabarro JDN (1983) The bioavailability of circulating antibody-bound insulin following insulin withdrawal in Type I (insulin-dependent) diabetes. *Diabetologia*, **24**, 355–358.

17 Oral Hypoglycaemic Agents

Donald WM Pearson BSc MB ChB MRCP ● **John M Stowers** MA MB BChir MD FRCP FRCOG

Oral hypoglycaemic drugs are clinically useful in Type II (non insulin-dependent) diabetic patients who have persisting hyperglycaemia despite appropriate dietary modifications; these drugs should only be used as adjuncts to dietary advice. The biochemical abnormalities of such patients are not very clearly understood and suggested explanations about the cellular mechanisms of action of glucose-lowering drugs are mainly based on *in vitro* experiments. In Type II diabetes, fasting hyperglycaemia results from excessive glucose production by the liver and diminished glucose uptake by the insulin-sensitive cells in muscle and adipose tissue (Fig. 17.1). This may occur despite normal or even high fasting insulin levels, particularly in overweight patients.

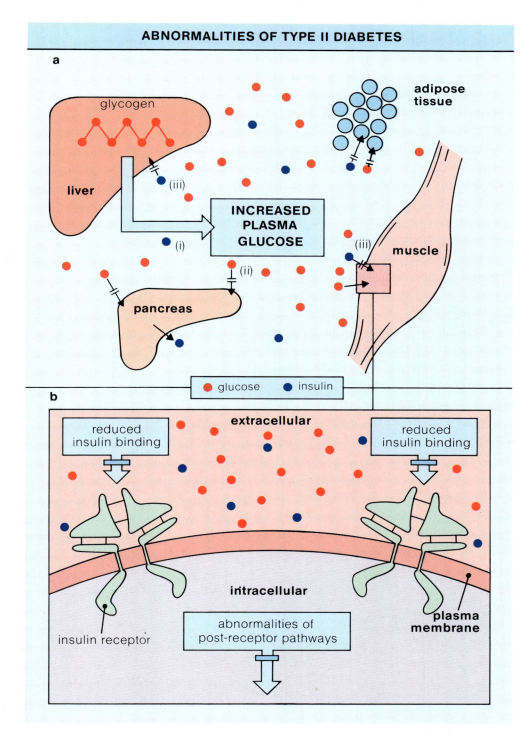

Fig. 17.1 Abnormalities in Type II diabetes. (a) the problems as illustrated here are: (i) fasting hyperglycaemia despite measurable circulating insulin; (ii) impaired pancreatic response to hyperglycaemia; and (iii) diminished degree and extent of the response of the liver and peripheral insulin-dependent tissues to insulin. (b) the cellular abnormalities are due to reduced insulin binding to membrane receptors and defects in post-receptor metabolic pathways.

ABNORMALITIES OF TYPE II DIABETES

Although the fasting insulin level may be elevated or normal, there is an impaired insulin response to an oral glucose load or a meal. Correction of the metabolic abnormalities would require both a direct pancreatic effect, to increase the sensitivity of the B cells to circulating glucose, and an effect on non-pancreatic tissue to give a normal physiological response to circulating insulin. The two groups of drugs most commonly used in clinical practice as glucose-lowering agents are the sulphonylureas and the biguanides (Fig. 17.2).

SULPHONYLUREAS
Mode of Action
Clinical studies have shown an improved insulin response to a glucose load when sulphonylureas are given in the acute situation to Type II diabetic subjects (Figs 17.3 and 17.4). However, early animal experiments revealed the need for an intact pancreas to ensure drug activity. This improved pancreatic response to hyperglycaemia is thought to be mediated by cyclic AMP. After chronic administration when a patient has normal pre- and post-prandial glucose levels, fasting insulin levels are similar to those of non-diabetic subjects and the longer term effect of these drugs appears to be mainly on non-pancreatic tissue. A direct hepatic effect of sulphonylureas has been suggested with a reduction of hepatic glucose output and also an increase in membrane insulin binding in adipocytes and lymphocytes (Fig. 17.4).

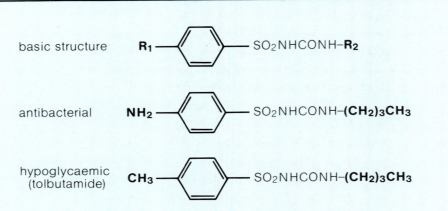

CHEMICAL STRUCTURES OF SULPHONYLUREAS

basic structure R_1 — ⬡ — $SO_2NHCONH$–R_2

antibacterial NH_2 — ⬡ — $SO_2NHCONH$–$(CH_2)_3CH_3$

hypoglycaemic (tolbutamide) CH_3 — ⬡ — $SO_2NHCONH$–$(CH_2)_3CH_3$

name	R_1	R_2
tolbutamide	CH_3	$(CH_2)_3CH_3$
chlorpropamide	Cl	$(CH_2)_2CH_3$
tolazamide	CH_3	$-N\bigcirc$
acetohexamide	CH_3CO	$\bigcirc$
glibenclamide	Cl / $-CONH(CH_2)_2-$ / OCH_3	$\bigcirc$
gliclazide	CH_3	$-N\bigcirc$
glipizide	N / $-CONH(CH_2)_2-$ / CH_3	$\bigcirc$
glibornuride	CH_3	$HO\bigcirc$
gliquidone	CH_3 CH_3 / $N-CH_2$ / CH_2- (dioxo-isoindoline)	$\bigcirc$

Fig. 17.2 Basic sulphonylurea structure and its derivatives. The hypoglycaemic effect of sulphonylureas was discovered by chance in the 1940's when Loubatières was assessing a sulphonamide derivative for its antibacterial action. If the amino group of the antibacterial sulphonamide is replaced by a methyl group (tolbutamide), the antibacterial properties of the sulphonylurea are lost but the substance retains its hypoglycaemic properties. Modifications of the side-chains R_1 and R_2 produce a range of drugs with varying chemical properties.

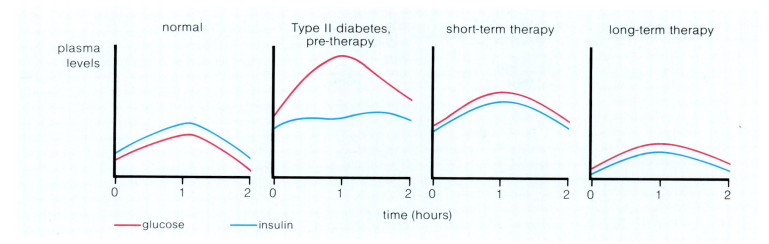

normal　　　Type II diabetes, pre-therapy　　　short-term therapy　　　long-term therapy

plasma levels

time (hours)

—— glucose　　　—— insulin

Fig. 17.3 Mode of action of sulphonylureas. The plasma insulin and glucose response to an oral glucose load in a non-diabetic individual, a newly diagnosed Type II diabetic subject and after both acute and chronic sulphonylurea therapy in Type II diabetic patients.

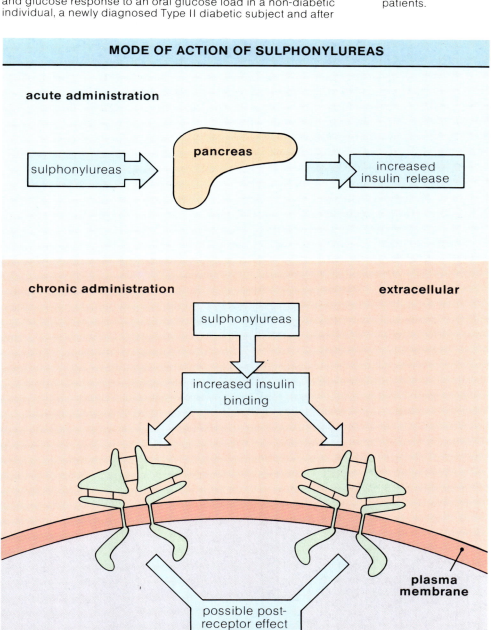

MODE OF ACTION OF SULPHONYLUREAS

acute administration

sulphonylureas → **pancreas** → increased insulin release

chronic administration　　　　　**extracellular**

sulphonylureas

increased insulin binding

possible post-receptor effect

plasma membrane

intracellular

Fig. 17.4 Mode of action of sulphonylureas after acute and chronic administration. With acute administration, sulphonylureas increase the output of insulin from the pancreas. After chronic administration, they appear to act mainly on non-pancreatic tissue by increasing membrane binding of insulin and possibly by acting at the post-receptor level.

SULPHONYLUREAS

name	duration of action (hours)	dosage range (mg)	tablet size (mg)	excretion/ metabolism	special features
first generation					
tolbutamide	6–8	500–3000	250, 500	hepatic	
chlorpropamide	36+	100–500	100, 250	renal	avoid in elderly or in renal failure
tolazamide	12–24	100–750	100, 250	hepatic	
acetohexamide	12–18	500–1500	250, 500	hepatic	
second generation					
glibenclamide	5–20	2.5–20	2.5, 5	hepatic	should be taken just before meals
glipizide	5–12	2.5–45	5	hepatic	
glibornuride	5–12	12.5–75	12.5	hepatic	
gliclazide	5–20	40–320	80	hepatic	antiplatelet action
gliquidone	5	15–180	30	hepatic	useful in renal failure
related compound					
glymidine	12–24	500–2000	500		no cross-allergenicity

Fig. 17.5 Characteristics of the sulphonylureas. All are metabolized in the liver, but only slightly in the case of chlorpropamide.

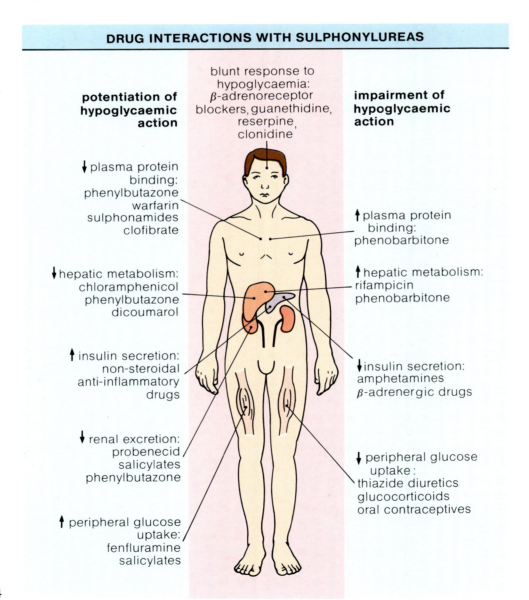

DRUG INTERACTIONS WITH SULPHONYLUREAS

potentiation of hypoglycaemic action

blunt response to hypoglycaemia: β-adrenoreceptor blockers, guanethidine, reserpine, clonidine

impairment of hypoglycaemic action

↓ plasma protein binding: phenylbutazone warfarin sulphonamides clofibrate

↑ plasma protein binding: phenobarbitone

↓ hepatic metabolism: chloramphenicol phenylbutazone dicoumarol

↑ hepatic metabolism: rifampicin phenobarbitone

↑ insulin secretion: non-steroidal anti-inflammatory drugs

↓ insulin secretion: amphetamines β-adrenergic drugs

↓ renal excretion: probenecid salicylates phenylbutazone

↑ peripheral glucose uptake: fenfluramine salicylates

↓ peripheral glucose uptake: thiazide diuretics glucocorticoids oral contraceptives

Fig. 17.6 Effects of various drugs on the action of sulphonylureas.

Characteristics

The main clinical indication for sulphonylurea therapy is in the non-obese Type II diabetic individual who has not responded to dietary advice. A selection of drugs is available, since modification of the basic structure (see Fig. 17.2) has produced a range of drugs with varying potency, duration of action, metabolic fate, route of excretion and side-effects (Fig. 17.5). The original (first generation) sulphonylurea compounds are still in widespread clinical use and can effectively control hyperglycaemia, but in some patients second generation drugs have clinical advantages, although they are more expensive.

The drugs are usually taken shortly before meals and are rapidly absorbed in the small intestine. They are transported in the plasma tightly bound to serum proteins, particularly albumin, which has almost limitless binding sites. Tolbutamide and chlorpropamide bind to albumin by ionic forces, whereas glibenclamide, glipizide and glibornuride bind by non-ionic forces. The drugs are transported to tissues where interaction with cell membranes produces the recognized biological effects. The route of degradation and excretion of sulphonylureas is shown in Fig. 17.5. Chlorpropamide virtually escapes hepatic metabolism and is only slowly eliminated from the body, especially in the presence of renal failure or in the elderly. It should therefore be avoided in these situations where it can produce profound and prolonged hypoglycaemia from unintentional overdosage. In contrast, drugs such as glibenclamide act quickly and can produce sudden onset of hypoglycaemia.

It has been suggested that gliclazide may have a beneficial effect on the haemostatic system of Type II diabetic subjects and thereby reduces the chances of developing micro- and macrovascular disease. It is uncertain, however, if this effect is due to the drug itself or is simply a result of the improved glycaemic control associated with it.

Drug Interaction with Sulphonylureas

Sulphonylureas can be displaced from binding proteins in the plasma by other protein-bound drugs leading to a potentiation of the hypoglycaemic effect (Fig. 17.6). Sulphonylureas, other than chlorpropamide, mainly undergo hepatic metabolism and certain drugs decrease hepatic metabolism leading to prolongation of the effective half-life of sulphonylureas. Sympathetic nervous system depressants as well as β-adrenoreceptor blockers may render the patient less aware of hypoglycaemia and, in addition, may impair compensatory responses to it, especially if non-selective β-blockers are used. However, in clinical practice the incidence of β-blocker associated hypoglycaemia is very low, but clinicians should be aware of this possibility. Rarely, non-steroidal anti-inflammatory drugs may potentiate the hypoglycaemic action of sulphonylurea drugs by increased insulin secretion or increased peripheral uptake of glucose. The former effect may be prostaglandin-mediated, but the mechanism of the latter effect is uncertain.

A number of drugs are known to antagonize the hypoglycaemic action of sulphonylureas and thus care should be taken to decrease sulphonylurea dosage when such interacting drugs are discontinued.

Side-effects

Side-effects are unusual and rarely serious (Fig. 17.7). Gastrointestinal disturbance with nausea, anorexia and vomiting may occur. Facial flushing after alcohol is also a well-recognized effect of tolbutamide or chlorpropamide (Fig. 17.8). The mechanism of the chlorpropamide-alcohol flush is uncertain. Initially the effect was thought to characterize patients who were less susceptible to diabetic retinopathy, but some recent evidence suggests that the trait does not distinguish groups having a low risk of complications.

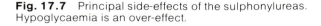

SIDE-EFFECTS OF SULPHONYLUREAS
alcohol flush
skin rash
anorexia
nausea
jaundice
exfoliative dermatitis (rare)
blood dyscrasias (rare)

Fig. 17.7 Principal side-effects of the sulphonylureas. Hypoglycaemia is an over-effect.

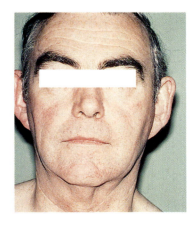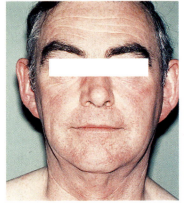

Fig. 17.8 Alcohol flush. Facial appearance of a patient on chlorpropamide before and after taking alcohol. A pronounced facial flush can be seen.

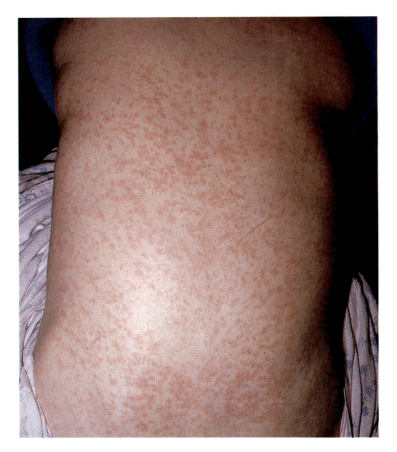

During the first two months of treatment, transient rashes (Fig. 17.9) may be noted and only rarely do these progress to erythema multiforme or an exfoliative dermatitis. Cholestatic jaundice has been recorded with chlorpropamide and this resolves after the drug is discontinued. Blood dyscrasias such as thrombocytopenia, agranulocytosis and aplastic anaemia are very rare side-effects. Dilutional hyponatraemia after chlorpropamide may occur due to increased renal sensitivity to vasopressin (antidiuretic hormone).

Indications for Substitution by Insulin Therapy

If a patient on sulphonylurea therapy develops an intercurrent illness, such as myocardial infarction or a severe infection, the drug should be temporarily discontinued and hyperglycaemia controlled by insulin therapy. During major surgical procedures it is prudent to use insulin rather than a sulphonylurea for control of hyperglycaemia in the perioperative period. If maximal doses of sulphonylureas and dietary adherence do not control hyperglycaemia, the addition of metformin will improve glycaemic control, but many such patients will later need insulin to achieve good results.

Fig. 17.9 Skin rash on back. Transient rashes may occur during the first few months of sulphonylurea treatment.

Fig. 17.10 Structure of guanidine, diguanidine and the biguanides.

STRUCTURE OF GUANIDINES AND BIGUANIDES

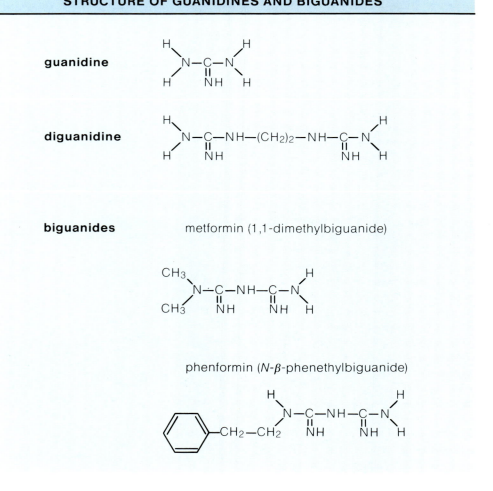

BIGUANIDES

The extract of the plant *Galega officinalis* was recognized to be useful in the treatment of diabetes many years ago due to the presence of galegin, a monoguanide, in the extract. In animals, guanidine (Fig. 17.10) has a hypoglycaemic effect but it is unsuitable for clinical use because of its toxicity. Diguanidine compounds are also toxic but substitution of the linking carbon groups with a nitrogen link produces a less toxic group of compounds, the biguanides. Metformin (1,1-dimethylbiguanide) is the only biguanide in widespread clinical use and at present it is regarded as the oral hypoglycaemic agent of choice in obese Type II diabetic individuals who have persisting hyperglycaemia after appropriate dietary modification.

Other biguanides have not been widely used since phenformin has been withdrawn due to its association with lactic acidosis. The tendency to lactic acidosis is much less with metformin and this difference can be explained by the chemical structure of the two biguanides. Metformin is bisubstituted and this ensures metabolic stability. Phenformin (*N*–β-phenylethylbiguanide) is monosubstituted and has a long lipophilic side-chain. This side-chain influences the type of membrane to which a biguanide will bind and phenformin is bound to mitochondrial membranes to a much greater extent than metformin. Binding to mitochondrial membranes interferes with oxidative phosphorylation and may favour the production of lactic acid by anaerobic pathways.

Cellular Mode of Action

In vitro, metformin will affect many metabolic processes not only in mammalian cells but also in bacteria, fungi, chloroplasts and chromatophores. It is unlikely that metformin exerts its effect by direct interaction with individual enzyme systems and its major effects seem to result from an alteration in the charge distribution or net charge on biological membranes. Properties of individual membranes depend upon the lipid/protein constitution of the membrane and metformin perhaps alters either the protein composition or relative protein/lipid conformation of various tissue membranes to allow, for example, increased insulin binding (Fig. 17.11). Increased insulin binding to erythrocytes which are unable to synthesize new protein has been demonstrated; increased binding to insulin-sensitive cells such as adipocytes has also been shown.

In mammalian tissues, addition of metformin *in vitro* can influence mitochondrial oxidation of succinate and NADH, the turnover of the citric acid cycle, incorporation of acetate into liver lipids, oxidative phosphorylation, gluconeogenesis in the liver and kidney and intestinal uptake of glucose. The drug inhibits cellular respiration *in vitro* and affects ATP production by a direct mitochondrial membrane effect.

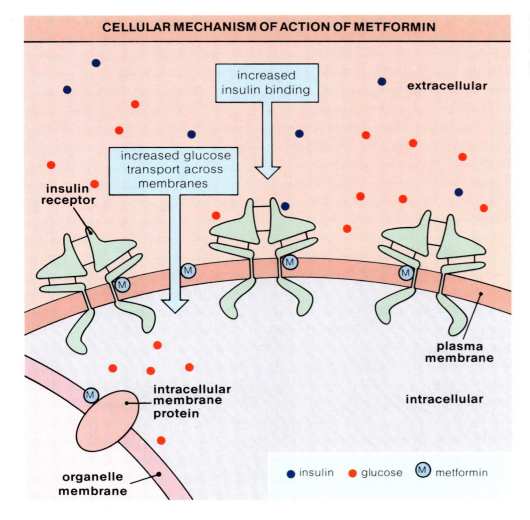

Fig. 17.11 Mechanism of action of metformin at the cellular level. It appears to bind to both plasma and organelle membranes and thus influences both the passage of glucose into the cell and its utilization by mitochondria.

Mechanism of Hypoglycaemic Effect

The biguanides have no hypoglycaemic effect in non-diabetic subjects. In Type II diabetic subjects, where the drugs have been clearly shown to reduce elevated blood glucose levels, the hypoglycaemic effect of biguanides is thought to result from a combination of reduced intestinal glucose absorption, decreased gluconeogenesis, increased anaerobic glycolysis and enhanced muscle uptake of glucose (Fig. 17.12). The hypoglycaemic effect is not caused by an increase of endogenous insulin secretion, although insulin is necessary for the therapeutic effect of the drug. The drug also reduces appetite. Since it does not have the lipogenic effect of sulphonylureas, it is useful in the management of Type II diabetic patients who are overweight.

Weight-reducing Effect

Clinical experience in several studies has shown that metformin therapy produces weight loss in obese people with Type II diabetes mellitus. There is often a marked initial fall followed by a period of stabilization (Fig. 17.13a). While anorexia may be part of the mechanism involved in weight loss, energy balance studies have revealed that the extent of weight loss is greater than would be expected purely on the basis of reduced energy intake

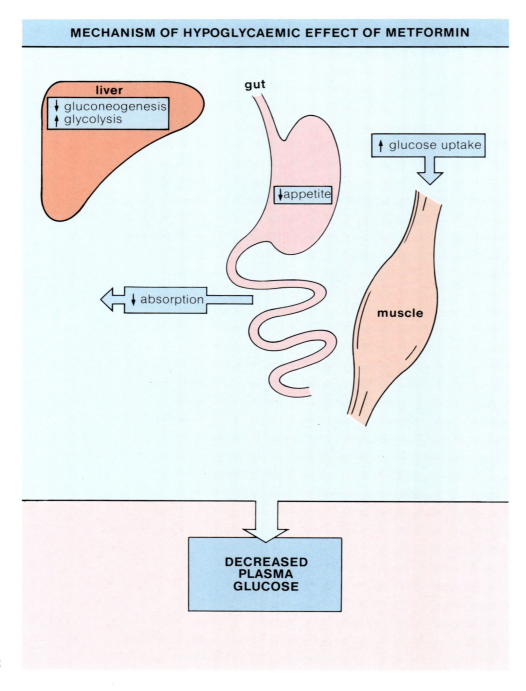

MECHANISM OF HYPOGLYCAEMIC EFFECT OF METFORMIN

liver
- ↓ gluconeogenesis
- ↑ glycolysis

gut

↑ glucose uptake

↓ appetite

↓ absorption

muscle

DECREASED PLASMA GLUCOSE

Fig. 17.12 Mechanism of the hypoglycaemic effect of metformin. Metformin suppresses appetite with the appropriate dose, reduces intestinal glucose transport, reduces gluconeogenesis and may enhance glycolysis, and increases the uptake of glucose by muscle.

(Fig. 17.13b). Weight reduction is not correlated with changes in blood glucose, but is related to the reduction of hyperinsulinaemia which follows the introduction of metformin therapy. Several studies indicate the role of malabsorption in weight loss, particularly at high dosages.

Patients are usually started on a small dose of metformin taking 500mg twice daily to minimize the incidence of gastrointestinal upset. This dose can be gradually increased at two-weekly intervals until blood glucose levels are controlled. In some patients, doses up to 3g daily may be required. In obese subjects, the dose may be adjusted not only according to blood glucose levels but also if there is a failure to lose weight. Hypoglycaemia is not associated with high doses of metformin unless used in association with either a sulphonylurea or insulin.

Effect on Glucose and Insulin Levels
The effect of biguanides on blood glucose and plasma insulin levels is shown in Fig. 17.14. Introduction of therapy produces a reduction of glucose and insulin in response to a glucose load. This would be in keeping with the mechanism of action proposed above suggesting an effect of metformin on glucose metabolism rather than on insulin secretion.

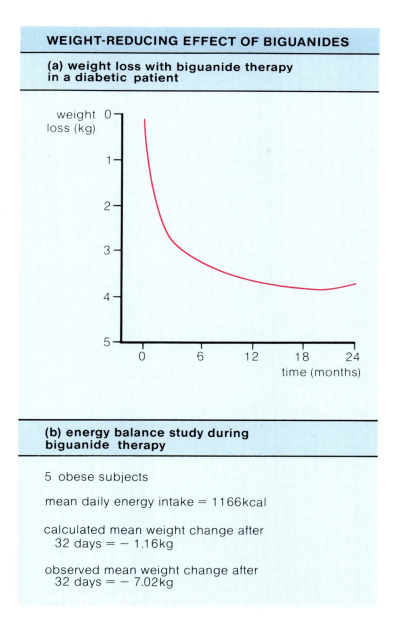

WEIGHT-REDUCING EFFECT OF BIGUANIDES

(a) weight loss with biguanide therapy in a diabetic patient

(b) energy balance study during biguanide therapy

5 obese subjects

mean daily energy intake = 1166kcal

calculated mean weight change after
   32 days = − 1.16kg

observed mean weight change after
   32 days = − 7.02kg

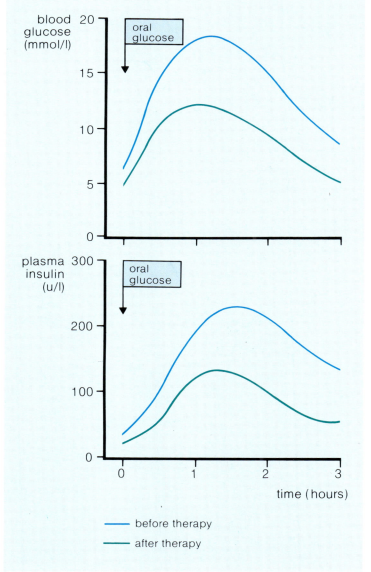

Fig. 17.13   Examples of the weight-reducing effect of biguanide therapy. (a) shows the weight loss in a patient which can occur once therapy is started. (b) shows the results of an energy balance study in five obese subjects which reveals that the weight loss which occurs with therapy is greater than would be expected purely on the basis of energy balance. The figures were obtained by comparing weight changes with and without sub-maximal doses of biguanide and taking into account food not eaten on the biguanide treatment.

Fig. 17.14   Effect of biguanides on blood glucose and plasma insulin levels. The responses before and after metformin therapy are shown.

Effect on Intestinal Absorption

Animal experiments have shown that metformin inhibits intestinal absorption of several substances and autoradiography has revealed that there is an accumulation of metformin in the intestinal mucosa. Serum vitamin B_{12} and folate concentrations may be significantly lower than normal in patients on long-term metformin therapy in a dose of at least 1.5g daily. In such patients, it is prudent to check regularly the full blood count, vitamin B_{12} and folate levels. Withdrawal of the drug shows a rise in vitamin B_{12} levels due to improved B_{12} absorption (Fig. 17.15). Neutrophil nuclear hypersegmentation also resolves when metformin is discontinued.

Route of Excretion

Metformin is rapidly absorbed and, as mentioned above, animal autoradiographic investigations have shown an accumulation of labelled metformin in the intestinal mucosa. Metformin is not protein bound in the plasma and is not metabolized but is excreted unchanged in the urine. Patients with impaired renal function have less rapid excretion of metformin and accumulation may occur in the presence of severe renal impairment.

Certain conditions will tend to predispose to enhanced action or toxicity of metformin and these include renal failure, hepatic failure, especially if there is alcoholic liver disease, and conditions predisposing to cellular ischaemia such as myocardial infarction or congestive cardiac failure.

Side-effects

Metformin reduces lactate elimination and affects mitochondrial oxidative phosphorylation and, in the presence of the various conditions discussed above, toxic levels of lactic acid may develop. The development of lactic acidosis in association with metformin therapy is very rare and in the majority of patients who have developed this complication there has been evidence of pre-existing marked renal impairment. Metformin should thus be avoided in the presence of renal failure especially in the elderly. It

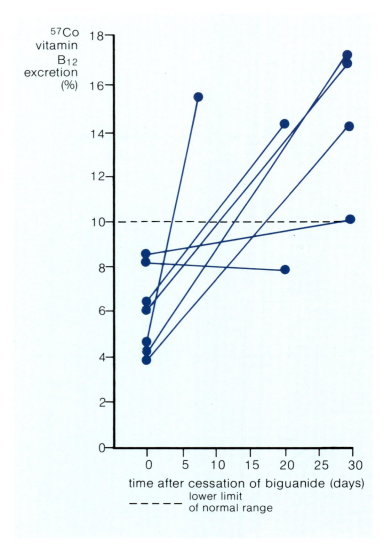

Fig. 17.15 Effect of withdrawal of biguanide on vitamin B_{12} absorption. The rate of absorption is measured indirectly by measuring the excretion of radioactively labelled cobalt in the urine.

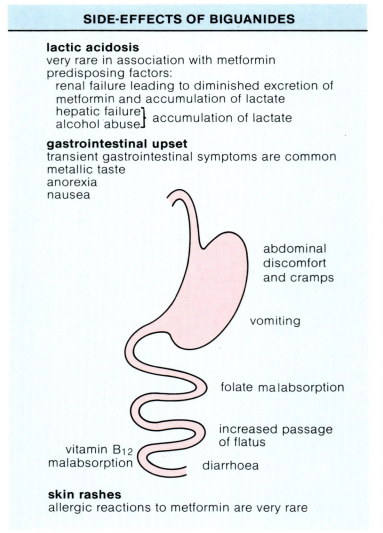

Fig. 17.16 Side-effects of biguanides.

should be remembered that the presence of severe diabetic retinopathy is usually associated with nephropathy and metformin should be avoided in this situation. Alcohol abuse and hepatic impairment predispose to the accumulation of lactic acid and metformin should be avoided here also. Lactic acidosis can arise in conditions of severe infection, dehydration or shock.

Apart from its major complications, side-effects such as anorexia, nausea, vomiting and transient diarrhoea are associated with biguanide therapy. These can usually be avoided if the patient is started on a low dose which can be increased gradually. When a patient is stabilized on long-term high doses of metformin, malabsorption of vitamin B_{12} and folate can occur as discussed above. Skin reactions and other allergic reactions to metformin are very rare. A summary of the side-effects of biguanides is shown in Fig. 17.16.

Biguanides and Lipid Metabolism

Metformin exerts an action on lipid as well as carbohydrate metabolism in diabetic individuals. The detailed molecular effect of metformin on lipolysis and lipoprotein metabolism is not well understood but elevated triglyceride and cholesterol levels may be reduced following the introduction of metformin therapy. This lipid lowering effect appears to be independent of changes in glucose tolerance, plasma insulin and body weight. In rabbit studies, metformin has a protective effect against the development of dietary induced atherosclerosis, but the significance of these findings in man is uncertain. Animal work suggests the effects on lipid turnover are related to changes in apoproteins and there is a reduction in low density lipoprotein with an increase in high density lipoprotein. Clinical studies have also shown a lipid lowering effect particularly in patients with Type IV hyper-lipoproteinaemia. A direct inhibitory action on triglyceride and cholesterol synthesis in addition to an action to reduce lipolytic rates in adipose tissue may contribute to the lipid lowering effect.

Potentiation between Sulphonylureas and Biguanides

Since there are differences in the cellular mechanism of action of sulphonylurea and biguanide drugs, it is not surprising that the drugs can be used successfully in combination if either drug fails on its own to control hyperglycaemia. Occasional patients, who would otherwise need insulin, respond to strict dietary control with a potent short-acting sulphonylurea drug and metformin. The predominant effect of sulphonylureas on fasting plasma glucose and the ability of the biguanide to reduce post-prandial hyperglycaemia is shown in Fig. 17.17.

LATEST DEVELOPMENTS

Methods which influence carbohydrate absorption have been developed to modulate post-prandial glycaemia, but unfortunately they do not correct a defect specific to Type II diabetes mellitus. Acarbose is an α-glucosidase inhibitor which blocks amylase and brush border intestinal sucrase. Although a reduction of glucose absorption occurs following ingestion of acarbose, increased quantities of disaccharides and polysaccharides reach the colon, and colonic metabolism of these carbohydrates produces a degree of flatulence and diarrhoea unacceptable to many patients.

Guar gum is derived from an Indian bean and is a high molecular weight polysaccharide, galactomannan. It is a soluble type of fibre which remains chemically unchanged until it reaches the colon, where bacteria break it down before its excretion. It has been shown to delay gastric emptying and delay the absorption of sugars, although it does not prevent their absorption; the effects occur especially when guar is mixed with food. In addition, it partially blocks the reabsorption of bile salts and this may partly explain its effect of lowering serum cholesterol in the low density lipoprotein but not the high density lipoprotein fraction. There has so far been no evidence of malabsorption of essential dietary components, such as minerals or trace elements, but guar may reduce the bio-availability of drugs such as sulphonylureas and

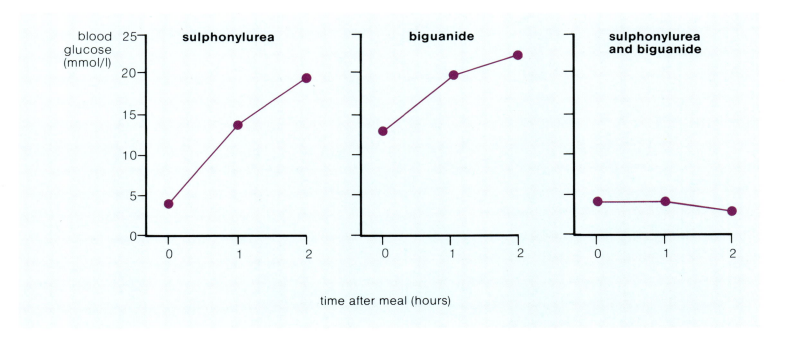

time after meal (hours)

Fig. 17.17 Potentiation between sulphonylurea and biguanide. Blood glucose responses to a meal in a Type II diabetic subject under three treatment regimens are shown. The combination of a sulphonylurea and a biguanide is most successful at preventing post-prandial hyperglycaemia.

possibly contraceptives. If there is concurrent treatment with drugs such as oral penicillins, these should be taken either one hour before or three hours after the administration of guar to ensure adequate peak levels of antibiotic.

The side-effects of guar products, as with other bulking agents, include nausea, a feeling of fullness, anorexia, flatulence and diarrhoea, but these are usually transient, especially if the dose is slowly increased. The combined use of acarbose and guar can greatly reduce post-prandial hyperglycaemia with fewer side-effects than is obtained with full dosage of either drug alone. If a diabetic diet high in fibre is adhered to, these drugs seem to have little extra to offer. It has been claimed, however, that guar can help patients who are resistent to voluntary dietary change.

CONCLUSION
If they are used with appropriate care and supervision, oral hypoglycaemic drugs are useful clinical tools in the management of obese and non-obese Type II diabetic individuals. A large study,

the University Group Diabetes Programme (UGDP), cast doubt upon the clinical use of oral hypoglycaemic agents and suggested that they may predispose to vascular complications. However, many other studies and re-examination of the original data from the UGDP have questioned such unfavourable conclusions and current evidence suggests that these drugs are useful in the long-term management of Type II diabetic patients.

The U.K. Prospective Diabetes Study has been in progress since 1978 and by January 1988 about 4000 Type II diabetic patients had been recruited in fifteen centres. Such patients are randomized to therapy with diet or diet plus either chlorpropamide, glibenclamide, or insulin, or, if the patient is overweight, metformin. Initial results have confirmed the ability of the therapeutic agents to reduce plasma glucose, but definitive information about the ability of these drugs and diet to reduce the large and small vessel disease associated with Type II diabetes is not yet available.

REFERENCES

Kilo C, Miller JP & Williamson JR (1980) The crux of the UGDP: spurious results and biologically inappropriate data analysis. *Diabetologia*, **18**, 179–185.

Lockwood DH, Gerich JE & Goldfine I (1984) Effects of oral hypoglycaemic agents on receptor and post-receptor actions of insulin. *Diabetes Care*, **7** (Suppl.1), 1–129.

Logie AW, Galloway DB & Petrie JC (1976) Drug interactions and long-term antidiabetic therapy. *British Journal of Clinical Pharmacology*, **3**, 1027–1032.

Lord JM, White SI, Bailey CJ, Atkins TW, Fletcher RF & Taylor KG (1983) Effect of metformin on insulin receptor binding and glycaemic control in Type II diabetes. *British Medical Journal*, **286**, 830–831.

Luft D, Schmülling RM & Eggstein M (1978) Lactic acidosis in biguanide-treated diabetics: a review of 330 cases. *Diabetologia*, **14**, 75–87.

Multi-centre Study (1983) UK prospective study of therapies of maturity-onset diabetes. I. Effect of diet, sulphonylurea, insulin or biguanide therapy on fasting plasma glucose and body weight over one year. *Diabetologia*, **24**, 404–411.

Multi-center Study (1985) UK prospective diabetes study II. Reduction in HbA$_{1c}$ with basal insulin supplement, sulfonylurea or biguanide therapy in maturity-onset diabetes. *Diabetes*, **34**, 793–798.

Paton RC, Kernoff PBA, Wales JK & McNicol GP (1981) Effects of diet and gliclazide on the haemostatic system of non-insulin-dependent diabetes. *British Medical Journal*, **283**, 1018–1020.

Peacock I & Tattersall RB (1984) The difficult choice of treatment for poorly controlled maturity onset diabetes: tablets or insulin? *British Medical Journal*, **288**, 1956–1959.

Stowers JM & Bewsher PD (1969) Studies on the mechanism of weight reduction by metformin. *Postgraduate Medical Journal Supplement*, **45**, 13–16.

University Group Diabetes Programme (1970) A study of the effects of hypoglycaemic agents on vascular complications in patients with adult-onset diabetes. II. Mortality results. *Diabetes*, **19**, 789–830.

18

Food and Diabetes

David R Hadden MD FRCPEd

Diabetes mellitus may be considered as a disorder of the metabolic disposal of food. The interaction of food and the diabetic state must be assessed from two aspects: first, whether food precipitates the diabetic condition and secondly, the type of food that is most appropriate for the person with established diabetes, whether it is insulin-dependent (Type I) or non insulin-dependent (Type II).

Although food science is often thought to be a difficult or obscure subject, for the diabetic patient it represents an intelligent interest in normal food and sensible eating, concepts also relevant to the general population. A proper knowledge of nutrition is essential for good diabetic management by doctor and nurse, as well as the patient. It is a great benefit to have a dietician available at a diabetic clinic, but this chapter is aimed at enabling the rest of the health care team to participate in this basic instruction.

FOOD AS A CAUSE OF DIABETES
Type I Diabetes
There is no definite evidence that any particular food can lead to

Type I diabetes, although research in Iceland has suggested that the consumption of contaminated smoked mutton during the Christmas and New Year period by pregnant women was both epidemiologically and experimentally linked with the subsequent development of Type I diabetes in their children. There was a significant excess of October births of male Type I diabetic children, nine months after the traditional smoked mutton feasting (Fig. 18.1). It was postulated that a streptozotocin-like nitrosamine compound produced in the smoking process may cause damage to the fetal pancreas with the later development of diabetes. However, the aetiology of Type I diabetes is complex and many other factors are known to be involved.

Type II Diabetes
The association of obesity with diabetes has long been known. The most extensive epidemiological studies were carried out by West and Kalbfleisch (1971) who showed that in ten populations from Asia and South and Central America there was a positive association between the prevalence of abnormal glucose tolerance

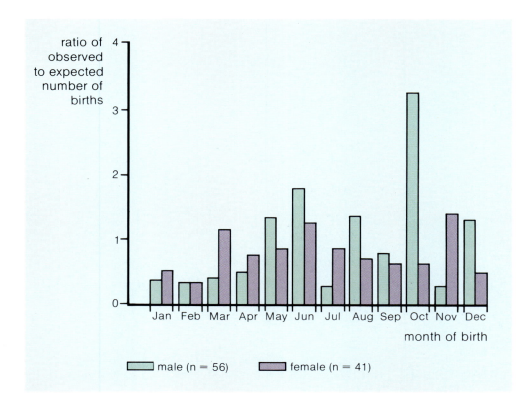

Fig. 18.1 Diet and onset of Type I diabetes. The seasonal distribution of births of ketosis-prone diabetic patients aged 0–14 years in Iceland is shown. The preponderance of male births in October is highly significant (p < 0.00001). From Helgason and Jonasson (1981), by courtesy of the *Lancet*.

and obesity (Fig. 18.2). A positive association between obesity and total carbohydrate consumption was also found.

Similar, more intensive studies among population groups with a high prevalence of diabetes, for example, the Pima Indians of Arizona and the Polynesian Pacific islanders of Nauru (see *Chapter 11*), showed the same trends. In the U.K., a very large study of government civil servants (the Whitehall Study) confirmed the association between obesity and impaired glucose tolerance.

One factor precipitating the onset of Type II diabetes is the change in eating habits related to population movement; this has been documented for Jewish immigrants to Israel from the Yemen, Italian and Irish immigrants to New York in the last century and, more recently, West Indian immigrants to London.

The most direct evidence that excess food intake is a cause of diabetes comes from Edinburgh, where careful dietary studies have shown that newly diagnosed Type II diabetic patients of all social classes eat up to 1000kcal (4.2MJ) daily more than their non-diabetic siblings.

DIETS AND FOOD PLANS FOR DIABETIC PATIENTS

The first fully documented diabetic diet was prescribed by Dr John Rollo for two patients in 1797. One patient refused to comply and soon died; the other kept meticulously to the diet and survived for many years. In retrospect, the main factor in Rollo's diet was to reduce the energy intake, but his prescription of rancid meat and suet puddings, 'as long as the stomach will bear', probably did much to suggest that diabetic diets were difficult to comply with and objectionable.

Before the discovery of insulin, eating less food was probably the only useful therapy for either type of diabetes. This might often have been curative for Type II diabetic patients and offered some temporary relief of symptoms for those who would now be termed 'insulin dependent'. The improvement in glycosuria among diabetic patients during the seige of Paris was recorded by

Bouchardat in 1875. Allen in New York in 1919, just before the discovery of insulin, went further than most experts in advising intentional undernutrition for the sake of short-term survival (the Allen 'starvation' diet). Intermittent fasting is still recommended by some authorities and certainly would not be detrimental to the diabetic state.

Goals of Dietary Modification

Following the discovery of insulin in 1921, it became possible to define rational dietary aims which are now widely accepted (Fig. 18.3). Current treatment also involves the use of either insulin or an oral hypoglycaemic agent where appropriate. The main approach is to encourage a sensible eating pattern within the framework of the food habits of the community. The first two goals, good nutrition and normal weight and growth, are applicable to everyone, whether diabetic or not. The third, to reduce the abnormality, can probably be achieved by attention to the total energy consumed without major adaptation of the types of food eaten. The fourth goal, prevention of diabetic complications, requires consideration of the proper balance of all the constituents of food (carbohydrate, protein, fat, fibre, alcohol, sweeteners, vitamins and salt).

The Food Plan

Principles

The most important consideration in the diet of a diabetic patient is the total energy intake, which is itself dependent upon age, occupation, sex and weight. On average, it is reasonable to propose an intake of 1500kcal for a moderately overweight Type II diabetic patient and 2500kcal for a normal weight Type I patient. The principles of the food plan are summarized in Fig. 18.4.

Carbohydrate content should supply close to fifty per cent of the total energy and fat less than forty per cent. Sucrose and sucrose-containing foods should generally be excluded in an energy-restricted diet, a concept which is readily understood by the

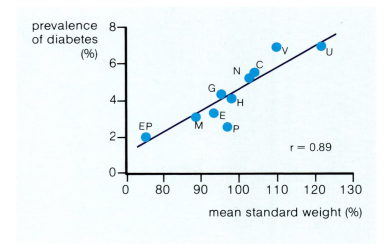

Fig. 18.2 Obesity and the onset of Type II diabetes. The data are from populations in East Pakistan (EP), Malaya (M), El Salvador (E), Panama (P), Guatemala (G), Honduras (H), Nicaragua (N), Costa Rica (C), Venezuela (V) and Uruguay (U). Only subjects over 34-years-old were included in the study. From West and Kalbfleisch (1971), by courtesy of the American Diabetes Association.

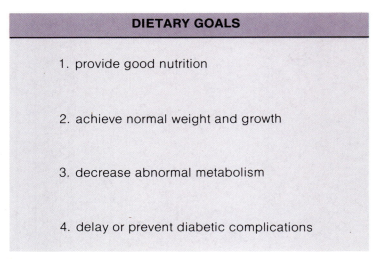

Fig. 18.3 Dietary aims for the control of diabetes.

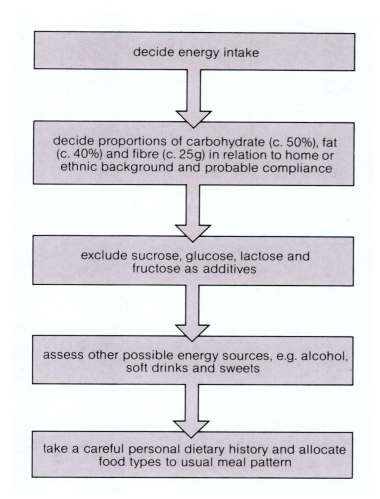

Fig. 18.4   Principles of the food plan.

patient. Likewise the use of glucose, lactose and fructose as additives is not sensible, although as constituents of normal foodstuffs they are certainly desirable. Fibre content should be approximately 25g daily. Alcohol is a major energy source and must be included in the energy calculations if the patient continues to drink it. On nutritional grounds, it is not a satisfactory foodstuff.

Guidelines for constructing a food plan are shown in Fig. 18.5. Protein should be allowed in usual amounts, unless restricted because of renal impairment. Fats and oils should only be allowed in moderation, except in total energy restriction; unsaturated fats are preferable. Most vegetables should be freely allowed and two or three portions of fruit daily are permitted. Milk intake should be restricted to 0.25–0.5 litres daily and low fat milk is preferred. Starch should be taken as measured quantities of bread (preferably with unrefined flour), cereals, plain biscuits and potatoes. Fibre can be obtained from natural sources. Estimation of quantities of the various foodstuffs may be difficult at first, but, with time, reasonably accurate judgement can be achieved.

The weighing of food is an essential part of the initial education of a newly diagnosed diabetic patient and it should be demonstrated and taught at the clinic, diabetes education centre and at home. The concept of 'carbohydrate exchanges', based on 10g portions is a convenient and helpful memory aid. Although there is some justification for considering 'energy exchanges', this concept is not yet fully accepted by clinicians. Complicated cookery books are only helpful to experienced cooks.

Carbohydrate intake

It is a reasonable and easily attainable goal to obtain fifty per cent of the daily energy intake from carbohydrate sources (Fig. 18.6). Although this is five per cent above the average U.K. diet in the 1980's, some advise the daily energy intake from carbohydrate to be increased further to sixty per cent. The main reason for this

CONSTRUCTION OF DAILY FOOD PLAN

protein foods	usual amount
fats and oils	moderate amount (unsaturated preferred)
vegetables	usual amount
fruit	2 or 3 portions
milk	0.25–0.5 litres (low fat preferred)
starches	weighed 10g portions
fibre	natural sources

Fig. 18.5   Make up of the food plan. Amounts refer to recommended daily intake.

MAJOR SOURCES OF CARBOHYDRATE

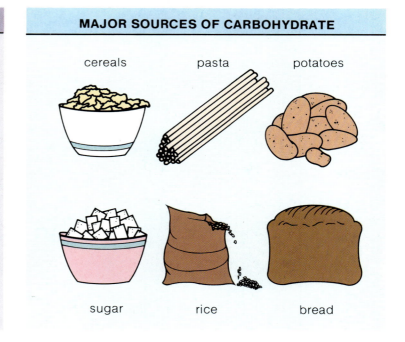

Fig. 18.6   Major sources of carbohydrate.

alteration is to allow the patient to reduce fat intake. The misconception that diabetic patients should eat a restricted carbohydrate diet arose from the over-simplification that 'carbohydrate control meant calorie control'. There is no evidence that such a relatively small increase in dietary carbohydrate alone will affect blood glucose control. Experimental studies with much higher or lower carbohydrate intakes are inconclusive, although they suggest some improvement in insulin sensitivity with the highest carbohydrate intakes.

The form of carbohydrate taken is more important than the quantity consumed, because different forms do not give the same plasma glucose or insulin responses (Fig. 18.7). Most carbohydrate intake should be as polysaccharides, such as bread, potatoes and cereals, and preferably as foods rich in fibre. Starch causes a lower plasma glucose and insulin response than equimolar quantities of glucose or sucrose and different forms of cooked starches are not identical. Although drugs which inhibit α-amylase or α-glucosidase enzymes in the intestine lower post-prandial glucose responses in diabetic patients, their usefulness is doubtful, since the therapeutic malabsorption produced by their use may lead to unpleasant gastrointestinal side-effects. It is preferable to achieve the same lowering of glucose response by correct food intake.

Most cookery books and guides for diabetic patients still concentrate on the carbohydrate content of foods and a change to energy-related food exchanges will be gradual. This change is part of a trend towards more health-conscious food habits in the general population.

Refined sugars, which at present contribute approximately twenty per cent of the total food energy in the U.K., are neither themselves less easily metabolized nor do they uniquely exacerbate diabetic hyperglycaemia, but it is customary and wise to exclude all added sucrose from a diabetic food plan. This is because of the

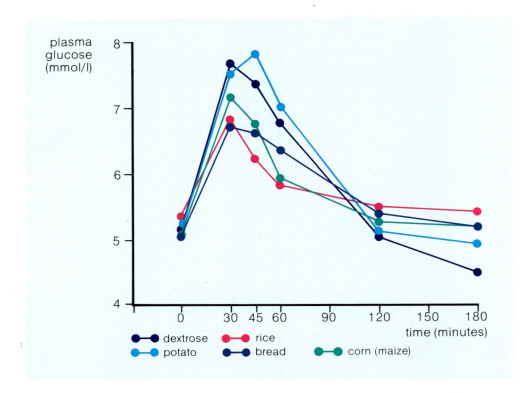

Fig. 18.7 Mean plasma glucose response to various carbohydrates in sixteen normal subjects. Each test dose contained 50g glucose and was given after an overnight fast. From Crapo *et al.* (1977), by courtesy of the American Diabetes Association.

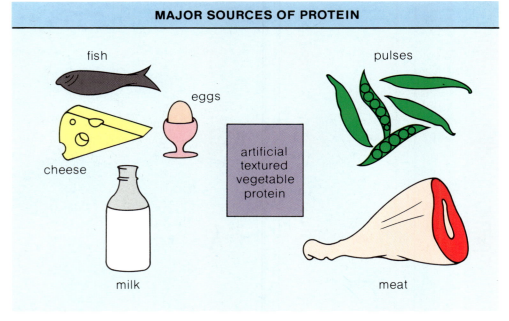

Fig. 18.8 Major sources of protein.

problem of compliance, particularly avoiding overconsumption of sucrose and glucose-containing drinks and confections. It is nevertheless possible for the well-controlled patient on insulin, or even on diet alone, to utilize a reasonable quantity of sucrose although proponents of high carbohydrate intake would not support this approach.

Protein intake
Although affecting many parts of the world, protein deficiency is not a problem in western Europe. The mean daily protein intake in the U.K. (Fig. 18.8) is between ten and twenty per cent of the total daily energy intake (60–120g/day). It is difficult to consider protein in isolation as it is often served with substantial quantities of saturated fats in dairy and meat products. An increase of vegetable-derived protein from whole-wheat cereals, peas and beans would therefore allow a reduced fat intake. In the future, various artificial vegetable protein products may be acceptable.

The average protein intake in the U.K. may be higher than is desirable (in India it is less than 40g/day) and there is increasing evidence that in diabetic patients a modest protein restriction to a maximum of 0.7g/kg body weight or 35–50g per day will delay the deterioration in renal function due to diabetic nephropathy. If this is confirmed in clinical practice, it may be useful to advise all diabetic patients to limit protein intake.

Fat intake
Fats can either be saturated or unsaturated (Fig. 18.9). Well-established nutritional and epidemiological evidence linking atheroma and heart disease to excess intake of saturated fats is now much more widely accepted by the consumer. There is no reason why a diabetic patient should not be at the forefront of the necessary change in eating customs which is, in essence, merely a reversion to older practices.

In the food plan, fat consumption should be limited to approximately thirty-five per cent of energy intake when linked to increased energy from carbohydrates. In conjunction with this, intake of foods rich in saturated fatty acids, such as meat fat, dairy fat and hard margarines, should be reduced. This does not mean that bread should be eaten dry or breakfast cereal taken without milk, but that unsaturated margarines and low fat milk products should be used in preference.

The concept of polyunsaturated to saturated fat ratio (P/S ratio) probably does have value in assessing which form of fat to eat (Fig. 18.10) and there are now many choices available. An average P/S ratio of 1.0 would be a considerable advance over the current U.K. value of 0.2, but it is unrealistic to try to obtain higher values which would require the excess consumption of corn and sunflower oils, or fish oils which are now becoming available.

A cholesterol intake of not more than 300mg per day (an egg contains 250mg cholesterol) would also be reasonable, but is a less important individual goal than the other modifications of fat intake.

Fibre intake
A high fibre diet has achieved some familiarity in the public mind as a current medical fashion. The clinical observations of Burkitt

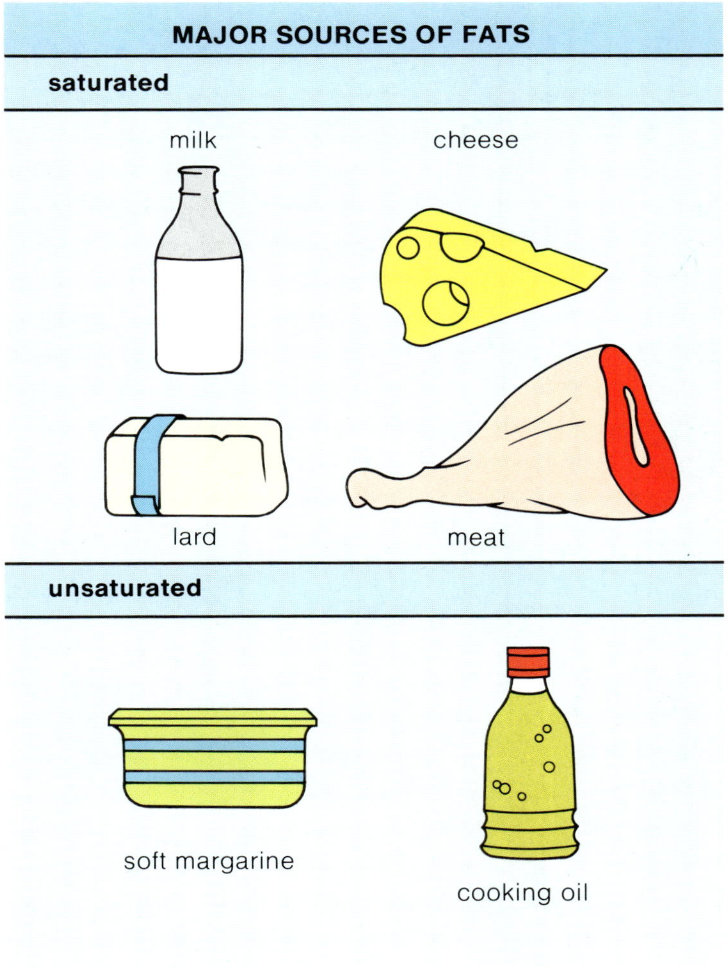

Fig. 18.9 Major sources of fat.

Fig. 18.10 Examples of typical polyunsaturated to saturated (P/S) ratios.

P/S RATIOS	
butter	0.04
cream	0.05
lard	0.08
hard margarine	0.26
olive oil	0.75
vegetable (groundnut) oil	1.07
soft margarine	1.15
polyunsaturated margarine	1.95
corn oil	3.26
sunflower oil	5.35

and his colleagues in East Africa led them to point out the deficiency of fibre in the Western diet. It is not clear what amount of fibre would be optimal, but by using whole-wheat bread and encouraging the consumption of more fruit and vegetables, a daily intake of about 30g fibre can easily be achieved. This compares with only 5–10g achieved with very refined white flour.

Numerous experimental dietary observations in Oxford (Fig. 18.11) and elsewhere have shown that blood glucose levels, both fasting and post-prandial, are reduced by ten per cent or more when the various fibre supplements are taken. Some of these fibre sources, such as guar and pectin, may be unpalatable and produce excess flatus and it is probable that natural cereal fibre is best taken in the amount found in coarsely milled flour. Beans of various types are very attractive to the fibre conscious nutritionist as a source of both vegetable protein and fibre, and a reasonable intake of beans is certainly desirable. Few would suggest that the relatively high intake of these pulses, as in a fully vegetarian diet, is obligatory, especially as public acceptability is poor.

The benefits of increased fibre also extend to bowel function, lipid absorption and satiety, and there is no doubt that public familiarity with the concept of natural foodstuffs is beneficial.

Alcohol and drinks

Although there is some justification on general grounds for a recommendation that diabetic patients should not drink alcohol, this is not based on any effect of moderate amounts of alcohol on plasma glucose values in a well-nourished person. If the problems of intoxication, facial flushing, occasional hypoglycaemia and simple over-indulgence are accepted as a price of civilization, it is possible to define advice on sensible drinking for the diabetic patient.

As an energy source, alcohol is second in efficiency only to fat and contains 7kcal/g. Many alcoholic drinks have additional carbohydrate energy (Fig. 18.12). A half a pint of beer, a glass of wine or sherry and a small measure of spirits all contain approximately 8g of alcohol which is 56kcal. The carbohydrate

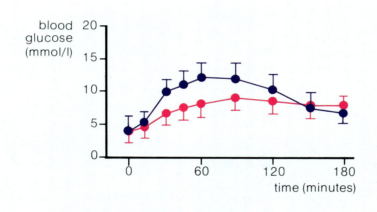

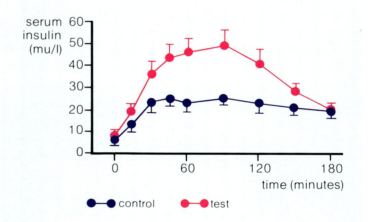

control   test

Fig. 18.11 Effect of dietary fibre on blood glucose and serum insulin levels. The results are from eight Type II diabetic patients after eating control and fibre-enriched test meals. Significant differences were found at 30–60min in blood glucose and at 30–120min in serum insulin levels (mean ± SEM). From Jenkins *et al.* (1976), by courtesy of the *Lancet*.

ENERGY CONTENT OF ALCOHOLIC DRINKS				
		carbohydrate (kcal)	alcohol (kcal)	total (kcal)
½ pint beer		28	56	84
1 glass wine		20	56	76
1 measure spirits		0	56	56

Fig. 18.12 Energy content of alcoholic drinks. The total energy content of a typical snack (48kcal carbohydrate, 12kcal protein and 36kcal fat) is approximately the same as one of these drinks.

content in mixers, wine or beer adds approximately 25kcal to the total energy intake. In all, this is equivalent to the energy value of a cup of tea and a wholemeal biscuit.

Soft drinks sweetened with sucrose or glucose are in the same category as refined sugars and are best avoided, although they do represent potential energy sources. There are many acceptable sugar-free drinks available and increasing interest is being taken in the various 'artificial' sweeteners in use. Natural fruit juices are probably the best beverages for diabetic patients.

An awareness of the problems of excessive alcohol intake and the circumstances which lead to it would benefit the diabetic population. As an energy source for healthy living, alcohol leaves much to be desired.

Sweeteners

'Sweeteners' are an established part of the Western diet. This may be an aspect of the excess use of refined sucrose already referred to, but must be considered in relation to dietary compliance. Some people can easily avoid any form of supplementary sweetener, a habit to be encouraged, and others only require minimal quantities of sucrose.

Fructose is the sweetest of the naturally occurring sugars and the average U.K. diet already provides approximately 50g daily. In the diabetic diet, fructose offers little advantage over glucose.

Sorbitol is only half as sweet as sucrose, is metabolized as fructose and has no particular merit. Xylitol is found in vegetables but is not widely available.

Aspartame, a synthetic dipeptide of aspartic acid and phenyl-alanine, is now available and is taking a major place as a sweetener. It is approximately two hundred times sweeter than sucrose, so its calorific value of 4kcal/g is insignificant and it may have a place in the therapy of overweight patients with a 'sweet tooth'. It does not have the identifiable taste of saccharine. A summary of the normal metabolic pathways for metabolism of glucose, fructose, sorbitol and xylitol is shown in Fig. 18.13.

Saccharine is widely consumed by the diabetic population. It is suggested that no more than 2.5mg/kg per day should be taken; this represents only ten to fourteen saccharine tablets per day. Although there is an increased risk of malignancy in rats following large doses of saccharine, there is no evidence for any toxicity in man. Fructose and aspartame are likely to become popular, but whether they have an advantage over a restricted quantity of sucrose for the diabetic patient is uncertain. Diabetic patients are better advised to take less of any form of sweetener than non-diabetic subjects.

A Typical 1500kcal Food Plan

It is more useful to remember the principles of this diet, since Type II diabetes is more prevalent than Type I. A 1500kcal food plan is shown in Fig. 18.14. Usually the task of writing out the diet is left to the dietician, but the doctor and nurse should also understand both the principles and the details.

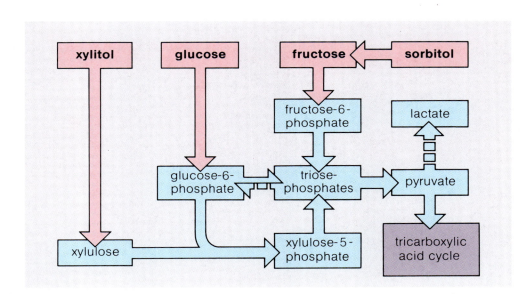

Fig. 18.13 Normal metabolic pathways for the cellular utilization of xylitol, glucose, fructose and sorbitol. Lactate can be produced after a marked increase in the triose-phosphate pool. With insulin deficiency, trioses are converted to glucose-6-phosphate and can exacerbate hyperglycaemia. There is a hexose monophosphate shunt between glucose-6-phosphate and xylulose-5-phosphate.

Fig. 18.14 1500kcal food plan. The figures given here are appropriate for a 70kg man.

A 1500kcal (6500kJ) FOOD PLAN				
	carbohydrate (CHO)	protein (P)	fat (F)	fibre
by weight	170g	56g	62g	27g
by energy	47%	15%	38%	0%
by body weight	2.4g/kg	0.8g/kg	0.9g/kg	0.4g/kg

1500kcal FOOD PLAN: BREAKFAST AND SNACK

breakfast						mid-morning snack			
	tea	whole milk (150ml)	branflakes (15g)	whole-wheat bread (60g), margarine	total	tea	whole milk (35ml)	1 digestive biscuit	total
CHO(g)		7	10	30	47		2	10	12
P(g)		5	1	4	10		1	2	3
F(g)		5	0	12	17		1	3	4
fibre(g)		0	2	5	7		0	1	1
energy (kcal)		93	44	244	381		21	75	96

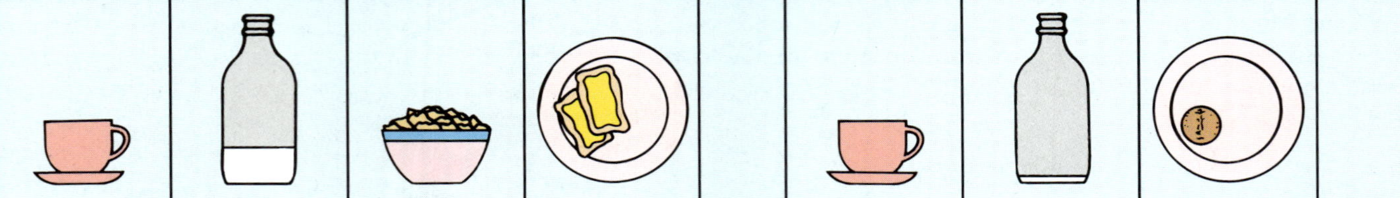

Fig. 18.15 Breakfast and mid-morning snack in the 1500kcal food plan. 26% of the day's food energy is present in the breakfast and 7% in the snack.

1500kcal FOOD PLAN: MIDDAY MEAL AND SNACK

midday meal						afternoon snack			
	lean meat or fish (60g)	vegetable (1 helping)	potato (180g)	fruit (1 portion)	total	tea	milk (35ml)	1 digestive biscuit	total
CHO(g)	0	0	30	10	40		2	10	12
P(g)	14	0	3	0	17		1	2	3
F(g)	8	0	0	0	8		1	3	4
fibre(g)	0	2	2	2	6		0	1	1
energy (kcal)	128	0	132	40	300		21	75	96

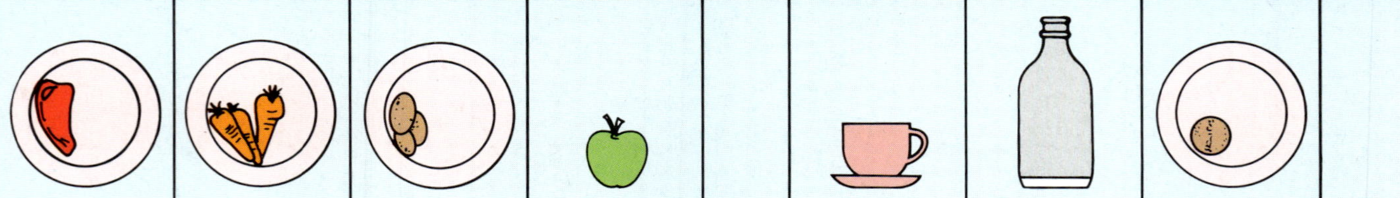

Fig. 18.16 Midday meal and afternoon snack in the 1500kcal food plan. 20% of the day's food energy is present in the midday meal and 7% in the snack.

Breakfast

It is surprising how many people now take no breakfast at all. There is no need for the traditional cooked breakfast and substitution of a glass of fruit juice for the cornflakes makes little difference to the energy supplied (Fig. 18.15).

Midday meal

The importance of a carbohydrate source at lunch time should be stressed if the higher carbohydrate intake is to be maintained (Fig. 18.16). The potato is an excellent choice although a sandwich lunch would be equally appropriate (high fibre bread). Afternoon tea and a biscuit is not essential but introduces an additional 100kcal.

Evening meal

In this example, this is more a 'high tea'. If a larger meal is envisaged, some of the energy allowance from the bedtime snack would give the possibility of cheese and biscuit or an extra vegetable (Fig. 18.17).

The most important aspect of the food plan is to try to establish how the patient will adapt to it and also how different it is from his normal diet; ideally it should be similar.

Dietary adherence

Poor adherence to a food plan usually means that an inappropriate diet has been inadequately and hurriedly explained to a nervous patient by a doctor who did not understand it and certainly did not know the energy content of common foodstuffs. All these factors can be improved upon.

1500kcal FOOD PLAN: EVENING MEAL AND SNACK										
evening meal							**bedtime snack**			
lean meat, fish or cheese (60g)	vegetable (1 helping)	whole-wheat bread (60g), margarine	fruit (1 portion)	tea	milk (60ml)	total	tea	milk (35ml)	whole-wheat bread (30g) margarine	total
CHO (g)	0	0	30	10		3	43		2	15	17
P (g)	14	0	4	0		2	20		1	2	3
F (g)	8	0	12	0		2	22		1	6	7
fibre (g)	0	2	5	2		0	9		0	3	3
energy (kcal)	120	0	244	40		38	442		21	122	143

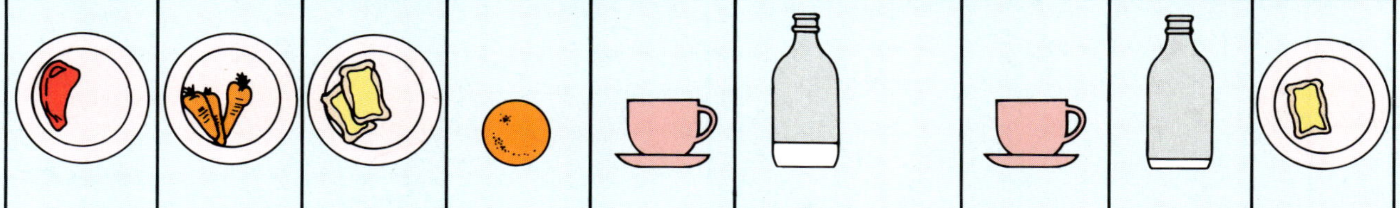

Fig. 18.17 Evening meal and bedtime snack in the 1500kcal food plan. 30% of the day's food energy is present in the evening meal and 10% in the snack.

REFERENCES

British Diabetic Association (1983) *Dietary Recommendations for Diabetics for the 1980's – A Policy Statement by the Nutrition Sub-Committee.* London: British Diabetic Association.

British Diabetic Association (1984) Dietary fibre in the management of the diabetic. *Proceedings of a British Diabetic Association Symposium.* Oxford: Medical Educational Services.

Crapo PA, Reaven G & Olefsky J (1977) Postprandial plasma-glucose and -insulin responses to different complex carbohydrates. *Diabetes,* **26**, 1178–1183.

Davidson S, Passmore R, Brock JF & Truswell AS (1979) *Human Nutrition and Dietetics.* 7th edition. Edinburgh: Churchill Livingstone.

Hadden DR (1982) Food and diabetes: the dietary treatment of insulin dependent and non-insulin-dependent diabetes. *Clinics in Endocrinology and Metabolism,* **11(2)**, 503–524.

Helgason T & Jonasson MR (1981) Evidence for a food additive as a cause of ketosis-prone diabetes. *Lancet,* **2**, 716–720.

Jenkins DJA, Goff DV, Leeds AR, Alberti KGMM, Wolever TMS, Gassull MA & Hockaday TDR (1976) Unabsorbable carbohydrates and diabetes: decreased post-prandial hyperglycaemia. *Lancet,* **2**, 172–174.

Keen H & Thomas B (1978) Diabetes mellitus. In *Nutrition in the Clinical Management of Disease.* Edited by Dickerson JWT & Lee HA. pp. 118–143. London: Edward Arnold.

Longstaff R & Mann J (1984) *The Diabetics' Cookbook.* London: Martin Dunitz.

Mann J & Oxford Dietetic Group (1982) *The Diabetics' Diet Book – a New High Fibre Eating Programme.* London: Martin Dunitz.

Metcalf J (1983) *Cooking the New Diabetic Way: The High Fibre Calorie-conscious Cookbook.* London: British Diabetic Association/Ward Lock.

Paul AA & Southgate DAT (1978) *McCance and Widdowson's The Composition of Foods.* 4th edition. London: Her Majesty's Stationery Office.

West KM (1973) Diet therapy of diabetes: an analysis of failure. *Annals of Internal Medicine,* **79**, 425–434.

West KM & Kalbfleisch JM (1971) Influence of nutritional factors on prevalence of diabetes. *Diabetes,* **20**, 99–108.

19 Diabetes and Surgery

Dai JB Thomas MD MRCP

THE PRE-INSULIN ERA

A quarter of a century before insulin was introduced clinically Sir Frederick Treves, a famous London surgeon, made a statement about the risks to the diabetic subject during surgery:

'Diabetes offers a serious bar to any kind of operation. A wound in the diabetic patient will not heal while the tissues appear to offer the most favourable soil for the development of putrefaction.'

At this time anaesthetic agents were relatively crude and there were no adequate intravenous fluids or antibiotics available. Treves stated that the poorly controlled diabetic subject had poor wound healing and that the affected tissues were prone to secondary infection. Since then there have been enormous advances in our understanding of diabetes and the metabolic changes produced in this disease when patients are subjected to surgery.

MORTALITY AND MORBIDITY OF DIABETIC PATIENTS DURING SURGERY

Fig. 19.1 shows data derived from a study of 12,000 diabetic subjects undergoing surgery between 1942 and 1969. The mortality rate varied between 1.3% and 3.7%, there being one hundred and three deaths during this period, forty-one of these resulting from arteriosclerotic heart disease (with myocardial infarction accounting for most). The mortality rates in diabetic patients are only slightly higher than those found in non-diabetic patients during general surgery, but are three or four times higher during specialist surgery such as renal transplantation .

Several surveys report an increased incidence of minor infections and septicaemia in diabetic patients but this is reduced by good glycaemic control. Although delayed wound healing has been demonstrated in animals with poorly controlled diabetes, it has been difficult to show in man.

There is little mention of loss of glycaemic control in most studies, presumably because hypoglycaemia and ketoacidosis are largely preventable and authors are reluctant to report their occurrence.

PERIOPERATIVE DIABETIC CONTROL

Perioperative control is very important in diabetic patients, mainly to prevent severe metabolic derangements. Hypoglycaemia should be recognized and corrected with glucose infusion. Minor degrees of ketoacidosis are surprisingly common postoperatively and it must be remembered that if severe ketoacidosis develops, mortality varies between five and ten per cent even in specialist diabetic centres. In addition to control of blood glucose levels, insulin also has important actions on electrolyte homoeostasis and there may be quite profound electrolyte abnormalities in the insulin deficient patient. Treves drew attention to the susceptibility of diabetic patients to secondary infection; this is supported by modern experimental work which suggests that poor glycaemic control results in a poor phagocyte action which in turn leads to susceptibility to infection.

Poor perioperative control of diabetic patients may also lead to substantially lengthened periods of inpatient treatment, with a subsequently raised cost of hospitalization, whilst metabolic normality is attained and related complications are treated.

Fig. 19.1 Mortality and morbidity of diabetic patients during surgery.

MORTALITY AND MORBIDITY OF DIABETIC SUBJECTS DURING SURGERY

mortality rate

1.3–3.7% in recent decades

40% of deaths due to arteriosclerotic heart disease

morbidity

minor infection and septicaemia increased

delayed wound healing

loss of glycaemic control (leading to hypoglycaemia and ketoacidosis)

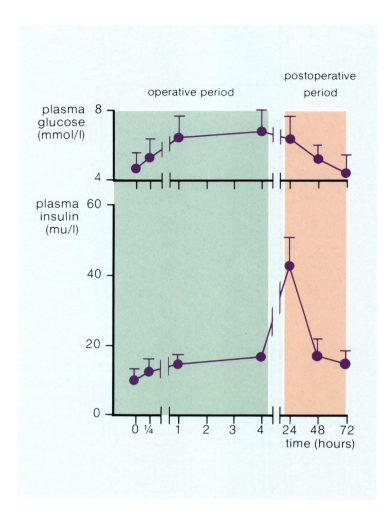

Fig. 19.2 Plasma glucose and insulin changes in non-diabetic patients during and after major surgery. Seven non-diabetic patients were followed for 72 hours from just before administration of anaesthetic (mean ± SEM).

GLUCOSE AND INSULIN CHANGES IN NON-DIABETIC PATIENTS DURING SURGERY

In order to provide the best control for diabetic subjects during surgery, it is essential to have a detailed knowledge of the relationships between glucose and insulin metabolism during the perioperative period in non-diabetic patients. Fig. 19.2 shows the perioperative period in seven non-diabetic patients. There was very little variation of plasma glucose with mean values increasing only slightly above 6mmol/l; initially insulin secretion remained at basal levels and did not increase until the first day of the postoperative period.

By comparing intravenous glucose tolerance tests before and after surgery it has been demonstrated that there is decreased glucose tolerance during the early postoperative period; glucose values are therefore higher after surgery and the insulin requirement is increased. In summary, there is always some measurable level of insulin present during the postoperative period. There is therefore no logical reason for stopping insulin therapy in the Type I (insulin-dependent) diabetic subject at this time.

RELATIONSHIPS BETWEEN ANABOLISM AND CATABOLISM IN VARIOUS STATES
The Non-diabetic Patient

The relationships between insulin, the only truly anabolic hormone, and the catabolic hormones, glucagon, corticosteroids and catecholamines, are shown in Fig. 19.3. The intermediary metabolism of carbohydrate, fat and protein is controlled by all these hormones. After feeding and the digestion of food, various substrates are absorbed which stimulate insulin release and

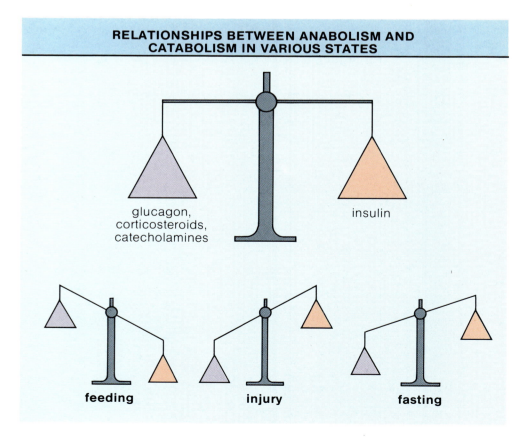

Fig. 19.3 Relationships between anabolism and catabolism in feeding, fasting and injury. Surgery, as injury, produces a higher catabolic state than fasting, where insulin levels are very low and the catabolic hormones glucagon, corticosteroids and catecholamines are elevated.

promote storage of glucose in the form of glycogen. Insulin also stimulates protein synthesis, lipogenesis and glycolysis, whilst inhibiting protein breakdown, lipolysis, ketogenesis and gluconeogenesis.

In the fasting state, insulin levels are reduced whereas the catabolic hormone levels are increased. This is important since it allows the release of substrate which is utilized as necessary. There is a certain absolute requirement of carbohydrate for the metabolism of the brain and various other tissues, but as fasting progresses ketone bodies become a more valuable source of fuel. In the analogous, but more disturbed, state of injury, insulin levels are more markedly decreased and levels of glucagon, corticosteroids and catecholamines are grossly elevated. This leads to extensive protein breakdown, gluconeogenesis, lipolysis and ketogenesis. This process probably allows release of a large amount of substrate which can be directed towards damaged tissues and utilized as either building blocks or energy releasing substances as required. In normal man, hyperinsulinaemia follows, and tends to restrict these catabolic processes. In the diabetic with no endogenous insulin secretion, this loss of insulin response leads to marked catabolism which can result in inanition or, in extreme circumstances, death.

Metabolic Response to Anaesthesia

The metabolic response to injury is a non-specific response to stress and is triggered by a wide variety of stimuli. Its level is dependent upon the degree of provocation. Modern anaesthesia alone, although having some minor biochemical consequences, has very little effect on the triggering of the overall response when compared to that of subsequent surgery or even the thought of it.

Historically, ether was used as an anaesthetic agent and this produced marked ketogenesis and hyperglycaemia in non-diabetic subjects, to the extent that insulin was often prescribed postoperatively. Modern anaesthetic agents, however, are much more sophisticated but do have some effects on the diabetic state, although these are probably minimal (Fig. 19.4).

Inducing agents such as propanidid and thiopentone have been demonstrated to be mildly glucogenic; the exact mechanism is, however, unknown. Cyclopropane increases catecholamine output but this is rarely sufficient to cause significant increases in hyperglycaemia. Halothane works in two ways: it inhibits insulin release directly from the pancreas whilst at the same time inhibiting oxidative phosphorylation. Some forms of anaesthesia, such as epidural anaesthetics, appear to decrease the cortisol, growth hormone and thyroid hormone responses normally associated with general anaesthesia. Thus, this form of anaesthesia is particularly valuable in conjunction with caesarean sections in diabetic subjects when it is most important to achieve good metabolic control.

Metabolic Response to Surgery

The magnitude of the metabolic response to surgery depends upon the severity of the operation (Fig. 19.5). Operations on the surface of the body, even those of long duration, have little effect on metabolic responses, for example, plastic surgery or skin grafting. However, with abdominal and thoracic surgery there is a marked injury response. The mechanism underlying the much higher levels of catabolic hormones found during these procedures

ACTION OF ANAESTHETIC AGENTS	
agent	action
induction agents, e.g. propanidid and thiopentone	mildly glucogenic
cyclopropane	increases catecholamine output
halothane	inhibits insulin release uncouples oxidative phosphorylation
epidural anaesthesia	decreases cortisol, growth hormone and thyroid hormone responses

Fig. 19.4 Effects of various anaesthetic agents on metabolism.

EFFECTS OF SURGERY ON METABOLIC RESPONSE TO INJURY		
mild	marked	very severe
surface operations routine minor surgery	abdominal surgery thoracic surgery	hypothermic cardiopulmonary bypass surgery

Fig. 19.5 Degree of metabolic response to various types of surgery.

remains unclear, but it is possible that splanchnic nerve stimulation and direct manipulation of the adrenal glands may lead to release of adrenal hormones. Splanchnic nerve stimulation causes glucagon release but there may be some central mechanism which also contributes to these changes.

The most severe surgical stress is certainly hypothermic cardiopulmonary bypass surgery. In this situation, there are tremendous increases in catabolic hormones and it is probable that maximum secretion rates of these hormones are obtained. This seems to be due to the combined effects of bypass procedure and hypothermia.

Associated Factors

The catabolic changes inherent in surgery predispose to hyperglycaemia and this becomes more pronounced when glucose-containing solutions are administered (Fig. 19.6). A five percent dextrose solution contains 25g of glucose in 500ml of solution and, if given rapidly, represents a substantial glucose load. Hartmann's solution, thought to be metabolically inert, contains small amounts of electrolytes which would appear to make it more like normal body fluids. Although this is a useful solution for diabetic patients, it contains lactate which is a glucogenic precursor and its use leads to hyperglycaemia. The transfusion of stored whole blood has been observed to increase plasma glucose levels, but this probably reflects the stress associated with hypotension and hypovolaemia rather than that associated with the constituents of the blood.

During the operative and postoperative period, a wide variety of drugs may be used if complications develop. Sympathetic agents, particularly beta-adrenergics, can lead to marked insulin resistance. Hydrocortisone and glucagon are catabolic hormones with predictable influences on carbohydrate metabolism.

MANAGEMENT OF TYPE I DIABETES IN SURGERY
Outmoded Forms

Since the clinical introduction of insulin, a wide variety of regimens have been recommended to control diabetes during the perioperative period (Fig. 19.7). The 'do nothing' regimen enjoyed a vogue in the mid-sixties and demonstrated the important point that, providing patients are well-controlled before surgery, there are likely to be few problems during the immediate perioperative period. However, if insulin withdrawal is continued indefinitely this will inevitably lead to ketoacidosis.

In the U.K. the use of short-acting insulins (soluble, regular insulins) has been favoured during the perioperative period. In the U.S.A., it has been advocated that isophane, with its intermediate length of action, might be of value if given preoperatively and postoperatively.

In 1968 it was seriously suggested that the plasma glucose concentration should be maintained above 22mmol/l. This was published in an anaesthetic journal and demonstrates the anaesthetist's irrational fear of hypoglycaemia. During anaesthesia, the natural response of the body is to increase the plasma glucose, not to decrease it. If the possibility of hypoglycaemia in

---

OTHER FACTORS INFLUENCING THE RESPONSE TO SURGERY

intravenous fluids
dextrose
Hartmann's solution
blood

drugs
adrenergic agents
corticosteroids
glucagon

Fig. 19.6 Factors other than the anaesthetic and type of surgery which affect blood glucose levels in surgery.

MANAGEMENT OF TYPE I DIABETES IN SURGERY: OUTMODED FORMS

do nothing

give isophane pre- and postoperatively

maintain plasma glucose above 22mmol/l

give short-acting insulin intramuscularly with intravenous glucose

Fig. 19.7 Outmoded forms of management for patients with Type I diabetes

an unconscious patient causes concern, the relatively simple process of monitoring blood sugar levels with blood glucose strips averts this problem.

Many regimens for the control of diabetes during surgery include a suggestion that a small amount of the daily insulin be given as short-acting insulin in conjunction with an intravenous glucose load, hopefully providing adequate insulin levels and at the same time minimizing the risk of hypoglycaemia.

Present-day Management: Comparison of Intramuscular and Intravenous Regimens of Insulin Administration

Insulin is always present in the circulation during the perioperative period in non-diabetic subjects and any proposed regimen for treating diabetes at this time should take this into account. One traditional regimen involved giving insulin intramuscularly. However, in the presence of hypotension due either to anaesthesia or to complications of surgery itself, insulin is poorly absorbed from peripheral sites; thus it is certainly more logical to deliver insulin intravenously.

Changes in blood glucose and other metabolites have been compared in diabetic patients having either standard intramuscular regimens or glucose/insulin infusions (Figs 19.8 and 19.9). Although it is traditional to measure glucose changes there are many other intermediary metabolites which may be affected during surgery, such as 3-hydroxybutyrate. Preoperatively there was very little difference between the two groups in mean 3-hydroxybutyrate concentration. During the infusion period

ketone body production appears to have been inhibited; this is not the case in patients treated with the intramuscular regimen. After completion of infusion there was no difference in the concentration of 3-hydroxybutyrate in either group of patients. It would therefore appear that short periods of intravenous insulin during surgery benefit control both immediately and also in the later postoperative period.

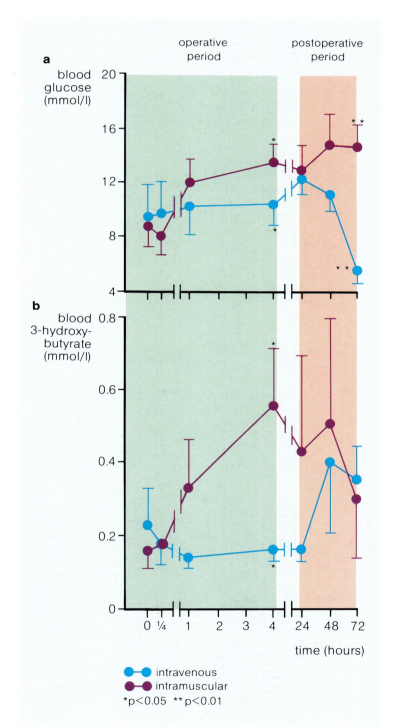

Fig. 19.9 Response to intramuscular and intravenous regimens in diabetic patients undergoing surgery. (a) shows the change in blood glucose and (b) the change in blood 3-hydroxybutyrate (mean ± SEM).

COMPARISON OF INTRAMUSCULAR AND INTRAVENOUS REGIMENS

intramuscular

half daily insulin dose given as short-acting insulin and 25g intravenous glucose given as 500ml of 5% dextrose over 4 hours

intravenous

500ml of 10% dextrose, with 10u short-acting insulin added, infused over 4 hours

Fig. 19.8 Comparison of intramuscular and intravenous regimens of diabetic control.

Postoperative Control

The important variations in postoperative care for different situations are outlined in Fig. 19.10. If the patient is able to eat soon after surgery, the infusion can be stopped shortly before the first meal and the patient then stabilized on short-acting insulin thrice daily. Once intravenous insulin infusion is terminated the circulating insulin levels fall off very rapidly and intramuscular insulin needs to be administered within half an hour. If the patient cannot eat, the infusion of insulin and dextrose can be continued for as long as is necessary, but in patients in a severe catabolic state and those who are infected it is important to consider parenteral nutrition as an alternative; this may substantially increase insulin requirements. Glucose results should be monitored and the insulin infusion increased or decreased as necessary. Blood-glucose strip results produce a useful guide and can initially be performed hourly with the test frequency being reduced when a stable state is reached. Occasionally this system should be calibrated with plasma glucose results estimated by standard laboratory methods to ensure both results correlate satisfactorily. If patients are in a severely catabolic state and have severe diabetes, it is important to measure bicarbonate levels since the plasma glucose result is sometimes divorced from ketone body production.

The Insulin Infusion Pump

The advantage of using an insulin infusion pump (see *Chapter 15*) is that the glucose and insulin can be infused as separate variables. This means that changes in insulin infusion can be adjusted almost immediately. It should be remembered, however, that although these pumps are extremely efficient they require constant supervision. For example, it is relatively easy for one of the intravenous lines to become disconnected from a restless patient and, unless this is noticed by vigilant nursing staff, insulin will not be infused into the patient.

PERIOPERATIVE MANAGEMENT IN TYPE I DIABETES

Good preoperative glycaemic control is of paramount importance for elective surgery. Ideally, patients should be admitted two days before planned surgery and an assessment of their glycaemic control

---

POSTOPERATIVE MANAGEMENT OF TYPE I DIABETIC SUBJECTS

if a patient will eat soon:
  continue insulin infusion until first meal
  stabilize on short-acting insulin thrice daily

if patient cannot eat:
  continue infusion for up to 8 days
  consider parenteral nutrition after 48–72 hours
  monitor glycaemic control 4-hourly with blood
    glucose strips
  periodically check venous plasma glucose in laboratory

N.B. sepsis increases insulin requirements; therefore
  add more insulin to dextrose infusion to maintain
  plasma glucose level under 10mmol/l

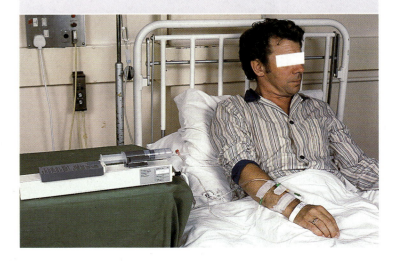

Fig. 19.10 Postoperative management of Type I diabetic patients. Treatment is dependent upon whether or not the patient is fasting after surgery. The insulin infusion pump is shown in use.

GUIDELINES FOR PERIOPERATIVE MANAGEMENT IN TYPE I DIABETES

good preoperative control

liaison between physician, anaesthetist and surgeon

perform surgery in the morning if possible

check preoperative plasma glucose

if plasma glucose >5mmol/l start: 5% dextrose,
  500ml 6-hourly, and insulin infusion pump 1–4u/h;
  or 10% dextrose, 500ml, and 16u short-acting insulin
  over 4 hours

check postoperative plasma glucose immediately after
  surgery is completed; increase insulin as necessary

continue infusion until first meal

stabilize on subcutaneous insulin when patient can eat

Fig. 19.11 Guidelines for perioperative management in Type diabetic patients. These guidelines are based upon the author's experience of diabetic control during surgery.

THE PREGNANT DIABETIC PATIENT

special features

metabolic control affects mother and fetus

rapidly changing situation

management

insulin/glucose mixture as for other diabetic patients
  in surgery

epidural anaesthesia favoured

Fig. 19.12 The pregnant diabetic patient. Treatment of pregnant diabetic patients during surgery, for instance caesarian section, requires a different approach because of a rapidly changing metabolic situation and because treatment affects not only the mother but also the fetus.

made. If diabetic control is poor, short-acting insulin should be given thrice daily before meals. It is important for the physician, surgeon and anaesthetist to liaise and surgery should be performed in the morning when more experienced staff are likely to be available to deal with any postoperative difficulties that might arise because of the diabetic state. It is prudent to measure the preoperative plasma glucose and if it is greater than 5mmol/l an insulin infusion should be started, unless the patient is only undergoing a very simple procedure, such as cystoscopy. Insulin requirements obviously vary enormously between patients and no single regimen can be dogmatically applied to all situations. A summary of useful guidelines is shown in Fig. 19.11.

With an insulin infusion pump the aim is to deliver 500ml of five per cent dextrose six-hourly; this supplies 100g per day. During this period one to four units of insulin infused hourly generally achieves good diabetic control. A modification of this regimen is to use a mixture of 500ml of ten per cent dextrose, with 16u of short-acting insulin added to it, and this is infused over four to six hours. It is very important to check the plasma glucose under anaesthesia; blood glucose strips provide a rapid result.

Postoperatively, the plasma glucose should be checked as soon as is practical and then compared with glucose strip results to assess correlation. Insulin should be increased as required and the infusion should be continued until the first meal. At the same time the patient should be started on short-acting insulin before meals. It is sometimes of value to add a small dose (4–8u) of intermediate-acting insulin to the last pre-meal injection of the day to maintain reasonable diabetic control throughout the night.

THE PREGNANT DIABETIC
Surgery in the pregnant diabetic has some unique features (Fig. 19.12). Poor metabolic control has an adverse effect on both mother and fetus. Although strict control of diabetes during pregnancy has undoubtedly reduced the incidence of most complications, unfortunately there are still some unexplained late intra-uterine deaths.

In labour there may be rapidly changing situations which require urgent surgery. It is therefore best to treat diabetic subjects in labour with a glucose/insulin infusion, using either of the two methods previously described. Close monitoring is most important, requiring hourly blood glucose reading. If caesarean section is required, this is best performed under epidural anaesthesia since it provokes less of a catabolic response than other types of anaesthetic. After the third stage of labour, there is a rapid return to pre-pregnancy insulin requirements and if the patient is a gestational diabetic she may not require further insulin after delivery.

It is also worth mentioning that Type I diabetic subjects treated with salbutamol to suppress premature labour will often develop insulin resistance because of the adrenergic agonist effects of this agent. In this situation diabetes can be extremely difficult to control and as ketosis has such a high mortality for the fetus it is probably better to avoid salbutamol in these patients.

CARDIAC SURGERY
This is another most unusual situation characterized by a much greater insulin resistance than in major general surgery. There is four times the normal catecholamine output and it is thought that maximal secretion rates of corticosteroids are reached. The effects of cardiopulmonary bypass itself and the priming agents which are used with it add to the problem, as does the fact that hypothermia appears to be associated with reduced pancreatic blood flow which will suppress any residual endogenous insulin secretion. The regimen shown in Fig. 19.13 has been found to be of value.

Clearly it is most important that these patients have good preoperative diabetic control. 500ml of five per cent dextrose should be infused with 16u of short-acting insulin added four-to-six hourly during the time of bypass; careful monitoring is necessary with blood glucose strips. After cardiac surgery has been completed, five per cent dextrose is continued at around 60–80ml/h and insulin needs to be delivered at between 5–10u/h. Flexibility is essential in this situation and control of diabetes is made much easier by using the insulin infusion pump which requires constant monitoring by highly skilled staff. Inotropic support, infection or renal failure with peritoneal dialysis will all increase insulin requirements.

PERIOPERATIVE MANAGEMENT IN TYPE II DIABETES
Guidelines for the care of Type II (non insulin-dependent) diabetic patients are given in Fig. 19.14. These patients should be

---

CARDIAC SURGERY AND DIABETIC CONTROL

begin with 500ml 5% dextrose with 16u short-acting insulin infused 4–6 hourly

postoperative insulin requirements vary between 5–10u hourly

inotropic support or infection further increases insulin requirements

Fig. 19.13 Control of diabetes during cardiac surgery.

GUIDELINES FOR PERIOPERATIVE MANAGEMENT IN TYPE II DIABETES

assess diabetic control:
  if poor, start on short-acting insulin thrice daily
  monitor with plasma glucose levels

minor surgery
stop oral agents on day of surgery (avoid chlorpropamide and metformin)
do not infuse large amounts of intravenous glucose

major surgery
as for minor surgery, although postoperative short-acting insulin thrice daily is often required for a few days (8–12u t.d.s.)

Fig. 19.14 Management of Type II diabetic patients during the perioperative period.

advantages: it is expensive to buy, it needs a continuous blood probably best to start them on short-acting insulin thrice daily before meals. If the patient is controlled on oral agents, these should be stopped on the day before surgery. Chlorpropamide and metformin should be avoided because the former can cause hypoglycaemia and the latter increases the risk of lactic acidosis. Ideally these drugs should be stopped just before surgery is planned. Infusion of large amounts of glucose should be avoided during the perioperative period as this may lead to quite marked degrees of hyperosmolality. After major surgery, postoperative insulin may be required for a few days. Most patients usually require 8–12u of short-acting insulin thrice daily.

An alternative method (Fig. 19.15) is to use an intravenous insulin and glucose mixture, as used for Type I diabetes. This should be avoided with simple surgical procedure as it complicates matters, but its use may be indicated in abdominal or thoracic surgery which is likely to be followed by prolonged fasting.

Hypotension due to shock will obviously make diabetic patients much worse and indeed insulin may have some inotropic action. A regimen with 5–10u of short-acting insulin in 500ml of ten per cent dextrose can be used; this mixture is infused over four to six hours. The insulin added can be adjusted as necessary.

ALTERNATIVE METHODS

A variety of more complex methods have been used to control diabetes during surgery. The method which provides the best control of diabetes perioperatively is the artificial endocrine pancreas (see *Chapter 15*). However, it also has many dis-

advantages: it is expensive to buy, it needs a continuous blood supply and is very labour intensive. Its use is effectively confined to very specialized units. Computer controlled insulin infusion pumps are also probably outside the budget of many hospitals. Other closed-loop insulin infusion systems have been used effectively but are not entirely satisfactory.

POSTOPERATIVE INSULIN INFUSION IN TYPE II DIABETES

indications

abdominal or thoracic surgery followed by
    prolonged fast
hypotension
infection
inotropic drugs

starting regimen

500ml 10% dextrose with 5–10u short-acting
    insulin added

Fig. 19.15 Insulin infusion in Type II diabetic patients.

REFERENCES

Alberti KGMM & Thomas DJB (1979) The management of diabetes during surgery. *British Journal of Anaesthesia*, **51**, 693–710.

Fletcher J, Langman MJS & Lellock TD (1965) Effect of surgery on blood sugar levels in diabetes mellitus. *Lancet*, **2**, 52–54.

Galloway JA & Shuman CR (1963) Diabetes and surgery. A study of 667 cases. *American Journal of Medicine*, **34**, 177–191.

Ryan NT (1976) Metabolic adaptations for energy production during trauma and sepsis. *Surgical Clinics of North America*, **56**, 1073–1090.

Taitelman U, Reece EA & Bessman AN (1977) Insulin in the management of the diabetic surgical patient: continuous intravenous infusion versus subcutaneous administration. *Journal of the American Medical Association*, **237**, 658–660.

Thomas DJB, Hinds CJ & Rees GM (1983) The management of insulin-dependent diabetes during cardiopulmonary bypass and general surgery. *Anaesthesia*, **38**, 1047–1052.

Wright PD, Henderson K & Johnson IDA (1974) Glucose utilization and insulin secretion during surgery in man. *British Journal of Surgery*, **61**, 5–8.

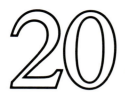

Management of Diabetes in Pregnancy

M Ivo Drury MD PRCPI FRCOG DSc (Hon) FACP (Hon)

NORMAL PREGNANCY AND GLUCOSE METABOLISM

Throughout normal pregnancy metabolic adaptations occur to provide a constant fuel supply for the life and development of the fetus. Initially, the pancreatic B cells of the mother, in response to rising levels of oestrogens and progesterone, become hyperplastic and secrete more insulin, causing greater utilization of glucose, increased glycogen storage and a reduction in the output of glucose from the liver (i.e. an anabolic state). The simplest evidence of this change is a reduction in fasting blood glucose levels.

Glucose is transferred across the placenta by facilitated diffusion whilst amino acids are actively transported by the placenta to the fetus. Consequently, the activity of the fetal pancreatic B cells is determined by the maternal blood glucose and amino acid levels. Giant islets indicative of overactivity are a common finding at autopsy in infants of diabetic mothers if diabetic control is inadequate (see Fig. 20.25d).

As pregnancy advances, further metabolic adaptations occur, with increasing maternal levels of oestrogens, progesterone, free cortisol and human placental lactogen (hPL), which lead to a progressive increase in tissue resistance to insulin at post-insulin receptor level (Fig. 20.1). This is counterbalanced by increased secretion of insulin from maternal B cells.

In summary, the metabolic adaptations of normal pregnancy result in a lowering of fasting blood glucose levels and an increasing output of insulin, the latter being particularly marked during the last twenty weeks of pregnancy. The practical considerations which arise from these changes include the following: (i) in some patients carbohydrate intolerance develops for the first time as pregnancy advances (gestational diabetes mellitus or GDM); (ii) the standard criteria for the diagnosis of diabetes mellitus are not applicable in pregnancy; (iii) there is an increase in insulin requirement as pregnancy advances; and (iv) the criteria of strict metabolic control are different during pregnancy. These considerations will be discussed individually.

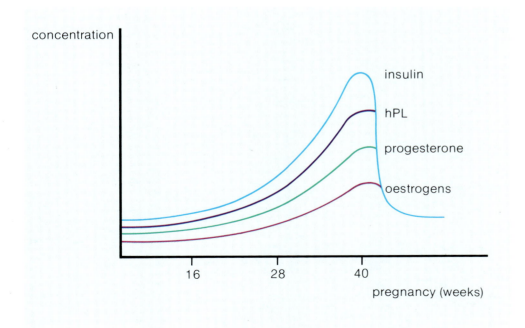

Fig. 20.1 Hormonal changes during normal pregnancy. As pregnancy advances, the output of insulin antagonists such as human placental lactogen (hPL), oestrogens and progesterone increases. This is counterbalanced by an increase in insulin secretion.

GESTATIONAL DIABETES MELLITUS (GDM)

As pregnancy advances, the increased demand for insulin is met by increased pancreatic B cell activity. If, however, B cell reserve is impaired, insulin resistance becomes dominant causing hyperglycaemia. The correct management of carbohydrate intolerance depends upon the degree of insulin deficiency. The intolerance may be either mild and difficult to detect, but easy to control by dietary restriction, or florid, requiring the administration of insulin to restore blood glucose to normal. It is important to detect carbohydrate intolerance even if it is mild because, if it is unrecognized, either macrosomia or perinatal death may occur (Fig. 20.2).

In the majority of cases, the carbohydrate intolerance develops in the last half and especially the last six weeks of pregnancy, at which time insulin resistance increases progressively until delivery when it rapidly disappears (Fig. 20.3). In a minority of cases, the carbohydrate intolerance persists after the puerperium.

Unrecognized gestational diabetes may result in fetal death, malformation or increased fetal size and weight (macrosomia), leading to difficulties at delivery, such as shoulder dystocia. The case history in Fig. 20.2 illustrates the importance of diagnosing gestational diabetes.

A number of clinical clues may suggest the presence of gestational diabetes; these include a family history of diabetes, unexplained problems with previous pregnancies and, particularly, large babies (Fig. 20.4). The reliability of these clinical pointers to the presence of gestational diabetes has been assessed (Fig. 20.5). Either glycosuria and a relevant obstetric or family history of diabetes or both of the latter together were important pointers to the presence of diabetes in this study.

Testing

As insulin resistance is maximal in the third trimester, the definitive oral glucose tolerance test (OGTT) should be performed near term in cases which come under suspicion at the antenatal clinic (see *Chapter 6*). However, in some patients, B cell inadequacy may be such that carbohydrate intolerance occurs at an early stage.

All suspect cases should be seen at three-week intervals when either a fasting or a random blood glucose measurement is taken. If the fasting value is 5mmol/l (90mg/dl) or lower or the random level 7mmol/l (126mg/dl) or lower, supervision should be continued at three-week intervals and the OGTT should be delayed until thirty-nine weeks of pregnancy. If these values are exceeded, the OGTT should be performed forthwith. The only validated, reliable OGTT criteria for the diagnosis of diabetes during pregnancy are those of O'Sullivan and Mahan (Fig. 20.6). However, the World Health Organization (WHO) recommends the same criteria as for non-pregnant adults.

OBSTETRIC HISTORY OF A PATIENT WITH UNRECOGNIZED GDM	
1945	neonatal death (spina bifida)
1950–1955	3 live infants
1956	neonatal death (birth weight 5kg)
1957	neonatal death (spina bifida)
1958	diabetes diagnosed

Fig. 20.2 Gross example of unrecognized GDM. This case illustrates the classical features: (i) malformations, (ii) neonatal death and (iii) macrosomia. A series of neonatal deaths occurred before diabetes was diagnosed.

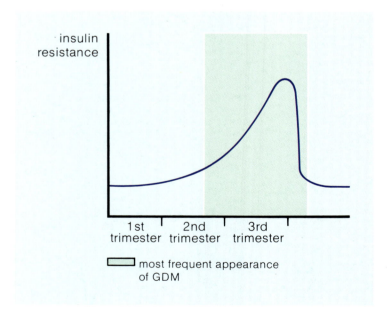

Fig. 20.3 Increase of insulin resistance and the appearance of GDM.

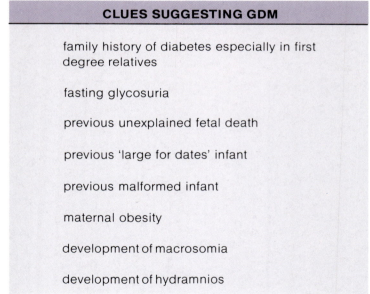

CLUES SUGGESTING GDM
family history of diabetes especially in first degree relatives
fasting glycosuria
previous unexplained fetal death
previous 'large for dates' infant
previous malformed infant
maternal obesity
development of macrosomia
development of hydramnios

Fig. 20.4 Diagnostic clues suggesting GDM.

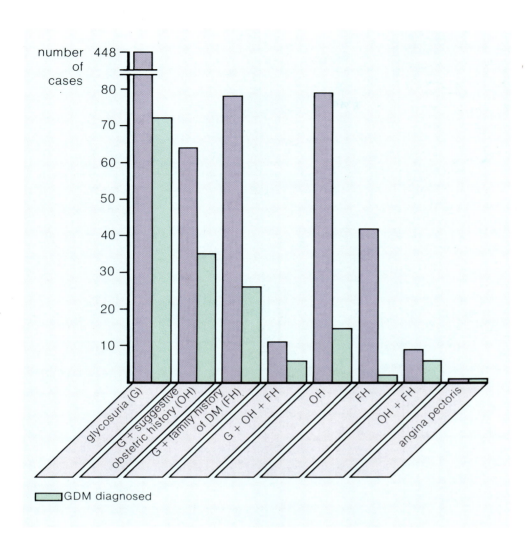

number of cases

GDM diagnosed

- glycosuria (G)
- G + suggestive obstetric history (OH)
- G + family history of DM (FH)
- G + OH + FH
- OH
- FH
- OH + FH
- angina pectoris

Fig. 20.5 Reliability of clues to the presence of GDM. 772 mothers were tested in this study. It was found that glycosuria (G) in combination with either a relevant obstetric history (OH) or family history (FH) of diabetes, is an important marker of GDM (Drury & Timoney, 1970).

100g OGTT DURING PREGNANCY	
time of sample (hours)	venous plasma glucose in mmol/l (mg/dl)
0 (fasting)	≥ 5.8 (105)
1	≥ 10.6 (190)
2	≥ 9.2 (165)
3	≥ 8.1 (145)

Fig. 20.6 The oral glucose tolerance test (OGTT) during pregnancy. The most reliable criteria for the diagnosis of GDM and those recommended by the National Diabetes Data Group (NDDG) of the USA, require a 100g oral glucose load and any two of the values shown in the table to be equalled or exceeded for the test to be positive (O'Sullivan and Mahan, 1964).

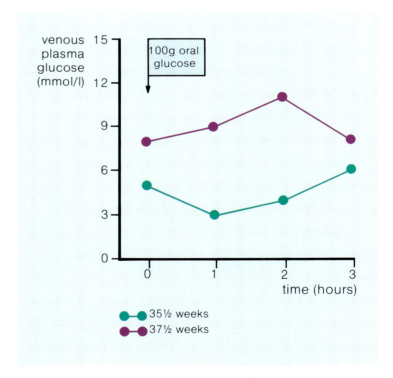

- 35½ weeks
- 37½ weeks

Fig. 20.7 Late diagnosis of GDM. The results of two OGTT's in a 38-year-old patient at 35½ and 37½ weeks of a pregnancy are shown. The patient had a family history of diabetes and the results show a rapid deterioration in glucose tolerance just prior to term.

The possibility that the B cell secretory reserve will fail increases as pregnancy advances. In a predisposed patient, a normal OGTT, even as late as thirty-six weeks, does not necessarily exclude gestational diabetes. This is illustrated in the case shown in Fig. 20.7 where glucose tolerance deteriorated over a period of two weeks just prior to term. Fig. 20.8 illustrates a case where glucose tolerance declined during pregnancy.

Medical Management

Most patients with gestational diabetes are able to control their condition with simple dietary restriction, although a small number require insulin. Insulin requirement during pregnancy does not preclude a return to normal after delivery (Fig. 20.9). All cases should therefore have an OGTT after the puerperium. The glucose tolerance has usually returned to normal but, if it continues to be abnormal, the condition should be classified as clinical diabetes mellitus. If the test is normal, the patient should be told that she has latent diabetes and that it may reappear later in life, in a subsequent pregnancy or during any episode of stress such as infection or trauma. She should be urged to maintain a normal body weight and to present at an early stage in subsequent pregnancies or ideally when a pregnancy is planned.

Obstetric Management

If blood glucose levels are controlled during pregnancy and there are no complications, full-term spontaneous delivery is awaited, but the possibility of macrosomia should be borne in mind. Unfortunately, typical macrosomic infants may be seen in the presence of a normal OGTT (Fig. 20.10). It is possible that macrosomia may develop from disturbances of intermediary metabolism and of amino acids in cases with normal glucose levels.

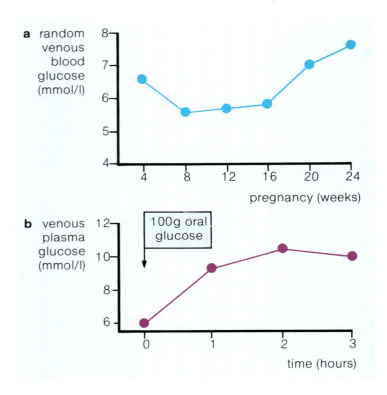

Fig. 20.8 Decline in glucose tolerance during pregnancy. These results are from a 28-year-old patient with a family history of diabetes. Because of this history, random blood samples were taken throughout the pregnancy to test glucose levels (a). When a rise in blood glucose was observed, an OGTT was performed at 22 weeks, which confirmed GDM (b).

MACROSOMIA AND NORMAL OGTT	
time of sample (hours)	venous plasma glucose in mmol/l (mg/dl)
0 (fasting)	3.8 (68)
1	8.1 (146)
2	8.2 (148)
3	7.2 (130)

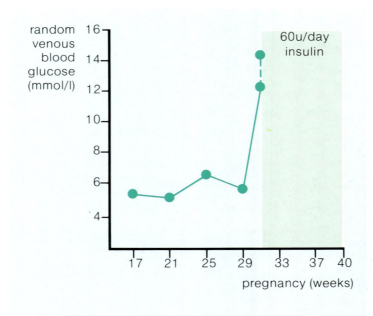

Fig. 20.9 Decline in glucose tolerance during pregnancy. These results are from a 29-year-old patient with a family history of diabetes and a previous pregnancy which produced a 4.5kg baby. Insulin was given for the last nine weeks of the pregnancy, but an OGTT after the puerperium was normal allowing discontinuation of the treatment. The correct classification is therefore GDM. Two random samples were taken in week 31.

Fig. 20.10 Macrosomic infant in the presence of a normal OGTT. The results shown in the table are for an OGTT performed at 38½ weeks in a pregnancy in a 40-year-old patient with a family history of diabetes. Two previous babies had weighed 4.5kg and 5.4kg. This pregnancy produced the baby shown which weighed 5.6kg.

PREGNANCY IN THE DIABETIC PATIENT

Most established diabetic patients will already be treated with insulin. For those on diet only, this may be continued only if glycaemic control is satisfactory (see below); if not satisfactory, insulin is needed. In patients taking oral hypoglycaemic therapy, it is essential to transfer to insulin for the duration of the pregnancy.

There are a number of complications associated with pregnancy in the diabetic woman. These affect the diabetes and its complications, the pregnancy and labour and the fetus (Fig. 20.11).

Strict glycaemic control from the earliest stage of pregnancy, if possible from before conception, reduces the incidence of problems during pregnancy. In particular, the incidence of ketoacidosis is reduced, hydramnios and macrosomia occur less frequently and delivery may safely be postponed to term.

White has proposed a classification of the severity of diabetes in pregnancy which may be useful in assessing the prognosis for the fetus (Fig. 20.12). However, the features in the White classification are not the only determinants of fetal prognosis. The following factors are of additional major importance for a successful outcome: pre-conception glycaemic control, compliance of the patient with strict glycaemic control during pregnancy, experience and dedication of the management team and avoidance of pre-term delivery.

The recommendation to defer delivery of well-controlled and uncomplicated cases to term is based on the author's experience since 1951 (Fig. 20.13). Dividing the experience into three time

---

PROBLEMS OF PREGNANCY IN THE CLINICAL DIABETIC PATIENT

ketosis more likely in diabetic mothers

possible worsening of diabetic complications, e.g. retinopathy

pre-eclampsia and hydramnios more common

malformations three times as common in infants of diabetic mothers

macrosomia may cause difficulties at delivery

further fetal problems may be produced by planned premature delivery

perinatal mortality exceeds normal

perinatal morbidity exceeds normal

Fig. 20.11 Problems of pregnancy in the diabetic patient.

A CLASSIFICATION OF THE SEVERITY OF DIABETES

class	definition
A	treated by diet alone
B	onset of DM when aged 20 or older, duration less than 10 years
C	onset at 10–19 years of age or duration 10–19 years
D	onset before 10 years of age or duration over 20 years; or with background retinopathy or hypertension
R	proliferative retinopathy or vitreous haemorrhage
F	nephropathy; more than 500mg/day proteinuria
R/F	both criteria fulfilled
H	arteriosclerotic heart disease
T	renal transplant

Fig. 20.12 Classification of the severity of diabetes. This system permits stratification of cases according to the duration and severity of diabetes (White, 1980).

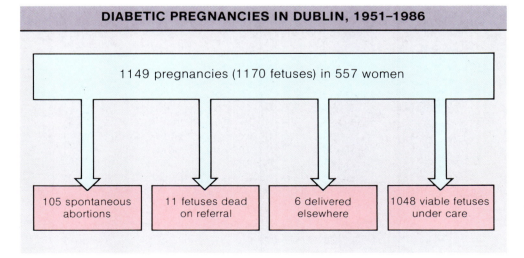

DIABETIC PREGNANCIES IN DUBLIN, 1951–1986

1149 pregnancies (1170 fetuses) in 557 women

| 105 spontaneous abortions | 11 fetuses dead on referral | 6 delivered elsewhere | 1048 viable fetuses under care |

Fig. 20.13 Diabetic pregnancies in Dublin. These data represent the author's experience between 1951 and 1986. There were no maternal deaths. The spontaneous abortion rate was 9.0% and there was a total perinatal mortality rate of 7.4% (42 intrauterine and 36 neonatal deaths).

phases, there was an improvement in perinatal mortality related to the introduction of very strict glycaemic control and the decision to allow uncomplicated, well-controlled cases to progress to term (Fig. 20.14).

Management of Diabetes during Pregnancy

Very strict blood glucose control is the key to successful management of diabetes during pregnancy. Before conception, the management policy should be agreed and introduced. This helps to reduce the frequency of fetal malformations. The degree of control that is aimed for is much more strict than that seen in most patients in routine clinics (Fig. 20.15). Glycaemic control is assessed by the patient performing intensive blood glucose home monitoring, preferably with a reflectance meter (Fig. 20.16). The results are seen at the clinic, initially every two weeks and later weekly, throughout pregnancy when glycosylated haemoglobin or fructosamine levels are checked to confirm the level of control.

There should be periodic checks on the optic fundi to assess any development or progression of diabetic retinopathy (Fig. 20.17). Insulin treatment should be given at least twice daily, usually using a mixture of an intermediate- and a fast-acting insulin. Occasionally, it may be necessary to use multiple daily injections;

DIABETIC PREGNANCIES IN DUBLIN		
period	viable fetuses	perinatal loss (%)
1951–1974	502	9.7
1975–1978	154	5.2
1979–1986	392	5.3 *

* perinatal loss was 3.1% if 9 cases of lethal malformations are excluded

Fig. 20.14 The three successive policies of management of diabetic pregnancies in Dublin between 1951 and 1986. In 1975 a policy of very strict glycaemic control was introduced and in 1979 it was decided to permit well-controlled, uncomplicated cases to go to term.

CONTROL OF DIABETES DURING PREGNANCY

fasting blood glucose levels should be
≤ 5mmol/l (≤ 90mg/dl)

post-prandial blood glucose levels should be
≤ 7mmol/l (≤ 126mg/dl)

glycosylated haemoglobin or serum fructosamine levels should be normal

Fig. 20.15 Aims of control of diabetes during pregnancy.

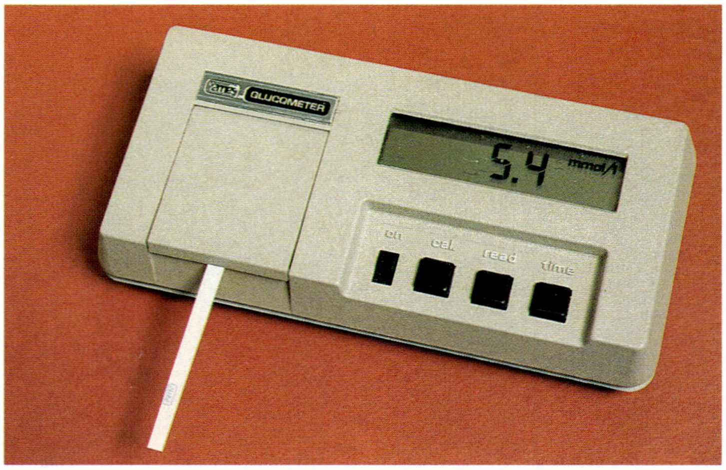

Fig. 20.16 Reflectance meter for blood glucose strips.

ASSESSMENT OF CONTROL OF DIABETES DURING PREGNANCY

home blood glucose profiles:
pre- and post-breakfast
pre- and post-lunch
pre- and post-dinner
late evening

home monitoring with meters

glycosylated haemoglobin or serum fructosamine levels checked every 2 weeks

periodic examination of optic fundi

Fig. 20.17 Measures needed to assess the success of control of diabetes during pregnancy.

for example, fast-acting insulin three or four times daily, with either a slow- or intermediate-acting insulin at bedtime (Fig. 20.18).

As insulin resistance increases during pregnancy, dose requirements for insulin will also increase. In a study of a personal series of fifty patients, the mean total daily dose requirements when not pregnant was 45 units compared with 88 units during pregnancy.

Monitoring Fetal Well-being

In selected cases where there is anxiety about fetal well-being, for example, if the mother shows signs of pre-eclampsia, certain measurements can be taken (Fig. 20.19). Twice-weekly oestriol levels provide some index of feto-placental function. Fetal growth can be assessed clinically and by ultrasonography; retarded growth indicates placental insufficiency and excess growth suggests inadequate glycaemic control. A reduction in liquor amnii suggests placental insufficiency and an increase suggests poor glycaemic control. Cardiotocography, twice-weekly, may also be used as an index of fetal well-being.

Maternal Hypoglycaemia during Pregnancy

Strict glycaemic control may cause maternal hypoglycaemia; however, this does not seem to be harmful to the fetus. Of one hundred and five cases studied, in which the mother was unconscious at least once during pregnancy, the perinatal mortality was only 3.5% and the perinatal deaths were not related in time to the episode of hypoglycaemia. Nevertheless, it is important to instruct the spouse or other relative in the use of glucagon injection for the treatment of severe hypoglycaemia.

Diabetic Retinopathy during Pregnancy

Careful examination will show that retinopathy is common at the onset of pregnancy. Thus, in a prospective study of fifty-three diabetic pregnancies supervised at Dublin, retinopathy was present in thirty-three (62%) at first examination, in contrast to eighteen (46.2%) of thirty-nine non-pregnant matched control subjects. As pregnancy advanced, eight other diabetic patients developed retinopathy, increasing the prevalence to 77.4%. Progressive changes also occurred. Four patients (7.5%) showed neovascularization, one for the first time; the condition of all four deteriorated during pregnancy. Six months after delivery background retinopathy had reverted to the level in the controls. Neovascularization also showed some regression.

Pregnancy should not be avoided because of the presence of proliferative retinopathy, but close observation is needed in case laser therapy is required.

Management at Home or in Hospital?

Previously, diabetic patients were admitted to hospital for long periods, often the whole of the third trimester, in order to achieve good glycaemic control. With the advent of blood glucose home monitoring systems, the trend has been towards outpatient management unless complications arise. The reasons for admission to improve diabetic control include poor compliance with therapy and infrequent attendance at clinic. Admission may be necessary in early pregnancy to establish control and to teach blood glucose home monitoring, and in late pregnancy if obstetric complications occur (Fig. 20.20).

STRICT CONTROL OF DIABETES DURING PREGNANCY

1. twice daily mixtures of fast-acting and intermediate-acting insulin; e.g. Actrapid and Monotard or Velosulin and Insulatard

2. multiple daily injections, e.g. Actrapid three times daily with meals, and slow- or intermediate-acting insulin at bedtime, e.g. Ultratard, Monotard or Insulatard

Fig. 20.18 Strict control of diabetes during pregnancy. These are two alternative regimens that can be used to attain strict control.

TESTS FOR FETAL WELL-BEING

oestriol levels checked twice weekly

clinical assessment twice weekly

ultrasonography for fetal size and liquor volume

cardiotocography

Fig. 20.19 Measurements used to monitor fetal well-being.

REASONS FOR ADMISSION TO HOSPITAL

early in pregnancy to educate patient

establish strict glycaemic control

familiarize patient with staff and with treatment targets

re-establish glycaemic control if lost

treatment of obstetric complications

Fig. 20.20 Reasons for the admission of pregnant diabetic patients to hospital. Admission may be required for any of the reasons given in this table.

Delivery

The well-controlled, uncomplicated case should not be delivered until term. If complications arise, a decision to deliver prematurely should be based on clinical judgement aided by assessments of fetal well-being and of placental function by, for example, cardiotocography and oestriol levels. In addition, the ratio of lecithin to sphingomyelin (L/S) in the amniotic fluid should be measured to determine the state of lung maturity and hence predict respiratory difficulties (Fig. 20.21). Previously, when premature delivery was standard practice, many neonatal deaths occurred from the respiratory distress syndrome. This condition is found more commonly in the offspring of diabetic mothers and is thought to be due to inadequate development of pulmonary surfactant leading to atelectasis.

Out of one hundred and fifty diabetic mothers whose infants were delivered in Dublin during the period August 1983 to December 1986, eighty-six per cent were delivered at thirty-eight weeks or later and forty-one per cent at term or later (Fig. 20.22). Two-thirds of these deliveries were vaginal (Fig. 20.23). In the

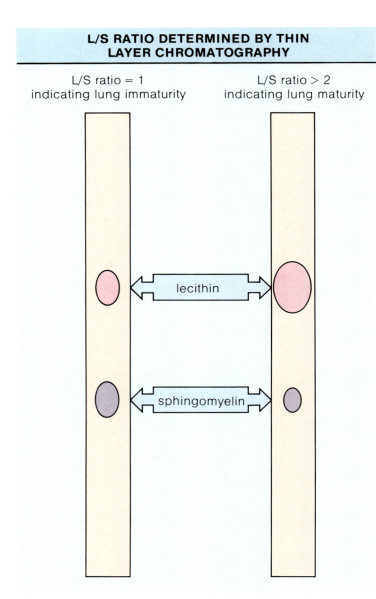

L/S RATIO DETERMINED BY THIN LAYER CHROMATOGRAPHY

L/S ratio = 1 indicating lung immaturity

L/S ratio > 2 indicating lung maturity

lecithin

sphingomyelin

Fig. 20.21 Measurement of the lecithin to sphingomyelin (L/S) ratio. This should be determined to predict respiratory difficulties.

MATURITY AT DELIVERY	
gestation (weeks)	number (%)
before 37	16 (10.6)
37–37 6/7	5 (3.3)
38–38 6/7	32 (21.3)
39–39 6/7	35 (23.3)
40–40 6/7	44 (29.3)
41 and following	18 (12.0)

Fig. 20.22 Fetal age at delivery. The data are of the 150 deliveries in Dublin between August 1983 and December 1986. 86% were delivered at 38 weeks or later.

MODE OF DELIVERY		
vaginal 100 (66.6%)		
caesarean section		
primary elective (1 for antepartum haemorrhage)	14	
for failed induction	20	50 (33.3%)
repeat operation	16	

Fig. 20.23 Mode of delivery in the 150 deliveries shown in Fig. 20.22.

U.K. survey, deliveries occurred much earlier (Fig. 20.24a) and this contributed to the different rates of perinatal morbidity (Fig. 20.24b). Benefits of late delivery include a high rate of spontaneous labour, a high rate of vaginal delivery with a correspondingly low caesarean section rate and a reduction in perinatal morbidity. As maturity is guaranteed, the lecithin to sphingomyelin ratio need not be estimated.

Management during Labour and Delivery

In uncomplicated cases, artificial rupture of the membranes at term may be performed. The patient should be fasting to permit general anaesthesia should problems arise.

If the liquor amnii is clear, breakfast is allowed and the usual insulin is administered. If the patient is not eating, five per cent dextrose solution should be infused intravenously, with 12–16 units of fast-acting insulin in each litre and run in over eight hours (i.e. 1.5–2u/h). Blood glucose should be monitored every two hours. If labour has not started within twenty-four hours,

oxytocin is given and if labour is not established six hours later, a caesarean section will be necessary. With a policy of delivery at term many infants may join their mother immediately without transfer to a neonatal unit.

Neonatal Mortality

With skilled paediatric care, neonatal mortality is rare unless delivery has been either very premature or a malformation exists; malformations now account for about one half of all perinatal loss. The only prospect of diminishing the malformation rate appears to lie in the strict control of diabetes at the time of conception.

Perinatal Morbidity in the Diabetic Patient

Unfortunately, perinatal morbidity is still a problem but it is largely determined by the timing of delivery. Thus, morbidity rates are much higher when early delivery is practiced (see Fig. 20.24).

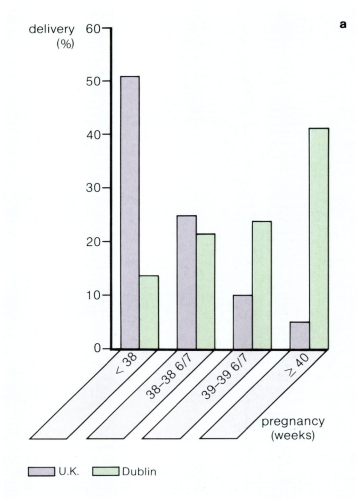

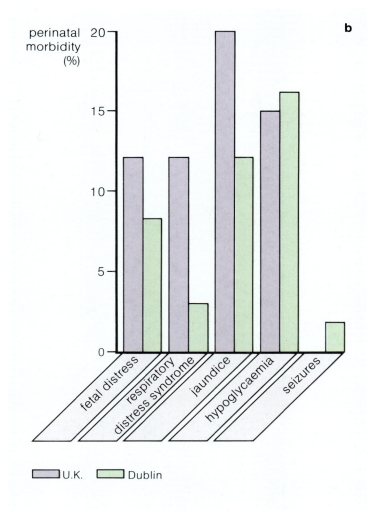

Fig. 20.24 Relationship between (a) gestational age at delivery and (b) perinatal morbidity. The results from a U.K. national survey and from the National Maternity Hospital, Dublin are shown. Perinatal morbidity is expressed as a percentage of all births to diabetic mothers.

Congenital Malformation

The malformations seen in infants of diabetic mothers are similar to those in infants of non-diabetic mothers except for a greater tendency towards cardiac and neural tube defects. Autopsy may disclose characteristic findings in the ovaries and testes of infants of diabetic mothers which are indicative of maternal diabetes (Fig. 20.25). Familiarity with these changes may draw attention to unrecognized gestational diabetes as a cause of perinatal death.

As it is possible that high levels of blood glucose may disrupt organogenesis, patients should be persuaded to report for special, intensive supervision when conception is contemplated. However, malformations have occurred in infants of mothers who had normal levels of glycosylated haemoglobin at conception.

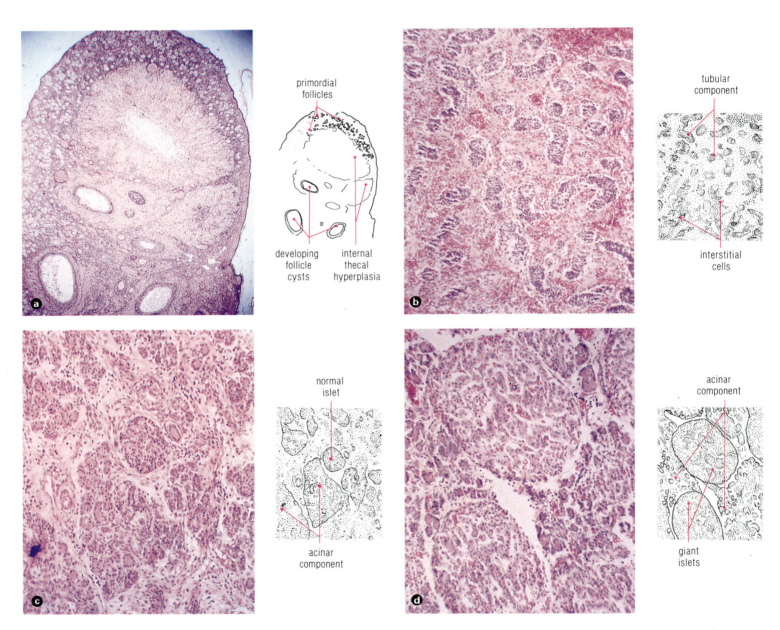

Fig. 20.25 Histological sections at autopsy of perinatal deaths. Section (a) is from the ovary of an infant of a diabetic mother. Section (b) shows an abnormal testis with hyperplasia of the interstitial tissue in maternal diabetes mellitus. It is essential that this feature is assessed in relation to the gestational age of the fetus. Sections (c) and (d) show normal and abnormal pancreatic tissue respectively, the latter showing marked islet hypertrophy in an infant of a patient with diabetes. H and E stain.

REFERENCES

Drury MI (1984) Diabetes in pregnancy – Matthews Duncan revisited. *Irish Journal of Medical Science*, **153**, 144–151.

Drury MI, Greene AT & Stronge JM (1977) Pregnancy complicated by clinical diabetes mellitus – A study of 600 pregnancies. *Obstetrics and Gynecology*, **49**, 419–522.

Drury MI, Stronge JM, Foley ME & McDonald DW (1983) Pregnancy in the diabetic patient: timing and mode of delivery. *Obstetrics and Gynecology*, **62**, 279–282.

Drury MI & Timoney FJ (1970) Latent diabetes in pregnancy. *Journal of Obstetrics and Gynaecology of the British Commonwealth*, **77**, 24–28.

Hare JW & White P (1980) Gestational diabetes and the White classification. *Diabetes Care*, **3**, 394.

O'Sullivan JB & Mahan CM (1964) Criteria for the oral glucose tolerance test in pregnancy. *Diabetes*, **13**, 278–285.

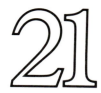

21 Diabetic Comas

Alan Rees MD MRCP ● **Edwin Gale** MB FRCP

A variety of metabolic emergencies may occur in the course of diabetes mellitus and its treatment (Fig. 21.1). Whilst all these comas may occur in patients with diabetes, the aetiology, pathogenesis, presentation and treatment of each may differ considerably. Only diabetic ketoacidosis, hyperosmolar non-ketotic coma and hypoglycaemic coma will be considered here.

DIABETIC KETOACIDOSIS

Diabetic ketoacidosis used to be known as 'diabetic coma', since diabetes almost inevitably progressed to coma and death in the days before insulin treatment. Nowadays less than ten per cent of new patients present initially with loss of consciousness. Severe diabetic ketoacidosis has been defined by Alberti as severe uncontrolled diabetes, requiring emergency treatment with insulin and intravenous fluids, and where the total blood ketone

concentration is greater than 5mmol/l. Schade and Eaton define it as a metabolic acidosis with an arterial pH less than 7.2, a blood glucose concentration greater than 16mmol/l and a plasma ketone concentration greater than 2mmol/l. The latter definition has the advantage of greater precision, but since measurement of ketone bodies is not readily available in most hospitals, and certainly not as an emergency, a simple definition in terms of severe uncontrolled diabetes (with an elevation of the plasma ketones), requiring emergency treatment with insulin and intravenous fluids, is usually sufficient.

Mortality from Ketoacidosis

Survival rates from diabetic ketoacidosis have greatly improved in the course of this century due to the introduction of insulin and other advances in medical care (Fig. 21.2). By 1950, most of the methods currently used in the treatment of diabetic ketoacidosis

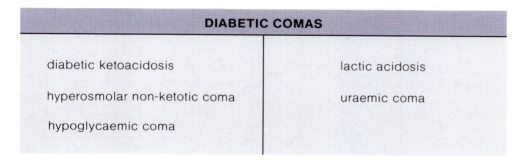

DIABETIC COMAS	
diabetic ketoacidosis	lactic acidosis
hyperosmolar non-ketotic coma	uraemic coma
hypoglycaemic coma	

Fig. 21.1 Causes of comas in diabetic patients.

Fig. 21.2 Milestones in the therapy of diabetic ketoacidosis. Each point represents mortality rates reported from individual centres in the U.S.A. and Europe. The dates at which the various improvements were endorsed are shown. Insulin revolutionized the treatment of this condition, but important supplementary advances have been made since then.

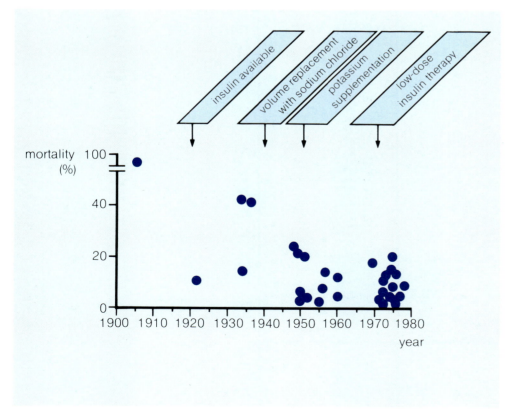

were available and overall mortality figures have changed little since then, with a present mean value of approximately nine per cent. There is, however, a wide range from zero to twenty per cent, even in major centres and in less specialized units the mortality may be as high as twenty to thirty per cent. This may reflect variability not only in patient care, but also in the methods used to calculate mortality rates. For example, some series have excluded patients who died soon after admission, or from a complication not directly related to the ketoacidosis. It seems likely therefore that a wide range in mortality will continue to be reported until uniform criteria are introduced.

Despite this variability, the death rate from diabetic keto-acidosis may be a useful indicator of adequacy of health care in a population. Indeed, the National Commission on Diabetes in the U.S.A. estimated that up to two-thirds of cases of diabetic ketoacidosis could be prevented. Different rates of incidence and mortality might reflect ethnic differences influencing the relative frequency of insulin-dependent (Type I) and non insulin-dependent (Type II) diabetes in the population, and may also be directly related to socioeconomic differences.

Age is one of the most important prognostic factors in diabetic ketoacidosis (Fig. 21.3). The incidence is considerably higher in

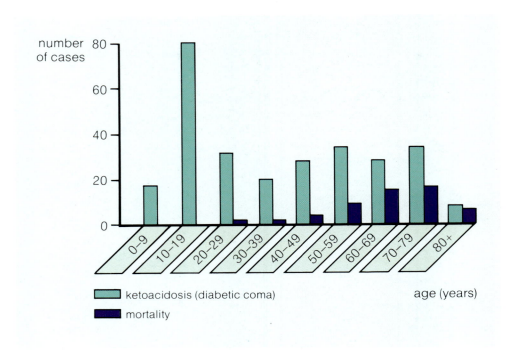

Fig. 21.3 Age and mortality from ketoacidosis. The results are from a series of 283 cases presenting between 1969 and 1975. From Gale *et al.* (1981), by courtesy of Springer Verlag.

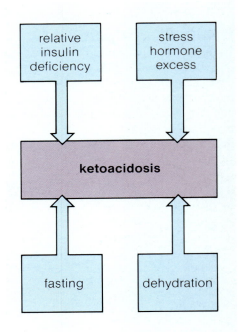

Fig. 21.4 Pathogenesis of diabetic ketoacidosis.

Fig. 21.5 Relative sensitivities of various metabolic processes.

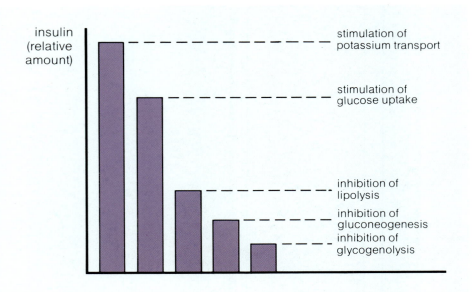

young patients, but a much higher mortality has been consistently reported in older people, possibly due to the greater frequency of associated disease. This is unlikely to be the whole explanation, however, and strategies of prevention and treatment of ketoacidosis should perhaps focus more on the elderly.

Pathogenesis

The pathogenesis of diabetic ketoacidosis is complex. A simple approach which may be helpful in understanding the condition is to consider the four main pathways which lead directly to increased ketogenesis and gluconeogenesis (Fig. 21.4).

Insulin Deficiency

The sensitivity of various metabolic processes to insulin varies considerably, resulting in a hierarchy of actions depending upon plasma insulin concentration (Fig. 21.5). Very low levels of insulin are necessary before lipolysis is fully stimulated and ketogenesis is unrestrained. This is consistent with the observation that ketoacidosis may take several days to develop after insulin withdrawal in an unstressed diabetic patient. Many Type I diabetic patients retain a limited capacity to produce endogenous insulin, thus delaying the development of hyperketonaemia and hyperglycaemia. If absolute insulin deficiency is defined as a plasma insulin concentration below 6mu/l, the majority of cases of ketoacidosis do not fall into this category. In fact, one series of one hundred and six cases showed no difference between the mean plasma insulin concentration in ketoacidotic patients and those of normal men after an overnight fast. However, relative insulin deficiency always exists in diabetic ketoacidosis and may be defined as a plasma concentration of less than 50mu/l when the concomitant blood glucose is greater than 14mmol/l.

Stress hormone excess

Many studies have emphasized the importance of increased secretion of stress hormones such as glucagon, cortisol, catecholamines and growth hormone (GH) in augmenting the rise in glucose and ketone bodies during insulin withdrawal. Indeed, whenever stress hormones have been measured, levels of at least one have been elevated. Plasma glucagon rises in parallel with the development of ketoacidosis and plasma catecholamine levels are directly related to the extent of the metabolic derangement. Thus diabetic ketoacidosis is characterized by relative insulin deficiency and stress hormone excess.

Dehydration

All patients with severe diabetic ketoacidosis are dehydrated with a fluid deficit usually ranging from five to seven litres. Several mechanisms contribute to dehydration including fever, vomiting, diarrhoea and hyperventilation. However, the most important factor is the osmotic diuresis which occurs when hyperglycaemia exceeds the renal glucose threshold. In a well hydrated patient, this permits the kidney to excrete glucose and, to a limited extent, hydrogen ions from the circulation. However, the severe hyperglycaemia associated with ketoacidosis causes an osmotic diuresis which contracts the intravascular volume. The patient is frequently nauseated and unable to replace this loss orally, with resulting severe dehydration and ultimately renal impairment. Thus the ability of the kidney to excrete glucose and hydrogen ions is compromised (Fig. 21.6). Rehydration is of fundamental importance in the therapy of diabetic ketoacidosis and will in itself lower plasma glucose and decrease stress hormone levels.

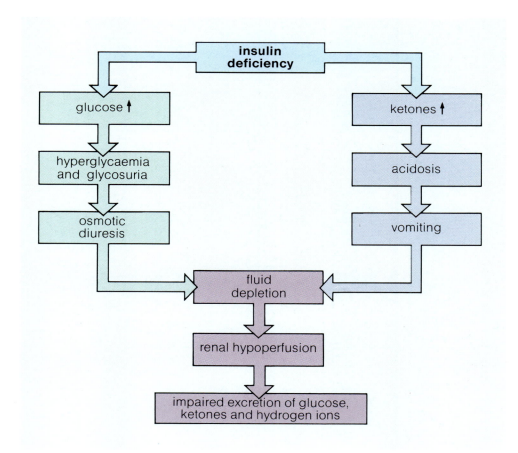

Fig. 21.6 Effects of osmotic diuresis. The combination of severe hyperglycaemia and ketoacidosis resulting from insulin deficiency leads to an osmotic diuresis and fluid depletion.

Fasting

Fasting induces ketoacidosis by several mechanisms including a gradual reduction of insulin levels and a simultaneous rise in counter-regulatory hormone concentrations. Fasting results in decreased peripheral utilization of ketone bodies, compounding the pre-existing hepatic ketogenesis in the decompensated patient and resulting in severe hyperketonaemia.

Ketosis and Ketonuria

Ketones are usually present in very small amounts in the blood (< 0.2mmol/l). During ketosis they accumulate in the circulation and are then excreted in the urine (ketonuria). Ketosis occurs when there is a deficiency of intracellular glucose metabolism as occurs in diabetes. The anabolic and catabolic phases of intermediary metabolism are hormonally controlled, with insulin as the main anabolic hormone and a rise in glucagon coupled with a fall in insulin characteristic of the catabolic phase. This can be induced by a twelve-hour fast and leads to stimulation of glycogenolysis and gluconeogenesis. In addition, hydrolysis of adipose tissue triglycerides to free non-esterified fatty acids (NEFA) is stimulated. These circulating free fatty acids are taken up by the liver at a rate dependent upon their plasma concentration. During catabolism they are transported to the mitochondria via fatty acyl CoA and fatty acyl carnitine. Acetyl CoA then undergoes condensation to acetoacetate which in turn may be reduced to β-hydroxybutyrate or decarboxylated to acetone (Fig. 21.7). Acetoacetate, acetone and β-hydroxybutyrate

are known as ketone bodies, although strictly speaking β-hydroxybutyrate is not a ketone and is not detected by bedside tests for ketones.

In diabetic ketoacidosis there is both increased lipolysis and hepatic ketogenesis coupled with decreased peripheral utilization of ketones. Circulating NEFA levels may be as high as 2mmol/l and contribute to the acidosis.

Clinical Presentation

Most of the symptoms and signs of diabetic ketoacidosis (Fig. 21.8) are easy to recognize and reflect the underlying metabolic disturbance. The classic deep-sighing (Kussmaul's) breathing, otherwise known as air hunger, is secondary to the acidosis and is quite different from the shallow rapid breathing of chest infections. It should, however, be noted that severe acidosis with a pH below 6.9 leads to inhibition of the respiratory centre and loss of this characteristic sign.

Conscious state

Fewer than ten per cent of patients are in true coma at presentation and this is usually associated with severe dehydration and a correspondingly poor prognosis. Hypoglycaemia is a much more common cause of loss of consciousness in patients with diabetes.

Gastrointestinal symptoms

Epigastric discomfort, nausea and vomiting are among the

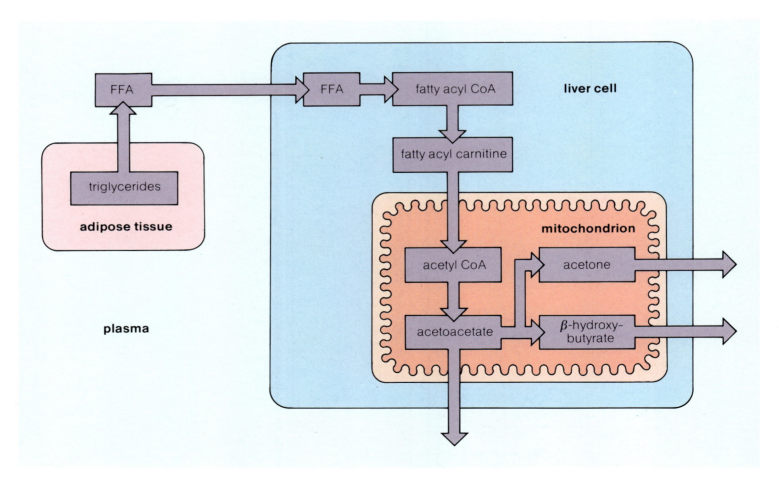

Fig. 21.7 Ketogenesis. The metabolic pathway which leads to an increase in ketone bodies (acetoacetate, acetone and β-hydroxybutyrate) in the plasma.

commonest symptoms of diabetic ketoacidosis. In one series, seventy per cent of patients had vomited at least once prior to admission. Gastric stasis and ileus may also be found in established diabetic ketoacidosis, possibly due to depletion of either potassium or magnesium. Acute abdominal pain has long been recognized as a presenting symptom and usually resolves rapidly as the ketoacidosis is treated. Such a presentation is one of the medical causes of the 'acute abdomen'.

Hypothermia
Although infection may precipitate diabetic ketoacidosis, fewer than ten per cent of patients are pyrexial on admission, many are mildly hypothermic and severe hypothermia is occasionally found. Ketoacidosis may, in addition, produce a leucocytosis and therefore both pyrexia and leucocytosis are unreliable indicators of infection. Pyrexia may be a late manifestation observed after correction of the ketoacidosis has taken place. It is thus important to check the temperature of patients admitted with ketoacidosis carefully, using a rectal thermometer if necessary. A meticulous search for possible sources of infection is always essential.

Investigations

Investigations are directed towards establishing the diagnosis of ketoacidosis, assessing its severity and seeking a possible underlying cause (Fig. 21.9). First-line investigation should include tests for glucose and ketones in both the urine and blood, using either tablets or reagent strips as appropriate. These should always be confirmed by laboratory measurements.

If the patient is severely hypotensive on admission, two units of blood should be cross-matched for transfusion. One of the most

PRESENTATION OF DIABETIC KETOACIDOSIS

symptoms	signs
vomiting (70%)	tachycardia
thirst (55%)	hypotension
polyuria (40%)	dehydration
weight loss (20%)	warm, dry skin
abdominal pain (15%)	hyperventilation
weakness (20%)	hypothermia
	impaired consciousness

Fig. 21.8 Symptoms and signs of diabetic ketoacidosis. The frequency with which each symptom occurs is given.

INVESTIGATIONS IN DIABETIC KETOACIDOSIS

assessment of severity	establishing cause
glucose	chest radiograph
urea and electrolytes	ECG
full blood count, packed cell volume and white cell count	blood and urine cultures
	throat swab
blood gases, including pH and bicarbonate	
blood ketones	

Fig. 21.9 Initial investigations in diabetic ketoacidosis. Investigations should be aimed at first assessing the severity and then establishing the cause.

important aspects of initial treatment is the maintenance of an accurate flow sheet. This makes for efficient management of the patient and ensures regular monitoring of progress.

Principles of Treatment

Diabetic ketoacidosis is a true medical emergency. The aim of treatment is smooth restoration to normal of the disordered clinical and biochemical state, with the least possible morbidity and mortality. This need not imply undue haste (Fig. 21.10). The metabolic decompensation may have taken days if not weeks to develop and over-rapid correction will lead to problems of its own. The average patient in ketoacidosis has lost approximately ten per cent of body weight with excessive loss of water over sodium (Fig. 21.11). Even so, plasma sodium may be low (67% of cases) or normal (26% of cases) on admission.

Fluid replacement

Adequate and rapid fluid replacement is probably the single most important factor in treatment. There is still some controversy about the nature of the replacement fluid to be used. The body is depleted of a hypotonic fluid and some advocate the use of hypotonic replacement solutions. However, rehydration with 75mmol/l (0.5N) sodium chloride has been linked, though not with certainty, with the development of cerebral oedema and with the onset of irreversible shock in some young patients. Most authorities now favour the use of isotonic saline to maintain the intravascular volume and to prevent rapid intracellular fluid shifts as the plasma glucose falls (Fig. 21.12).

Rehydration should normally be vigorous, particularly in the early stages of treatment. Thus 1–1.5 litres of normal saline should be given as quickly as possible once the diagnosis is established, the second litre in one hour and so forth. In shocked patients or in patients with ischaemic heart disease, a central venous line is invaluable as a guide to fluid therapy.

On occasions there is a place for the use of hypotonic saline. Hypernatraemia may compromise cerebral function and, if the plasma sodium is in excess of 150mmol/l after the first few hours of therapy, hypotonic saline (75mmol/l; 0.5N) may be used.

Potassium

All patients admitted in diabetic ketoacidosis are depleted of potassium, although the plasma potassium concentration may be high, low or normal. The principal aim of potassium replacement in the early stages of therapy is to maintain normal plasma levels, since the combination of rehydration and insulin may potentially result in severe hypokalaemia.

Plasma potassium should be measured as soon as possible following admission. The addition of 13–20mmol KCl (1–1.5g KCl) to each litre of isotonic saline is recommended, provided the initial potassium level is below 6.0mmol/l. If the initial potassium concentration is very low (below 3.0mmol/l), as much as 39–50mmol/l of KCl may be needed. A suggested potassium supplement regimen is shown in Fig. 21.13. Ideally, the potassium level should be kept at 4–5mmol/l and regular measurement of plasma levels is essential in the early stages of therapy. Continuous ECG monitoring is also recommended to indicate plasma potassium changes. Oral potassium supplements may be given for between seven and ten days after normal feeding resumes. One practical point in the interpretation of reported plasma levels of potassium is that the laboratory should always report if haemolysis is present, since release of intracellular potassium can cause a serious overestimation of plasma levels.

Insulin therapy

The aim is to correct relative insulin deficiency. When this has been achieved, lipolysis, ketogenesis and gluconeogenesis will be inhibited. At the same time peripheral utilization of glucose and ketone bodies will be restored towards normal, as will the normal transmembrane electrolyte balance. An example of a low-dose regimen is shown in Fig. 21.14. At an intravenous dosage of 6u/hour an average plasma free insulin level of 100mu/l is achieved in adults, which is more than sufficient to meet these requirements.

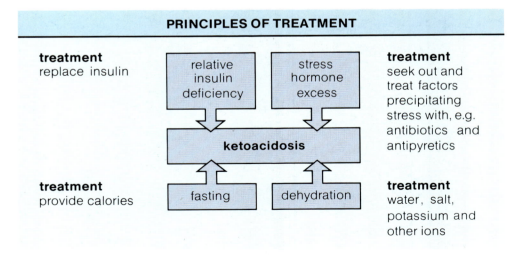

Fig. 21.10 Principles of treatment of diabetic ketoacidosis.

WATER AND ELECTROLYTE DEFICITS	
water	5–11 litres
sodium	300–700mmol
chloride	350–500mmol
potassium	200–700mmol

Fig. 21.11 Water and electrolyte deficits in diabetic ketoacidosis. All values are approximate.

FLUID REPLACEMENT REGIMEN	
use normal saline (0.9% NaCl; 150mmol/l)	
1st hour	1.5 litres
2nd hour	1.0 litre
3rd & 4th hours	1.0 litre over 2 hours
5th hour onwards	2.0 litres every 8 hours
monitor state of hydration throughout	

Fig. 21.12 Regimen for fluid replacement in diabetic ketoacidosis.

POTASSIUM SUPPLEMENTATION IN DIABETIC KETOACIDOSIS

principles

measure plasma potassium concentration on admission

aim to maintain concentration at 4–5mmol/l

estimate concentration frequently

recommended regimen

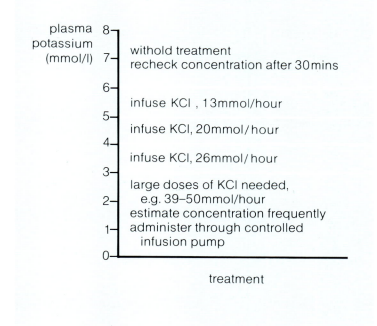

Fig. 21.13 Principles and recommended regimen for potassium supplementation in diabetic ketoacidosis.

Since insulin given as an intravenous bolus has a circulating half-life of only approximately five minutes, intermittent intravenous dosage will result in fluctuating insulin levels. It is therefore more rational to give insulin as a continuous infusion.

As a rough guide, each unit of insulin given per hour provides an increment in plasma free insulin levels of 20mu/l in adults. The relatively low infusion rate of 6u/hour is sufficient to produce a steady smooth fall in blood glucose, with considerably less risk of hypoglycaemia and hypokalaemia than the high-dose regimens. No loading dose is required when the intravenous route is used, since effective insulin concentrations are rapidly achieved. In rare instances, a patient will exhibit insulin resistance. If, after one hour, the plasma glucose is still rising and the pH falling, the pump, intravenous lines and connections should all be checked and the insulin dose doubled until a significant response is observed.

While continuous intravenous infusion is the treatment of choice, a low-dose intramuscular regimen has been developed as a simple alternative. It has the important advantage of simplicity and, in practice, it may also be safer outside an intensive care environment, since pumps sometimes fail, and this failure may pass unnoticed by inexperienced nursing staff. The method works extremely well, but extra care is needed when patients are either severely dehydrated or in shock, since circulatory failure may prevent adequate absorption of the insulin. This should not be a problem if early, adequate rehydration is used. Needles used for routine subcutaneous insulin injections are not long enough for intramuscular injections.

INSULIN REPLACEMENT
continuous intravenous infusion (soluble insulin)
children: 0.1u/kg/hour
adults: 6u/hour
intermittent intramuscular infusion
children: 0.25u/kg at once, then 0.1u/kg/hour
adults: 20u at once, then 6u/kg/hour

Fig. 21.14 Low-dose insulin regimen for the treatment of insulin deficiency in diabetic ketoacidosis. No loading dose is required with the intravenous route.

The acidosis takes longer to correct than the hyperglycaemia and ketones may remain elevated when the blood glucose has returned to normal. Continuation of the insulin infusion is thus essential. One system is to continue rehydration with normal saline until the blood glucose has fallen to below 14mmol/l. Thereafter, the infusion is changed to glucose, given as 500ml of ten per cent dextrose four-hourly. The insulin infusion is then adjusted to maintain blood glucose levels of around 10mmol/l. The plasma glucose should be checked frequently as a precaution against hypoglycaemia and as a guide to insulin dosage. The glucose infusion is useful as a source of calories and the continued glucose and insulin infusion serves to inhibit ketogenesis. Potassium supplements should also be maintained, at a rate dictated by frequent plasma potassium estimation. The intravenous infusion can be stopped and subcutaneous injections resumed when the patient is able to eat normally.

Problems of Management
Complications of diabetic ketoacidosis may occur either as the condition develops or in the course of hospital treatment (Fig. 21.15). Most are preventable, but constant clinical observation and frequent biochemical testing are necessary if this is to be achieved.

PROBLEMS OF MANAGEMENT	
problem	corrective measure
cerebral oedema	mannitol and steroids
gastric dilatation with or without ileus	nasogastric tube and aspiration
no urine produced in first 4 hours	catheterize
Po_2 less than 80mmHg on air	oxygen
blood pressure less than 80mmHg	plasma expanders
disseminated intravascular coagulation	heparinization

Fig. 21.15 Complications of treatment in diabetic ketoacidosis and the measures needed for their correction. All these problems also occur in hyperosmolar coma.

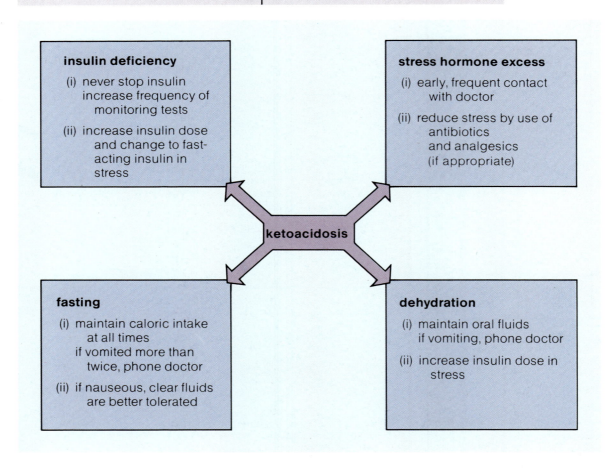

insulin deficiency
(i) never stop insulin increase frequency of monitoring tests
(ii) increase insulin dose and change to fast-acting insulin in stress

stress hormone excess
(i) early, frequent contact with doctor
(ii) reduce stress by use of antibiotics and analgesics (if appropriate)

ketoacidosis

fasting
(i) maintain caloric intake at all times if vomited more than twice, phone doctor
(ii) if nauseous, clear fluids are better tolerated

dehydration
(i) maintain oral fluids if vomiting, phone doctor
(ii) increase insulin dose in stress

Fig. 21.16 Prevention of diabetic ketoacidosis. Preventative measures under each condition are divided into (i) advice to the patient and (ii) therapeutic measures.

Can Ketoacidosis be Prevented?

As has already been described, most episodes of ketoacidosis are potentially preventable. For example, a newly-presenting patient should have been diagnosed and treated long before the stage of ketoacidosis. Similarly, many episodes would be avoided if patients were trained to continue or increase their insulin dose during periods of intercurrent illness or vomiting. Even when severe physical stress is present, for example, during myocardial infarction, prompt and efficient supervision should ensure that ketoacidosis is never allowed to develop. In other words, most problems could be avoided by better patient education, better education of hospital staff at all levels and better communication. A summary is given in Fig. 21.16. If in doubt, the only safe course is to admit patients early to hospital. Although some of these admissions may prove unnecessary, the alternative is development of a life-threatening emergency.

HYPEROSMOLAR NON-KETOTIC COMA
Pathogenesis

Hyperosmolar non-ketotic diabetic coma forms part of a spectrum of metabolic disorders in diabetes. Its proposed pathogenesis is shown in Fig. 21.17. It occurs at only ten per cent

of the frequency of ketoacidosis, but has a mortality approaching fifty per cent. Although it can occur at any age, the median age at presentation is between sixty and seventy years. A variety of precipitating causes have been reported, but the most common is perhaps uncontrolled Type II diabetes mellitus. The cause may be partly due to patients satisfying their thirst with glucose containing drinks such as lemonade or cola. These worsen hyperglycaemia and, in turn, provoke further osmotic diuresis. Antihypertensive drugs may also aggravate the condition.

At presentation, there is marked dehydration with severe hyperglycaemia and glucose levels are often over 50mmol/l. Most patients have had symptoms of polyuria and polydipsia for many days, or even weeks. Patients who are mentally alert complain of extreme thirst, weakness and fatigue. Confusion, stupor or coma may supervene and may cause diagnostic problems. Several studies have shown that the most common misdiagnosis is stroke. Convulsions are occasionally seen. Complications include stroke, myocardial infarction, peripheral gangrene and renal failure, and death can ensue.

The altered state of consciousness is probably due to plasma hyperosmolality and a strong correlation exists between the two (Fig. 21.18). In normal subjects, the level is approximately

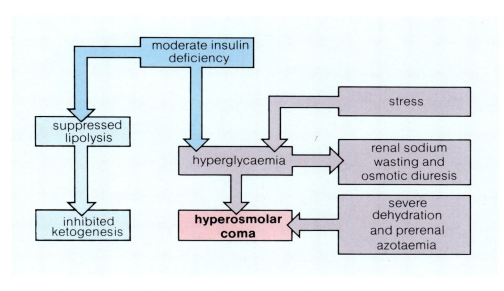

Fig. 21.17 Proposed pathogenesis of hyperosmolar non-ketotic coma (HONKC). This develops when there is a relative insulin deficiency. Circulating levels of insulin are sufficient for partial suppression of lipolysis and inhibition of hepatic ketogenesis, but insufficient to prevent hyperglycaemia.

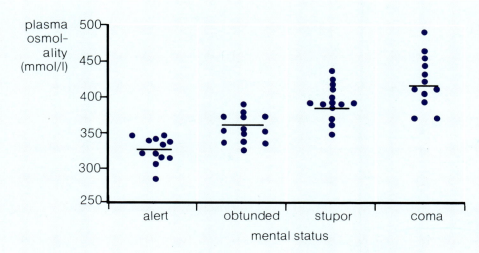

Fig. 21.18 Conscious level and plasma osmolality in hyperosmolar non-ketotic coma. Mean values are indicated.

288mmol/kg and progressive changes in the level of consciousness develop as the plasma osmolality exceeds 350mmol/kg. While it is best measured directly, the plasma osmolality can be calculated from the following formula:

$$\text{plasma osmolality (mmol/kg)} = 2 \times (Na^+ + K^+) + glucose + urea$$

The reason why some patients develop hyperosmolar coma and others develop ketoacidosis is not always clear. It may be that plasma insulin concentrations in the former condition are sufficient to suppress lipolysis and ketogenesis, but insufficient to promote effective glucose transport into the cell. Severe hyperglycaemia results from increased glucose production together with a marked decrease in glucose disposal. The osmotic diuresis causes marked dehydration which in turn causes the glomerular filtration rate to fall by more than fifty per cent. Since large quantities of glucose can be excreted rapidly by a normal kidney, compromised renal function makes an important contribution to this condition.

Treatment

Treatment is broadly similar to that outlined for diabetic ketoacidosis. Rehydration is the mainstay of therapy, but there has been considerable argument concerning the best fluid to use. It is suggested that isotonic saline (0.9%) is used during the first three hours, and thereafter hypotonic saline (0.45%), if the plasma sodium level is still greater than 150mmol/l. If the fluid deficit is large, then ten litres may need to be given over a twenty-four-hour period. However, since the majority of these patients are elderly, great care must be taken to prevent volume overload. Careful clinical observation is often sufficient, but in severe cases central venous pressure or pulmonary wedge pressure may need to be monitored. Insulin is given according to the low-dose regimen previously described (see Fig. 21.14). Potassium is administered with the start of insulin therapy and a rate of 13–20mmol/hour is usually necessary. Plasma potassium levels should be followed by regular measurement to judge adequacy of therapy.

As the high mortality rate is often associated with multiple microinfarction in the brain and severe peripheral gangrene, some authorities recommend routine anticoagulation with heparin with the initial treatment. Prostacyclin has been used in the treatment of peripheral arterial insufficiency. As always in elderly patients, multiple disease processes may be present and a careful search for underlying or associated illness is essential.

HYPOGLYCAEMIA

This is the commonest complication of insulin therapy and, for some patients, the most severe practical problem associated with the diabetic state. The term 'hypoglycaemia' is often used rather loosely in clinical practice. Strictly speaking, it is a biochemical definition of a deviation below a normal fasting range of plasma glucose. Clinicians, however, tend to use the term to describe the symptom complex produced by the neurohumoral response to

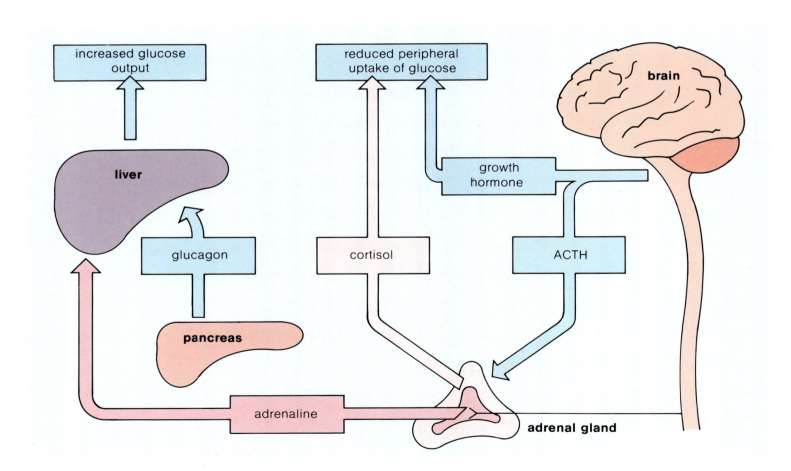

Fig. 21.19 Humoral responses to acute insulin-induced hypoglycaemia. The counter-regulatory response involves the anterior pituitary, adrenals (both cortex and medulla) and the A cells of the pancreatic islets. Glucagon and adrenaline produce a rapid increase in hepatic glucose output. Cortisol and growth hormone have a delayed effect in reducing peripheral glucose uptake.

neuroglycopenia. This complex is highly variable in patients with diabetes, partly because of adaptation to recurrent hypoglycaemia and partly because the neurohumoral response itself may change in patients who have had diabetes for many years. The humoral response to hypoglycaemia is shown in Fig. 21.19.

Clinical Features

Two main variants of the symptom complex are recognized. First, non-diabetic subjects and recently diagnosed patients typically show an adrenergic pattern of response. As the term implies, the typical features of sweating, tachycardia, pallor and tremor are partly due to catecholamine secretion and are sufficiently marked and characteristic to alert the patient to the need for glucose. With the passage of time, however, the second variant develops and insulin-treated patients often find that symptoms become variable and sometimes idiosyncratic. Symptoms of this type include blurring of vision or diplopia, circumoral paraesthesia, difficulty in concentration and impaired coordination. If these are not perceived in time the neuroglycopenia progresses to irrational behaviour, automatism or coma.

Causes

Three major factors are usually involved in hypoglycaemia, but these may be modified by a variety of other circumstances. The major factors are insulin, counter-regulation and perception of hypoglycaemia (Fig. 21.20).

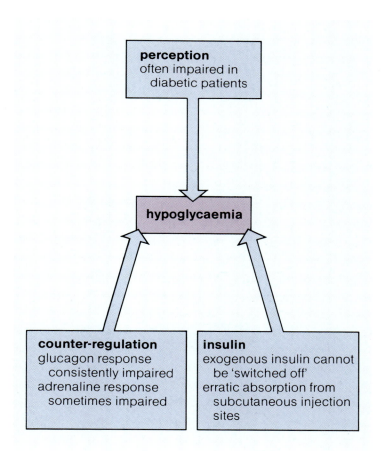

Fig. 21.20 Causes of hypoglycaemia.

Insulin absorption from injection sites is often extremely variable and for this reason alone hypoglycaemia may develop in careful patients whose diabetes is usually well-controlled. The periods of greatest risk are before meals, especially lunch, and in the early hours of the morning.

Blood glucose recovers more slowly from insulin-induced hypoglycaemia in diabetic patients than in normal subjects. One reason for this is that the glucagon response to hypoglycaemia fails progressively in the course of diabetes, so that patients then come to depend entirely upon the catecholamine response. This in turn may become impaired, leaving the patient almost defenceless against the challenge of exogenous insulin and unable to counteract its hypoglycaemic effect.

The outcome of untreated hypoglycaemia largely depends upon the balance between insulin absorption and counter-regulatory responses. However, hypoglycaemia is only an important clinical problem because many patients fail to either perceive or recognize its onset. This loss of warning may be related to failure of catecholamine secretion or autonomic neuropathy, but may prove hard to explain in individual patients.

The response to hypoglycaemia may be modified by a number of circumstances. These include age; the young and the elderly are particularly sensitive to hypoglycaemia. The risk, as indicated, also increases with longer duration of diabetes. Exercise increases the speed of insulin absorption and promotes peripheral glucose uptake in the presence of insulin. Alcohol inhibits hepatic gluconeogenesis and masks the warning symptoms of hypoglycaemia, which may be mistaken by others for simple intoxication. β-blocking drugs may modify warning symptoms, but more selective agents such as atenolol or metoprolol may safely be given.

Other problems arise because of inappropriate or excessive therapy prescribed by either a doctor or adopted by a patient striving to achieve an unrealistic level of glycaemic control. Improved control itself influences the threshold for hypoglycaemic response; in other words, the glucose level falls further before symptoms and hormonal responses are triggered. This may be the reason why intensified therapy is usually associated with more frequent, severe hypoglycaemia.

Frequency of Hypoglycaemia

Intermittent biochemical hypoglycaemia is an almost inevitable consequence of insulin therapy in adequate doses. The extent to which this is reflected in clinical symptoms varies widely. Several recent European surveys have revealed an unexpectedly high incidence of hypoglycaemic coma in patients on conventional insulin therapy; approximately one patient in three experiences coma at some time during insulin therapy, about one in ten experiences coma in the course of an average year and about one in thirty experiences recurrent problems with severe hypoglycaemia.

Recurrent hypoglycaemia

Undue sensitivity to insulin may be due to undiagnosed pituitary or adrenal insufficiency, delayed gastric emptying (a feature of autonomic neuropathy), coeliac disease or renal impairment. An unrecognized low renal threshold may be important in patients who rely on urine tests, since inappropriate amounts of insulin will be given in an attempt to abolish glycosuria. Failure of glucagon and adrenaline secretion in response to hypoglycaemia may be present, but many instances are due to mismanagement by the doctor or patient.

Management of Hypoglycaemic Coma

Hypoglycaemic coma has a relatively good prognosis when compared with other causes of non-traumatic coma, with a mortality of perhaps one in five hundred episodes. Treatment is by intravenous glucose (50ml of 50% dextrose) or by 1mg glucagon intramuscularly. The latter treatment has the advantages that it can be administered by non experts when a doctor is not available and that it avoids the technical problems of intravenous injection in a confused and restless patient. Oral glucose should always be given following recovery of consciousness, which usually occurs within five to ten minutes.

Occasionally, patients fail to respond to either therapy. In these cases a constant dextrose infusion should be given, with the aim of maintaining glucose concentrations in the 10–15mmol/l range. Cerebral oedema may be present and some authorities advocate mannitol infusion. Other causes of coma need to be considered and these will include alcohol, drug overdose and cerebral haemorrhage. Full recovery of mental function is unlikely in patients who do not regain consciousness within a few hours of treatment.

Other Presentations of Severe Hypoglycaemia

Hypothermia is a frequently overlooked complication of hypoglycaemia, which inhibits shivering. This response is rapidly restored by intravenous glucose and passive rewarming is the only other measure usually needed. Hypoglycaemia may also present with hemiplegia which may persist for several hours beyond the restoration of normoglycaemia, but full recovery of function usually occurs within twenty-four hours. Other patients, especially children, may present with convulsions. Since idiopathic epilepsy is not more common in diabetic patients, unexplained fits should be considered hypoglycaemic until proved otherwise, particularly if they occur during the night.

Prevention of Hypoglycaemia

The treatment of severe hypoglycaemia is incomplete until the cause has been identified and measures taken to prevent its recurrence. The possibility of attempted suicide may need to be considered when an episode of severe hypoglycaemia appears otherwise inexplicable. In other cases it is important to realize that many patients, and their families, fear hypoglycaemia more than any other aspect of diabetes. Improved metabolic control will have little appeal to such patients until this fear can be recognized and alleviated.

REFERENCES

Felts PW (1983) Ketoacidosis. *Medical Clinics of North America*, **67**, 831–843.

Gale EAM, Dornan TL & Tattersall RB (1981) Severely uncontrolled diabetes in the over-fifties. *Diabetologia*, **21**, 25–28.

Johnson DG & Alberti KGMM (1980) Diabetic emergencies: practical aspects of the management of diabetic ketoacidosis and diabetes during surgery. *Clinics in Endocrinology and Metabolism*, **9**(3), 437–460.

Schade DS & Eaton RP (1983) Diabetic ketoacidosis – pathogenesis, prevention and therapy. *Clinics in Endocrinology and Metabolism*, **12**(2), 321–338.

Schade DS, Eaton RP, Alberti KGMM & Johnson DG (1981) *Diabetic Coma*. Albuquerque: University of New Mexico Press.

Diabetic Macrovascular Disease

R John Jarrett MD MB BChir FFCM

The term 'macrovascular' in contrast to 'microvascular' disease is used to describe diseases of the cerebral, coronary and peripheral circulations. Accompanying disorders are based on atherosclerosis with potential contributions from abnormal platelet behaviour and increased blood coagulability. Diabetic patients on average have quantitatively more atherosclerosis than appropriate non-diabetic controls but qualitatively the atherosclerosis does not differ. There is a difference in anatomical distribution since diabetic patients are more likely to have atherosclerosis affecting vessels below the knee. These vessels are also more likely to become calcified.

MORBIDITY AND MORTALITY

Whatever the type or geographical location of diabetes, potential morbidity arises from disorders of the kidney and urinary tract, from peripheral and autonomic neuropathy and from eye disorders. With cardiovascular disease, in particular coronary artery disease, the position is more complex. Excess mortality in Type I diabetic patients arises principally from renal failure, often complicated by cardiovascular disease, and the patterns of mortality may be affected by the use and availability of dialysis and transplantation programmes. The excess mortality of older diabetic patients, however, is due principally to cardiovascular disease, similar in kind to that prevalent in the non-diabetic population.

Mortality Rates

Fig. 22.1 shows mortality rates from all causes in diabetic patients from Edinburgh compared with the general population. There are relatively higher excess rates in younger and in female diabetic patients over most of the age range, findings typical of several reported series, though the sex difference was not found in Warsaw (Poland; Fig. 22.2), Erfurt (East Germany) nor in Tecumseh (U.S.A.), for coronary heart disease mortality.

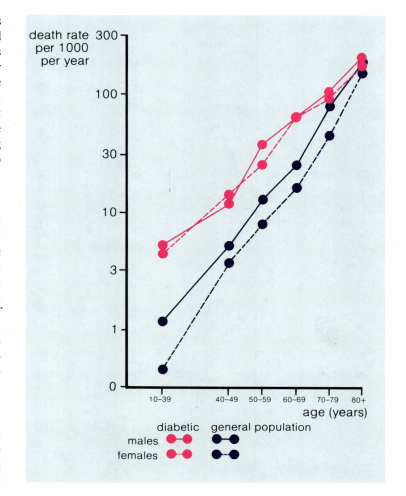

Fig. 22.1 Death rates (all causes) in diabetic males and females compared with those from the general population in Edinburgh. From Shenfield *et al.* (1979), by courtesy of Masson Editeur.

MACROVASCULAR CAUSES OF MORTALITY IN DIABETES IN WARSAW									
	deaths from CHD			deaths from CVD			all deaths		
age at diagnosis of diabetes mellitus	observed	expected	o/e ratio	observed	expected	o/e ratio	observed	expected	o/e ratio
30–49 M	18	5.3	3.40	4	1.0	4.00	52	24.4	2.13
F	6	1.8	3.33	3	0.8	3.75	21	13.2	1.61
50–68 M	67	38.2	1.75	27	9.5	2.84	171	145.1	1.17
F	31	19.3	1.60	13	10.1	1.30	126	102.9	1.22
total M	85	43.5	1.95	31	10.5	2.95	223	169.5	1.31
F	37	21.1	1.75	16	10.9	1.47	147	116.1	1.27

Fig. 22.2 Mortality rates in Warsaw from coronary heart disease (CHD), cerebrovascular disease (CVD) and from all causes in diabetic patients compared with those which would be expected if age- and sex-specific rates from the general Warsaw population were applied. There are similar excess ratios in diabetic patients of both sexes. From Królewski *et al.* (1977), by courtesy of Springer Verlag.

Reports from the U.S.A. and U.K. indicate that the incidence of either strokes or mortality rates from cerebrovascular disease, or both, are higher in diabetic patients. Fig. 22.3 presents results from a cohort study of members of the British Diabetic Association followed for thirteen years. Below the age of sixty-five years, there was an increase of seventy-five percent in the excess mortality rate of female diabetic patients, but this was not statistically significant from that of controls; male diabetic patients had rates similar to those of the general population. However, above the age of sixty-five years, diabetic patients of both sexes had significantly increased standardized mortality rates. However, two reports on Japanese populations, from Osaka and Hawaii, found no significant excess of deaths attributed to cerebrovascular disease.

Data from three prospective studies, Framingham and Honolulu (U.S.A.), and Whitehall (U.K.; Fig. 22.4), indicate that risk factors for either all causes of death or those resulting from coronary heart disease, or both, have similar predictive power in diabetic and non-diabetic subjects. These risk factors include high blood pressure/hypertension, total cholesterol and cigarette smoking. There are no satisfactory prospective data on high density lipoprotein (HDL) cholesterol, though in prevalence studies, the level of HDL cholesterol has been shown to be inversely related to the prevalence of macrovascular disease. Thus, the excess mortality rates in diabetic patients do not appear to be due to a greater effect of a particular risk factor, but might be due to clustering of risk factors within individuals.

Causes of Increased Morbidity and Mortality

Several hypotheses have been advanced to explain the excess rates of macrovascular disease in diabetes, including a greater frequency of hypertension, lipid abnormalities and hyperinsulinaemia. In insulin-dependent subjects, there is increasing evidence of an association between levels of blood pressure and serum cholesterol and increased urinary albumin excretion, most evident when clinical proteinuria develops. Those who escape proteinuria have only a modestly increased risk of vascular disease. In Type II diabetes, the literature is inconsistent, with some studies finding an increased prevalence of hypertension and others no increase. Some of the inconsistencies may be explained by obesity; if the diabetic population contains a higher proportion of obese persons, then blood pressure levels would tend to be higher. Type II diabetic patients are more likely to have apparently deleterious lipid profiles, with lower levels of HDL cholesterol and higher levels of triglycerides than matched control subjects.

STANDARDIZED MORTALITY RATIOS FOR CEREBROVASCULAR DISEASE			
age (years)	15–44	45–64	65+
male	392	102	145
female	541	175	138

Fig. 22.3 Mortality due to cerebrovascular disease in diabetes. These results are from a cohort study of 5971 members of the British Diabetic Association followed from 1966–1979. Standardized mortality ratios were calculated by comparison with the general population of England and Wales. Above the age of sixty-five years, both sexes with diabetes had significantly increased standardized mortality ratios. From Fuller et al. (1983a), by courtesy of Springer Verlag.

LOGISTIC COEFFICIENTS RELATING MORTALITY DUE TO CORONARY DISEASE TO SPECIFIED CHARACTERISTICS	diabetic		non-diabetic	
characteristic	β	SE(β)	β	SE(β)
age (years)	0.165	0.062	0.077	0.007
systolic blood pressure (mmHg)	0.021	0.016	0.014	0.002
body mass index (kg/m^2)	−0.124	0.101	0.022	0.014
cholesterol (mmol/l)	0.003	0.219	0.227	0.032
smoker (1=smoker) (0=otherwise)	1.053	1.370	0.684	0.170
number of cigarettes per day in smokers	0.008	0.060	0.012	0.006
ECG abnormalities (1=positive) (0=negative)	−0.312	0.929	1.112	0.108
population at risk	145		16,130	
number of deaths	15		642	

Fig. 22.4 Comparison of coefficients (β) derived from logistic analyses relating death from coronary heart disease over a ten-year follow-up in male diabetic and non-diabetic civil servants in Whitehall, U.K. There are no statistically significant differences, implying similar predictive values from putative risk factors in diabetic and non-diabetic subjects alike. From Jarrett & Shipley (1985), by courtesy of Periodica.

The evidence for insulin as a risk factor comes largely from two prospective studies in Finnish and French policemen, not confirmed in a general population study in Australia. In none of these studies was HDL cholesterol measured; as this is inversely related to plasma insulin levels, it is not possible to determine, in the Finnish and French studies, whether the positive relationship between plasma insulin level and cardiovascular morbidity/mortality might have been confounded by a common association with HDL cholesterol levels. In addition, fasting plasma triglyceride and HDL cholesterol levels tend to be inversely associated, so the interpretation of any or all of these associations with macrovascular disease is difficult.

Glucose Intolerance and Cardiovascular Disease

An increased mortality rate from both coronary heart disease and cerebrovascular disease is not confined to those fulfilling the World Health Organization's (WHO) criteria for Type II (non insulin-dependent) diabetes. In the 'Whitehall Study' of men aged 40–64 years, ten-year mortality rates from coronary heart disease and stroke were significantly increased in glucose intolerant men (those with blood glucose values above the 95th centile; Fig. 22.5). Furthermore, several studies have shown electrocardiographic abnormalities to be more frequent among people with glucose intolerance. The latter also have an increased risk of progressing to diabetes, the risk being directly related to the degree of glucose intolerance.

The frequency and degree of atherosclerosis and coronary heart disease vary considerably between different populations of diabetic patients (Figs 22.6 and 22.7). While ethnic differences may play a part, environmental differences seem more probable as

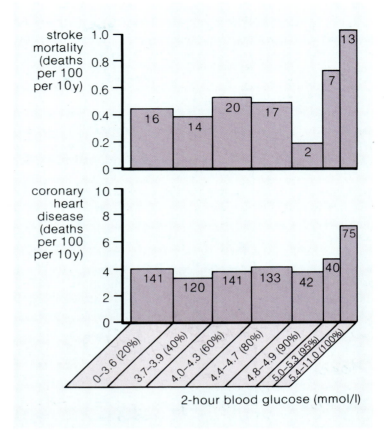

Fig. 22.5 Relationship between mortality due to stroke or coronary heart disease and blood glucose concentration, two hours after a glucose load in non-diabetic males. Mortality was measured over ten years and age adjusted in this study from Whitehall. The figures in the columns are the numbers of deaths; percentages are centile points. There is a significant increase in mortality above the 95th centile. From Fuller *et al.* (1983b), by courtesy of the British Medical Journal.

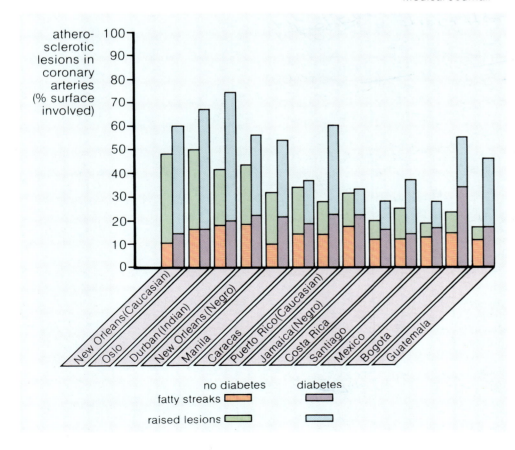

Fig. 22.6 Atherosclerosis in diabetes. In this study (International Atherosclerosis Project), standardized examinations were made of aortas and coronary arteries removed post-mortem from people in countries with widely different frequencies of coronary heart disease. The mean extent of atherosclerotic lesions in diabetic and non-diabetic males is shown. In general, populations with low mean values for the extent of coronary atherosclerosis in non-diabetic subjects also had low mean values for diabetic patients, and vice versa. However, even in populations with generally low levels of coronary atherosclerosis, the extent of raised lesions was usually greater in diabetic patients. From Robertson and Strong (1968), by courtesy of Williams and Wilkins Company.

an explanation. Thus, Japanese migrants with diabetes on the island of Hawaii showed a pattern of cardiovascular disease morbidity and mortality similar to that of Caucasian diabetic patients but this was very different from Japanese with diabetes remaining in their homeland (Fig. 22.8).

CONCLUSION

In Type I diabetes, much, if not all, of the increased risk of macrovascular disease appears to be secondary to diabetic renal disease. Thus prevention of the macrovascular disease in this form of diabetes requires two approaches: prevention of the renal disorder in addition to control of conventional risk factors for macrovascular disease. In Type II diabetes, hyperglycaemia itself may be less important in determining the macrovascular disease risk. Although there is no evidence from clinical trials in diabetic populations to justify any particular therapy, the similarity of risk factor prediction in diabetic and non-diabetic populations would support any attempt to make lipid profiles normal, control blood pressure and discourage cigarette smoking in Type II diabetic subjects. However, as the excess risk diminishes with age of onset, the energy of therapeutic intervention might, with reason, be similarly modified.

FREQUENCY OF ECG ABNORMALITIES PROBABLY INDICATIVE OF ISCHAEMIA IN DIABETIC SUBJECTS		
region	male (%)	female (%)
London	3.1	5.8
Switzerland	6.8	5.5
Brussels	4.2	5.4
Moscow	3.1	2.9
Warsaw	5.4	1.2
Berlin	5.3	10.5
Zagreb	3.6	3.9
New Delhi	6.6	3.0
Hong Kong	1.5	0.4
Tokyo	1.7	1.5
Havana	3.9	3.5
Oklahoma (Indians)	9.6	8.9
Arizona (Pima Indians)	4.6	1.3
Bulgaria	4.1	3.6

Fig. 22.7 Regional variations in the prevalence of ECG abnormalities in diabetes. In this WHO study of vascular disease in diabetes, similarly constructed samples of diabetic patients in several countries were studied. Electrocardiograms were read centrally and the prevalence of those with changes indicative of probable ischaemia is shown. Particularly low frequencies were found in Hong Kong and Tokyo in both sexes. From Jarrett (1986), by courtesy of Croom Helm.

FREQUENCY (%) OF VASCULAR DISEASE IN DECEASED DIABETIC SUBJECTS					
	Hawaii		Japan		
	Caucasians (n=128)	Japanese (n=251)	clinical diagnosis* (n=1917)	clinical diagnosis† (n=1885)	autopsy cases (n=4421)
total	75.8	74.5	47.3	51.0	48.8
brain	18.0	21.9	18.8	18.3	19.1
IHD	32.8	32.7	13.3	9.7	13.5
other cardiac	15.6	8.8		6.9	1.8
renal	8.6	10.6	16.4	16.1	14.4

*from Goto et al. (1973)
† from Hirata et al. (1973)
IHD = ischaemic heart disease

Fig. 22.8 Effect of environment on frequency of vascular disease in diabetes. The frequencies from Hawaii, obtained by autopsy, show that Japanese diabetic patients in Hawaii have a frequency of vascular disease similar to other local inhabitants rather than Japanese still in Japan. From Kawate et al. (1979), by courtesy of the American Diabetes Association.

REFERENCES

Fuller JH, Elford J, Goldblatt P & Adelstein AM (1983a) Diabetes mortality: new light on an underestimated public health problem. *Diabetologia*, **24**, 336–341.

Fuller JH, Shipley MJ, Rose G, Jarrett RJ & Keen H (1983b) Mortality from coronary heart disease and stroke in relation to degree of glycaemia: the Whitehall Study. *British Medical Journal*, **287**, 867–870.

Goto Y, Sato S & Masuda M (1973) Causes of death in diabetics and its vascular complications. *Sogorinsho*, **22**, 779–786.

Hirata Y, Mihara T, Sakasegawa K, Ando Y, Nishimura H, Mori M, Kasahara T, Nagaoka K, Tominaga M, Takeda A & Toyota T (1973) Statistical studies of 1885 death cases of diabetes in Japan. The relation between causes of death and therapeutic methods of diabetes. *Journal of the Japanese Diabetic Society*, **16**, 290–299.

Jarrett RJ (1984) The epidemiology of coronary heart disease and related factors in the context of diabetes mellitus and impaired glucose tolerance. In *Diabetes and Heart Disease*. Edited by Jarrett RJ. pp. 1–23. Amsterdam: Elsevier Science Publishers B.V.

Jarrett RJ (1986) *Diabetes Mellitus*. London: Croom Helm.

Jarrett RJ & Shipley MJ (1985) Mortality and associated risk

factors in diabetes. *Acta Endocrinologica*, **110** (Suppl. 272), 21–26.

Kawate R, Yamakido M, Nishimoto Y, Bennett PH, Hamman RF & Knowler WC (1979) Diabetes mellitus and its vascular complications in Japanese migrants on the island of Hawaii. *Diabetes Care*, **2**, 161–170.

Królewski AS, Czyzyk A, Janeczko D & Kopczyński J (1977) Mortality from cardiovascular diseases among diabetics. *Diabetologia*, **13**, 345–350.

Pyörälä K & Laakso M (1983) Macrovascular disease in diabetes mellitus. In *Diabetes in Epidemiological Perspective*. Edited by Mann JI, Pyörälä K & Teuscher A. pp. 183–247. Edinburgh: Churchill Livingstone.

Robertson WB & Strong JP (1968) Atherosclerosis in persons with hypertension and diabetes mellitus. In *Geographical Pathology of Atherosclerosis*. Edited by McGill HC Jr. pp.78–84. Baltimore: Williams and Wilkins Company.

Shenfield GM, Elton RA, Bhalla IP & Duncan LJP (1979) Diabetic mortality in Edinburgh. *Diabete et Metabolisme*, **5**, 149–158.

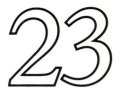

23 Diabetic Retinopathy

Eva M Kohner MD FRCP

INTRODUCTION

During the last three decades, diabetic retinopathy, previously uncommon, has become the single most common cause of blindness in the developed countries in patients between the ages of twenty and sixty-five years. This complication is now largeiy preventable by photocoagulation which, if applied adequately and at an early stage, can reduce the threat of blindness in some groups by as much as eighty per cent. Recognition of the lesions of diabetic retinopathy has therefore become important. Both diabetologists and ophthalmologists should be aware of those lesions which respond to treatment and also the stage at which they should be treated. This chapter will therefore emphasize the problems of clinical diabetic retinopathy, its manifestations, indications for treatment and treatment results. It does not aim to be a comprehensive review of all aspects of diabetic retinopathy.

The Problem of Diabetic Retinopathy

Whilst there are many reports on the prevalence of diabetic retinopathy in different countries and communities, none are adequate. Even prevalence studies frequently suffer by representing very highly selected hospital populations and by rarely standardizing the methods of examination. Previous studies have been well reviewed by L'Esperance and James (1983).

The most important study was by Klein and co-workers (1984) who used standardized methods of examination, including retinal photography. The prevalence of 'any retinopathy' reached a staggering 97.5% after fifteen years of diabetes in insulin-treated patients, with forty per cent suffering from proliferative lesions after twenty years. The non insulin-treated patients fared better; in these the prevalence never exceeded sixty-five per cent and proliferative

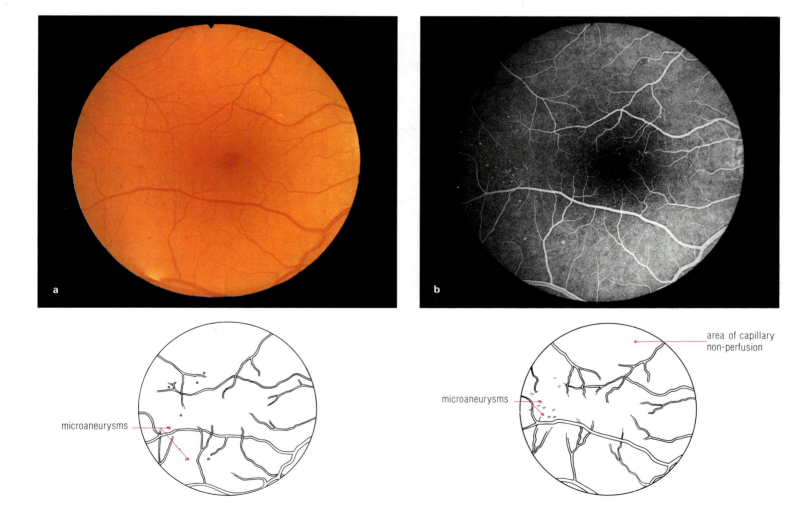

Fig. 23.1 Case 1. (a) minimal retinopathy with very few microaneurysms (MA). However, the fluorescein angiogram (b) of the same macula reveals many more MA's compared with normal colour photography. Also shown are small areas of capillary non-perfusion in the perifoveal area and also the area lateral to the macula.

retinopathy was only recorded in at most twenty per cent. Klein's work was important since it showed a much higher prevalence of diabetic retinopathy, especially proliferative retinopathy, than hitherto expected. It thus emphasized the importance of screening for diabetic retinopathy and of the provision of adequate facilities for treatment.

Evolution of Diabetic Retinopathy

The earliest clinically recognizable abnormality in diabetic retinopathy is the occlusion of individual capillaries, which can be recognized on good quality fluorescein angiograms (Figs 23.1b and 23.2b). Capillary occlusion precedes all other lesions and as these lesions increase in size they lead to ophthalmoscopically-visible lesions. Later, arteriolar and arterial occlusions occur. Once the larger vessels become occluded, capillary non-perfusion is always extensive.

The pathogenesis of capillary non-perfusion is unknown. Many possible mechanisms have been postulated, such as abnormal coagulation of the blood, endothelial cell damage by increased blood flow and accumulation of sorbitol in the vessel wall. Endothelial cell damage is a prerequisite, since only when endothelial cells disappear is there complete non-perfusion of capillaries. Arteriolar occlusion is preceded by narrowing of the origin of the vessel, which later progresses to complete occlusion.

When capillary occlusion alone is present, the resulting clinical picture is 'background diabetic retinopathy' without, or if more severe, with macular oedema, which progresses to 'diabetic maculopathy'. When arteriolar and arterial lesions are also present, the condition can be recognized as 'pre-proliferative diabetic retinopathy' which proceeds to the development of new vessel formation with glial proliferation at a later stage. This leads to an advanced stage of diabetic eye disease.

BACKGROUND DIABETIC RETINOPATHY

Background diabetic retinopathy, in its milder form, is characterized by microaneurysms (MA) which are the earliest unequivocal features which can be observed clinically (Fig. 23.1a). They are first seen at the posterior pole of the retina, most commonly in the macular area. Only the larger microaneurysms (over approximately 30μm in diameter) are recognized using ophthalmoscopy. Fluorescein angiograms, however, are more revealing since they also demonstrate the smaller MA's (Fig. 23.1b). MA's alone rarely cause visual loss; however, their walls often become leaky, allowing the escape of plasma constituents which then give rise to hard exudates (Fig. 23.2a). Whilst MA's represent localized dilatation of the capillary wall, generalized dilatation (usually irregular) is associated with more widespread, but still discrete, capillary occlusion. As some capillaries become occluded neigh-

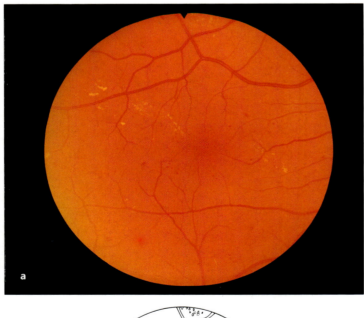

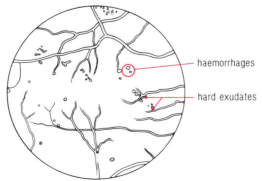

haemorrhages —
hard exudates —

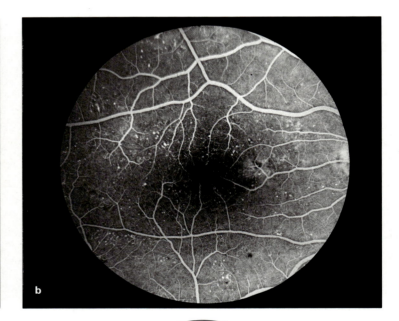

microaneurysms —
area of haemorrhages —
blush —
capillary non-perfused retina —

Fig. 23.2 Case 2. (a) mild background retinopathy which is more advanced than in Fig. 23.1a. In addition to MA's, there are also scattered hard exudates suggesting focal leakage and

haemorrhages. The haemorrhages can be seen on the fluorescein angiogram (b) as black areas; many more MA's are also visible.

bouring ones become dilated. The dilated capillaries are always leaky and can be recognized clinically by the presence of hard exudates, which usually form rings around focal capillary dilatations (Fig. 23.3). More extensive leakage leads to the formation of hard exudate plaques (Figs 23.3a and 23.4a). The focal abnormalities and capillary leakage result in the appearance of a 'wet' retina which can affect any part of the posterior pole. This is of clinical importance only when it approaches the macula and gives rise to diabetic maculopathy.

Since mild background retinopathy is not associated with visual loss, no specific treatment is required. Several studies have examined the effect of various treatments aimed at preventing progression of the retinopathy. These include agents which inhibit platelet aggregation, aldose reductase inhibitors and the effect of optimized diabetic control using continuous subcutaneous insulin infusion. At present, no study yields conclusive results.

DIABETIC MACULOPATHY

In diabetic maculopathy, the two key pathological processes are capillary closure and hyperpermeability of the remaining capillaries. The commonest early sites for such lesions are the capillaries lateral to the fovea. These lesions then gradually encroach on the fovea. Depending upon the extent of leakage and occlusion, three types of diabetic maculopathy can be recognized: exudative, ischaemic and oedematous.

Exudative Maculopathy

Exudative maculopathy is the commonest and most easily recognized form, being characterized by microvascular abnormalities and hard exudates (Figs 23.3a and b). The exudates arise lateral to the macula and, as the leakage extends into the foveal area, visual loss occurs. Hard exudate plaques follow and when they extend into the fovea, visual loss is permanent.

Ischaemic Maculopathy

In ischaemic maculopathy, non-perfusion is more important than leakage. This form of maculopathy is characterized ophthalmoscopically by the presence of certain features of ischaemia, such as clusters of haemorrhages (Fig. 23.4a) and venous and arterial abnormalities. Fluorescein angiograms also demonstrate a markedly enlarged area of perifoveal non-perfusion (Fig. 23.4b). In the middle-aged and elderly, the ischaemia is associated with oedema at the macula concomitant with large areas of peripheral non-perfusion (Figs 23.4a and b). The visual acuity is always poor and there is a danger of development of proliferative changes.

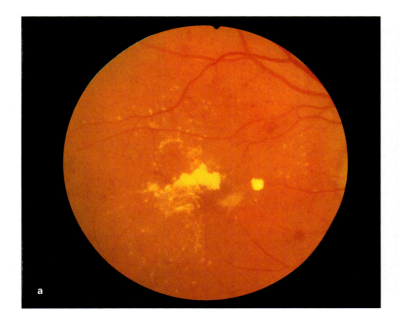
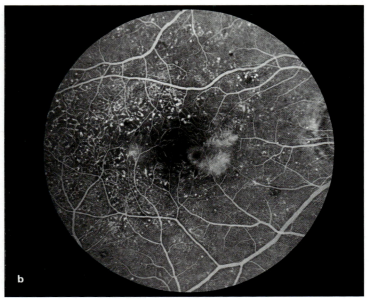

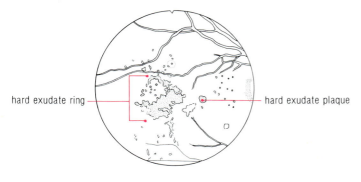
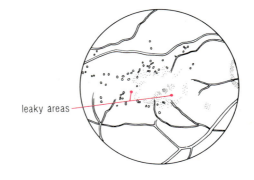

Fig. 23.3 Case 3. This diabetic patient had background retinopathy with macular oedema (diabetic maculopathy). (a) a hard exudate ring lateral to the macula can be seen as well as a hard exudate plaque near the fovea. The fluorescein angiogram (b) shows the very coarse capillary bed, especially lateral to the macula. None of the capillaries are normal and there is extensive leakage from some of these capillaries both lateral and medial to the fovea.

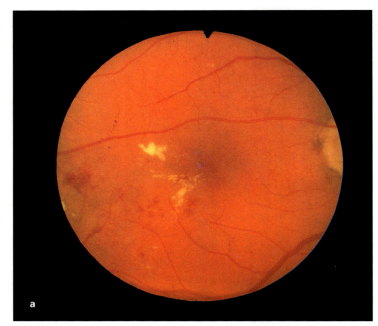

a

Fig. 23.4   Case 4. In this retina of a 42-year-old patient with visual acuity of 6/24, only a few hard exudates are seen near the macula. In (a), many haemorrhages are seen in clusters lateral to the macula and indicate ischaemic areas. The fluorescein angiogram (b) indicates the cause of poor visual acuity which is the large area of capillary non-perfusion surrounding the fovea. Irregularity of the superior macular artery together with narrowing of the origins of side branches is clearly shown. The larger branches have 'pruned-off' side branches. There are large areas of non-perfusion lateral to the macula indicating that proliferative retinopathy may develop. (c) was taken two years later and shows development of new vessels on the disc. As a result, photocoagulation therapy was given and the scars can be seen.

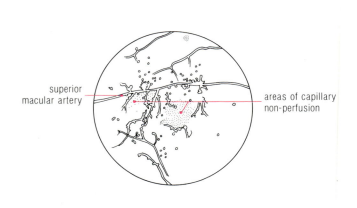

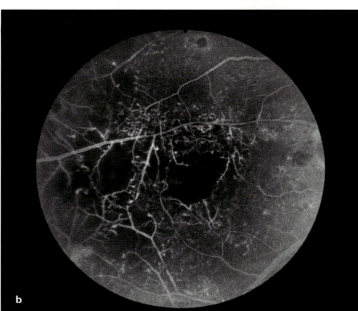

b

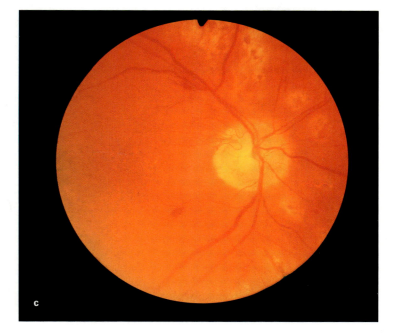

c

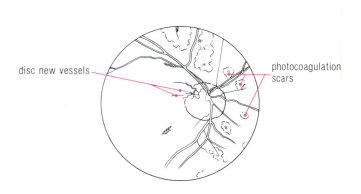

Oedematous Maculopathy

In oedamatous maculopathy, all the remaining capillaries in the posterior pole become leaky, with extensive oedema involving the entire area between the superior and inferior temporal vessels (Figs 23.5a and b). Occasionally, long-standing oedema results in the formation of small cysts surrounding the fovea. This cystoid

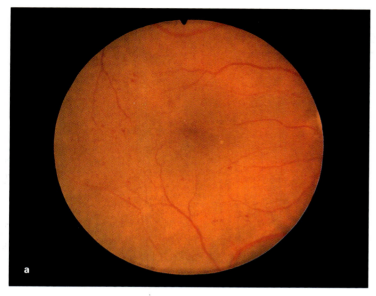

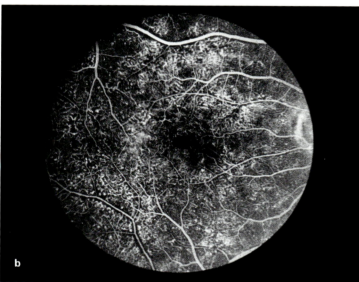

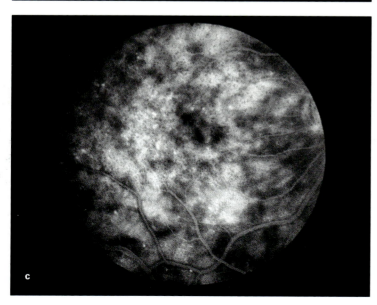

Fig. 23.5   Case 5. This 52-year-old patient complained of blurring of vision. Although on direct ophthalmoscopy (a) very few abnormal features were seen, slit lamp biomicroscopy showed extensive oedema. The fluorescein angiogram (b), in the capillary phase, shows the coarse capillary network. All the remaining capillaries are dilated and leaky. The angiogram (c), taken in the late phase, shows extensive leakage extending into the fovea. This accounts for the oedema and associated visual symptoms.

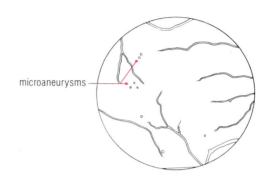

microaneurysms

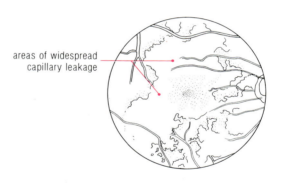

areas of widespread capillary leakage

oedema is usually associated with severe visual loss and, even if it disappears, there is often persistent pigment epithelial damage (see Fig. 23.12d).

Treatment of Maculopathy

Of all the methods used in treating diabetic maculopathy, only photocoagulation has been found to be effective in maintaining

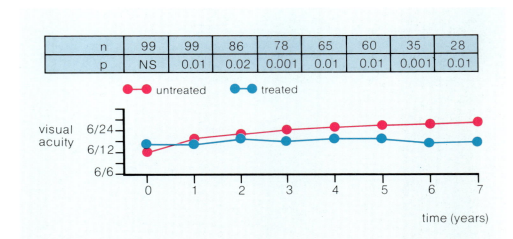

| n | 99 | 99 | 86 | 78 | 65 | 60 | 35 | 28 |
| p | NS | 0.01 | 0.02 | 0.001 | 0.01 | 0.01 | 0.001 | 0.01 |

Fig. 23.6 Mean visual acuity of treated and control eyes of patients with diabetic maculopathy in the British Multicentre Study of photocoagulation. The treated eyes maintained their initial visual acuity, whilst the untreated eyes gradually deteriorated.

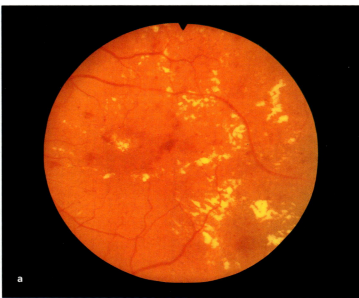

Fig. 23.7 Case 6. (a) diabetic maculopathy in a patient with a visual acuity of 6/18. There are many hard exudates forming rings and also marked microvascular abnormalities, such as haemorrhages and microaneurysms, in the centre of the rings. View (b) shows the same areas as (a), but six months after argon laser photocoagulation. The visual acuity improved to 6/9 and most lesions have disappeared. The very light laser burns do not cause visual field loss.

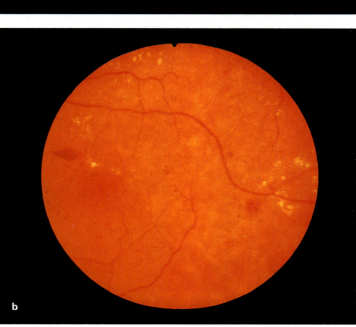

vision in a significant number of patients. The largest of the studies reported is that by the British Multicentre Study Group in 1983. In this study, ninety-nine patients with symmetrical maculopathy (visual acuity between the two eyes within two lines on the Snellen chart and retinopathy of similar severity) were studied. Each patient had one of their eyes (chosen randomly) treated by xenon arc photocoagulation, whilst the other eye remained untreated and served as a control.

The results after five years indicate that treatment is better than no treatment and at each yearly interval the treated eyes deteriorated less than the untreated ones. In the treated eyes, the mean visual acuity was maintained throughout the period of study, whilst in the control eyes there was steady deterioration. This difference in deterioration between treated eyes and controls was significant at each yearly interval (Fig. 23.6). Fewer treated eyes became blind than untreated controls and again the difference was significant when all eyes were considered. The difference was greatest in those with initially good vision (6/6 to 6/12); out of twenty such patients, only one became blind in the treated eye, whilst ten patients (50%) became blind in the control eye. In those with initially poor vision (6/36 and worse) treatment made little difference.

Xenon arc therapy was used in this study, which was carried out before the subdivision of diabetic maculopathy into various clinical subgroups was available (Whitelocke et al., 1979). Today, only laser therapy would be used for the treatment of diabetic maculopathy since the lighter burns and the smaller spot size allows burns to be made close to the fovea as well as producing more accurate treatment of lesions.

Laser treatment, similar to xenon arc therapy, is most effective in the exudative type of maculopathy. Treatment of microvascular abnormalities in the centre of hard exudate rings or those associated with hard exudates is almost always effective in reducing the oedema and allowing the clearance of hard exudates

(Fig. 23.7). Treatment is less effective if widespread oedema, especially cystoid oedema, is present. This is probably because long-standing oedema causes permanent damage to the visual elements. Treatment of exudative maculopathy is often effective, contrasting with treatment of ischaemic maculopathy which is rarely effective in maintaining vision. In these patients, complete blindness resulting from complications of proliferative retinopathy can be avoided by panretinal photocoagulation of the peripheral ischaemic areas (Fig. 23.4c).

PRE-PROLIFERATIVE DIABETIC RETINOPATHY

Pre-proliferative lesions are those in which there is closure of arteries in addition to capillaries. These lesions should be recognized, since approximately fifty per cent of patients with such lesions will develop new vessels within a year and some within three months. The lesions are cotton wool spots, clusters of large blot haemorrhages, intraretinal microvascular abnormalities (Fig. 23.8) and venous abnormalities such as dilatation, loops, beading and reduplication. Arteries are irregular, sheathed or replaced by white lines, and the peripheral retina has a featureless 'empty' appearance. The irregularities of the arterial wall are even easier to see on fluorescein angiograms, with the origin of side-branches constricted and, at times, branch arterioles 'pruned-off' altogether (Fig. 23.4b). Fluorescein angiograms also clearly delineate the large non-perfused areas in the retinal periphery.

Although pre-proliferative retinopathy is not associated with visual loss, adequate treatment by photocoagulation may prevent the development of new vessels.

PROLIFERATIVE DIABETIC RETINOPATHY

Proliferative lesions arise as a result of a stimulus from large areas of ischaemic retina. New vessels develop from the optic disc or from the retinal periphery. The earliest proliferative lesions are

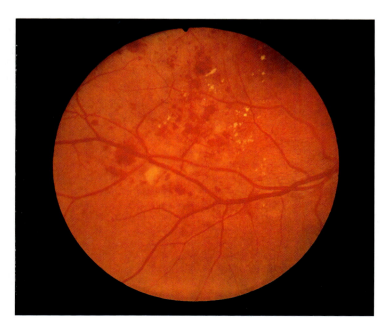

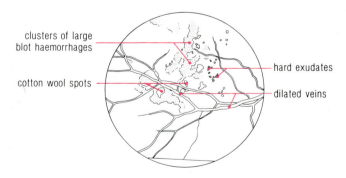

Fig. 23.8 Case 7. Pre-proliferative diabetic retinopathy showing large blot haemorrhages grouped in clusters. Cotton wool spots, dilated veins and intraretinal microvascular abnormalities are also present.

fine new vessels which may arise from intraretinal microvascular abnormalities (Fig. 23.9) or, more commonly, from large veins (Fig. 23.10a). The new vessels, initially naked, rapidly develop fibrous tissue cover, break through the internal limiting membrane of the retina and form dense adhesions with the cortical vitreous.

New vessels themselves are not associated with visual symptoms even when severe (Fig. 23.11b). However, the extensively-leaking, intraretinal microvascular abnormalities can cause

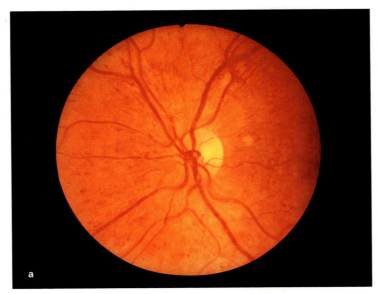

Fig. 23.9   Case 8. Retina of a young woman without retinopathy prior to pregnancy who was found to have proliferative changes during the second month of pregnancy. (a) proliferative lesions can be seen as well as cotton wool spots, intraretinal microvascular abnormalities and early new vessels. During pregnancy the patient received argon laser photocoagulation to decrease the number of new vessels present; however, they did not disappear completely because the treatment was incomplete. (b) was taken in the fourth month of pregnancy and (c) in the ninth month. As a result of more extensive photocoagulation the majority of new vessels have now disappeared. During a second pregnancy, no further treatment for retinopathy was necessary and her vision remained normal.

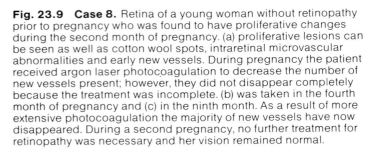

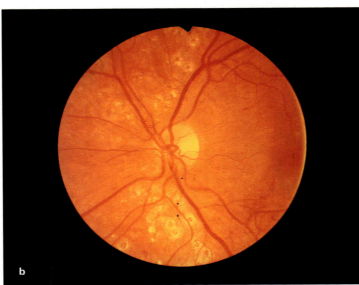

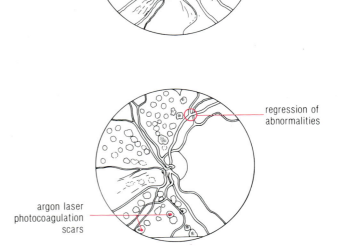

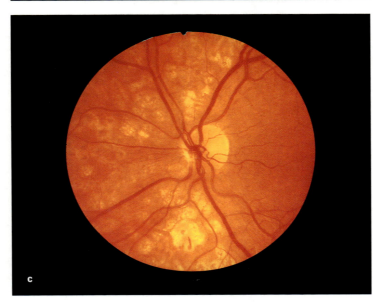

macular oedema and visual loss (Figs 23.12b and c). Profound and complete visual loss resulting from the complications of new vessels is associated with contraction of the fibrovascular membrane adherent to the posterior vitreous surface. Shrinkage of this tissue or the vitreous will result in elevation, and eventually a break in the vessels, causing vitreous haemorrhage. This haemorrhage may absorb rapidly if it is in the retro-vitreal space, but will remain for a long time if it breaks into the vitreous gel. As the fibrovascular membrane shrinks and vitreous detaches, there is stress on the retina. If the vector of the stress is tangential, traction lines will form and cause distortion or dragging of the macula nearer the disc (Fig. 23.13) with severe visual loss. If the vector is anteroposterior, the result is detachment of the retina which can be focal or may involve the macula (Fig. 23.14a). Macular detachment is always associated with catastrophic deterioration of vision.

All these complications are more common, and occur sooner, in patients with new vessels arising from the disc. Thus, in the first large study of the natural history of new vessels, Deckert and co-workers (1967) found that, five years after the first diagnosis of disc new vessels, fifty per cent of patients were blind.

Treatment of Proliferative Diabetic Retinopathy

The aim of treatment is to prevent the complications of new vessels, all of which result in advanced diabetic retinopathy. This can be achieved by photocoagulation. Once advanced diabetic retinopathy is present, the treatment is operative and is aimed at relieving vitreo-retinal traction (by vitrectomy, division or stripping of fibrous tissue with or without scleral buckling, see Fig. 23.11b) or at removing vitreous haemorrhage by vitrectomy.

Of all the treatments for proliferative lesions tried over the years, photocoagulation has been found to be the most successful. Whether xenon arc or argon laser is used, the results achieved are similar since it is the adequacy and timing of the treatment which matter. Treatment should therefore be given early, before tractional complications are present.

Two multicentre, randomized, controlled studies have confirmed the efficacy of photocoagulation for proliferative retinopathy. The larger of these studies, the Diabetic Retinopathy Study Research Group (1976 and 1981), reported on over 1700 patients recruited in the United States. Both eyes of each patient were either treated or remained as untreated controls using a randomization procedure. There was a highly significant benefit

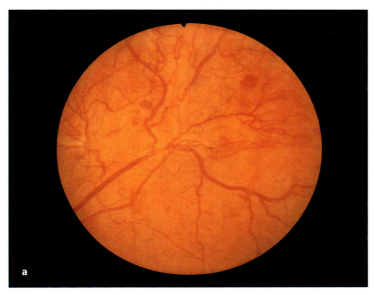

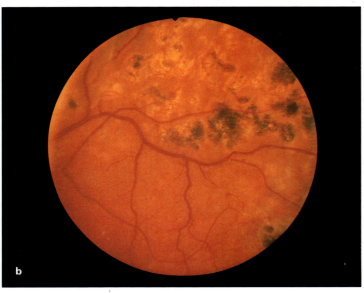

Fig. 23.10 Case 9. Retinopathy showing extensive peripheral new vessels arising from the large superior temporal vein in the right fundus. (a) large well-established new vessels have a fibro-glial covering seen as the white tissue associated with the new vessels. (b) shows the same area as (a) but two years after photocoagulation. The new vessels have disappeared and vision is maintained at 6/9.

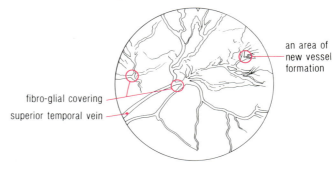

an area of new vessel formation

fibro-glial covering

superior temporal vein

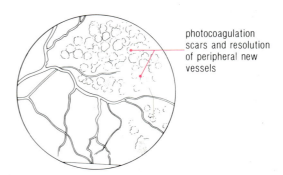

photocoagulation scars and resolution of peripheral new vessels

from treatment within the first two years in all groups except those with pre-proliferative retinopathy. The difference was greatest in those showing 'high-risk' characteristics which included new vessels on the disc of more than minimal severity, with or without new vessels in the retinal periphery and with or without vitreous haemorrhage. Eyes with peripheral new vessels

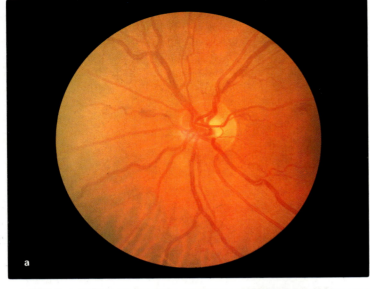

Fig. 23.11 **Case 10.** (a) left disc of a diabetic patient with relatively few lesions. There was, however, some ischaemia in the retinal periphery not shown in the photograph. (b) shows the retina fifteen months later. There has been extensive development of disc new vessels. (c) was taken five years later after panretinal photocoagulation. All the new vessels have disappeared and the vision has been maintained at 6/9, but with a reduced visual field.

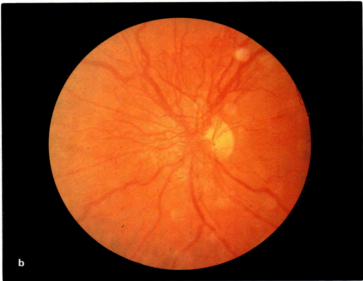

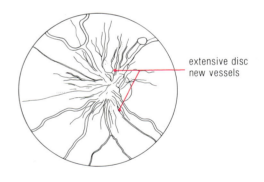

extensive disc new vessels

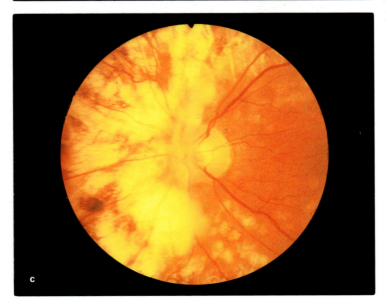

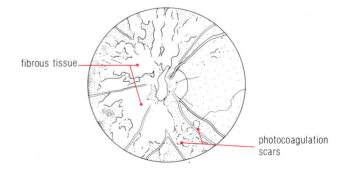

fibrous tissue

photocoagulation scars

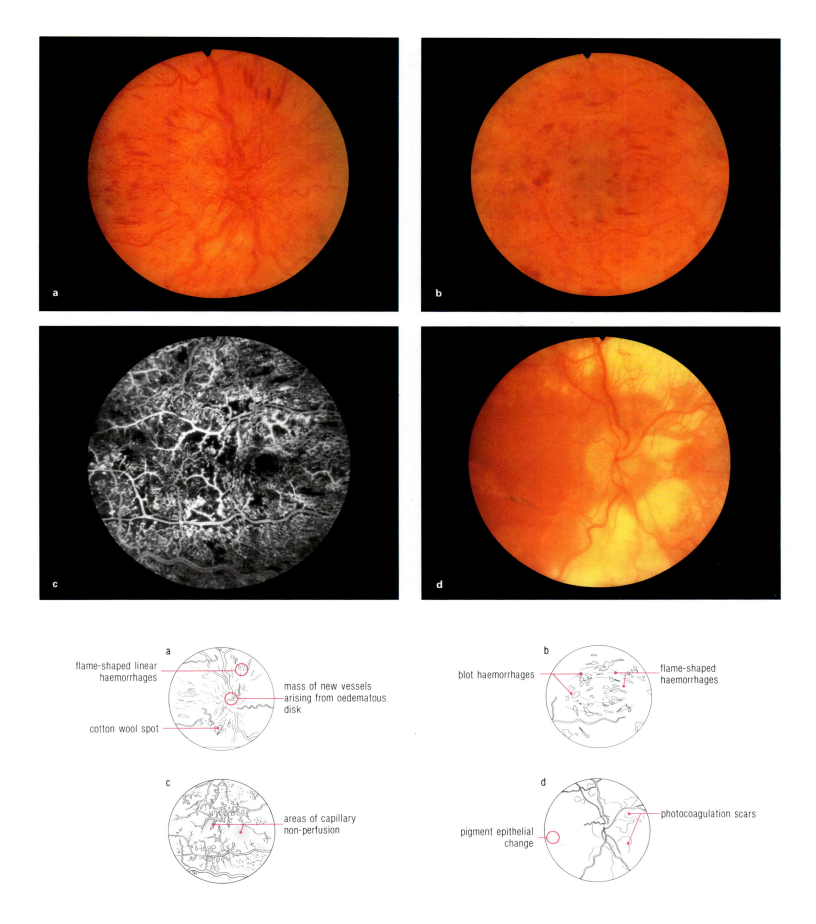

Fig. 23.12 Case 11. (a) right disc area of a very active 'florid' diabetic retinopathy. This 16-year-old girl had extensive disc new vessels with disc oedema. This type of retinopathy is most common in patients between 15 and 25 years of age. (b) shows the right macula area of the same patient. The macular oedema, resulting from leakage from many abnormal intraretinal vessels, caused vision to be reduced to 6/60. The fluorescein angiogram (c) of the same area reveals that all the remaining capillaries are abnormal, dilated and leaky. Many small areas of capillary non-perfusion are present. (d) the same right disc three years after photocoagulation shows that the retinopathy is now quiescent and there is complete regression of new vessels. The vision, however, was only improved to 6/24 because of a pigment epithelial change at the fovea, secondary to the oedema.

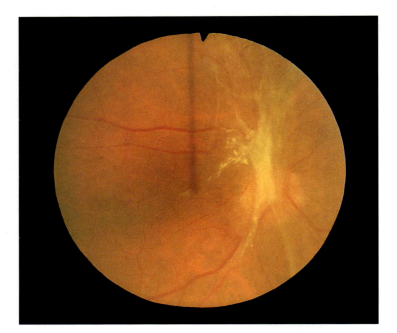

Fig. 23.13 Case 12. Retinopathy with fibrous tissue formation at the disc causing macular traction. The fovea, normally approximately 1.5 disc diameters from the disc, is pulled in towards it, as indicated by the fixation target which overlies the macula.

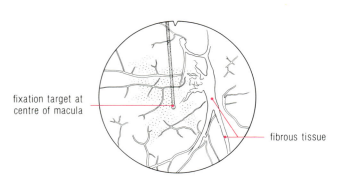

fixation target at centre of macula

fibrous tissue

Fig. 23.14 Case 13 (a) the right eye with detachment of the macula caused by traction arising from the development of new fibrous tissue at the disc. Haemorrhages were also present. The macula was detached for less than 1 month, when vitrectomy and endophotocoagulation were performed. (b) was taken eighteen months after successful vitrectomy. The remaining fibrous tissue could not be peeled off because of its attachment to the vessels. Some traction lines arising from the fibrous tissue are causing the increasing tortuosity of the vessels. Visual acuity improved to 6/18.

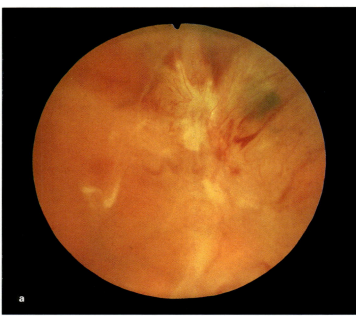

a

fibrous tissue

disc

detached retina

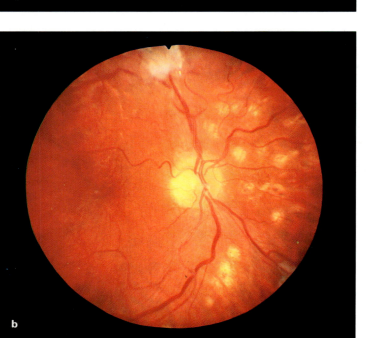

b

remains of fibrous tissue

tortuous vessels

endophotocoagulation scars

alone were considered at high-risk only if they had associated vitreous haemorrhage. Of those eyes which had high-risk characteristics, twenty-five per cent of untreated but only ten per cent of treated eyes, lost vision to 5/200 or less over a three year period.

The much smaller British Study (1984) reported on 107 patients. In this study, patients with two similarly affected eyes had one treated whilst the other remained untreated as a control. In this study, similar to the American one, treatment was better than no treatment, the mean visual acuity deteriorating by less than one line on the Snellen chart in treated eyes but by over two lines in the untreated ones. When patients with new disc vessels were considered separately the difference was greater, mean deterioration in the control eyes reaching nearly four lines on the visual acuity chart.

At each yearly interval, there was a significant difference in deterioration between treated and control eyes (Fig. 23.15). There was no significant difference in mean visual acuity between treated and untreated eyes in those with peripheral new vessels alone. In those with disc new vessels, only fifteen per cent of those treated, but fifty per cent of the control patients, deteriorated to legal blindness. The British Study, however, unlike the American study, did not specify the amount of treatment given. Knowing this it could be demonstrated that those who had more extensive treatment fared better and that, if they had peripheral new vessels only at the start of the study, they were less likely to develop new vessels on the disc.

The method of treatment for disc new vessels is panretinal photocoagulation which involves between two thousand and five thousand argon laser burns of 500μm in diameter in the periphery. The disc margin is approached outside the temporal vessels and all ischaemic areas are treated whilst avoiding only the perimacular area (Figs 23.9b, 23.11c and 23.12d). For peripheral new vessels there is no such firm agreement on the method of treatment. All agree that the new vessels can be treated directly and that the entire retinal segment in which the new vessels are present should be treated (Fig. 23.10b). In diabetic retinopathy most researchers now believe that even if new vessels are only seen in one quadrant usually most of the retinal periphery is ischaemic. Therefore panretinal photocoagulation should also be used for this type of retinopathy.

Photocoagulation has now been shown to be effective in all forms of proliferative retinopathy. Patients can be treated during pregnancy (Figs 23.9a and b) and, once treated adequately, are unlikely to develop further new vessels in subsequent pregnancies. Photocoagulation has also been shown to be effective in the rapidly advancing 'florid' retinopathy of the young (Fig. 23.12). However, these patients must be treated as emergencies and often require very extensive photocoagulation.

Treatment of the tractional complications of proliferative retinopathy requires not only specialized equipment, but also highly skilled and specially trained ophthalmologists. Only under the best circumstances are good results achieved (Fig. 23.14). Nevertheless, even the best results obtained do not approach those of photocoagulation.

The best results in proliferative retinopathy are obtained before the onset of visual symptoms and, in maculopathy, before severe visual loss. Diabetic patients should have their eyes tested regularly to find early and treatable retinopathy. Thus doctors in charge of such patients must be able to recognize early lesions.

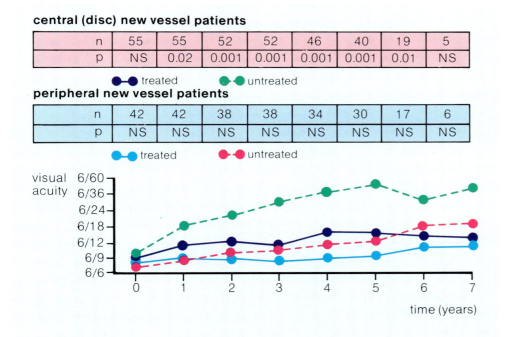

central (disc) new vessel patients

| n | 55 | 55 | 52 | 52 | 46 | 40 | 19 | 5 |
| p | NS | 0.02 | 0.001 | 0.001 | 0.001 | 0.001 | 0.01 | NS |

treated   untreated

peripheral new vessel patients

| n | 42 | 42 | 38 | 38 | 34 | 30 | 17 | 6 |
| p | NS | NS | NS | NS | NS | NS | NS | NS |

treated   untreated

Fig. 23.15 Mean visual acuity of treated and control eyes of patients with new vessels in the British Multicentre Study on photocoagulation. There was marked deterioration in those with disc new vessels when untreated, whilst the treated eyes deteriorated by less than one line on the Snellen chart. In patients with peripheral new vessels only, the difference between treated and untreated eyes was less, but the treated eyes still fared better.

REFERENCES

British Multicentre Study Group (1983) Photocoagulation for diabetic maculopathy. A randomized controlled clinical trial using the xenon arc. *Diabetes*, **32**, 1010–1016.

British Multicentre Study Group (1984) Photocoagulation for proliferative diabetic retinopathy. A randomized controlled clinical trial using the xenon arc. *Diabetologia*, **26**, 109–115.

Deckert T, Simonsen SE & Poulsen JE (1967) Prognosis of proliferative retinopathy in juvenile diabetes. *Diabetes*, **16**, 728–733.

Diabetic Retinopathy Study Research Group (1981) Photocoagulation treatment of proliferative diabetic retinopathy. DRS report nr. 8. *Ophthalmology*, **88**, 583–600.

Diabetic Retinopathy Study Research Group (1976) Preliminary report on the effects of photocoagulation therapy. *American Journal of Ophthalmology*, **81**, 383–396.

Engerman R, Kern TS & Madison WI (1982) Experimental galactosemia produces diabetic-like retinopathy. *Diabetes*, **31** (suppl. 2), 26A.

Klein R, Klein BEK, Moss SE, Davis MD & DeMets DL (1984) The Wisconsin epidemiological study of diabetic retinopathy: 2. Prevalance and risk of retinopathy when age at diagnosis is less than 30 years. *Archives of Ophthalmology*, **102**, 520–526.

Klein R, Klein BEK, Moss SE, Davis MD & DeMets DL (1984) The Wisconsin epidemiological study of diabetic retinopathy: 3. Prevalance and risk of retinopathy when age at diagnosis is 30 years or older. *Archives of Ophthalmology*, **102**, 527–532.

L'Esperance FA Jr & James WA Jr (1983) The problem of diabetic retinopathy. In *Diabetic Retinopathy*. Edited by Little H, Jack RL, Patz A & Forsham PH. pp.11–20. New York: Thieme-Stratton Inc.

Whitelocke RAF, Kearns M, Blach RK & Hamilton AM (1979) The diabetic maculopathies. *Transactions of the Ophthalmological Societies of the United Kingdom*, **99**, 314–320.

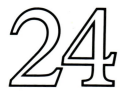

24 Diabetic Neuropathy

John D Ward BSc MD FRCP

The complications of diabetes help to make it such an unhappy and unpleasant disease, and damage to the peripheral nervous system contributes considerably to its morbidity. Diabetic neuropathy has a wide variety of manifestations which include sensory abnormalities, muscle weakness and wasting, foot ulceration and impotence.

Clinical surveys suggest that about ten per cent of diabetic patients have overt neuropathy, while another ten per cent have abnormal physical signs indicating nerve damage. Thus, about one in five diabetic subjects has evidence of neuropathy.

AETIOLOGY

Controversy surrounds the mechanism by which diabetes leads to nerve damage. Some authorities consider that nerve function is compromised by metabolic changes, while others favour interference with nerve blood supply. It is likely that both are involved (Fig. 24.1).

Metabolic Hypothesis

Peripheral nerves in diabetic patients accumulate sorbitol and fructose in large quantities (Fig. 24.2), in direct relationship to the blood glucose level. This is associated with depression of electrical conduction velocities. Probably of greater importance is the reduction of myo-inositol levels associated with depression of the enzyme system, Na$^+$/K$^+$ ATPase (Fig. 24.3). It has been suggested that, due to hyperglycaemia, a vicious circle is set up in which phosphoinositide metabolism is depressed, this being an important energy source for nerve metabolism and function. Abnormalities of these pathways have been well substantiated in peripheral nerve tissue from diabetic animals.

AETIOLOGY OF DIABETIC NEUROPATHY

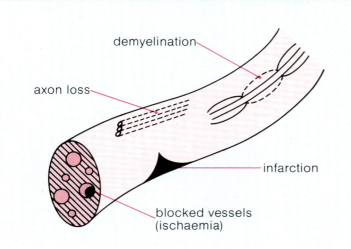

nerve metabolism
glucose ↑
sorbitol ↓↑
myo-inositol ↓

Fig. 24.1 Aetiology of diabetic neuropathy. Metabolic and vascular changes may both contribute to the aetiology.

SORBITOL AND FRUCTOSE SYNTHESIS

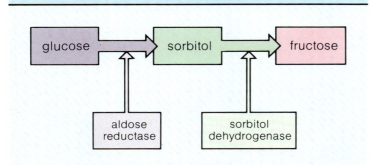

Fig. 24.2 Conversion of glucose to fructose via sorbitol. Fructose and sorbitol accumulate in large quantities in the peripheral nerves of diabetic patients.

REDUCTION OF MYO-INOSITOL LEVELS BY HYPERGLYCAEMIA

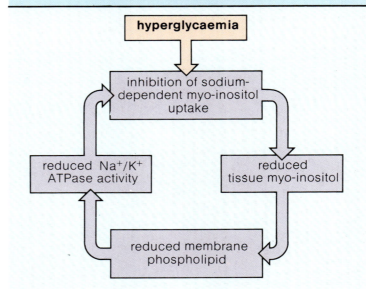

Fig. 24.3 Effect of hyperglycaemia on the Na$^+$/K$^+$ ATPase enzyme system. Hyperglycaemia leads to a depression of myo-inositol which reduces membrane phospholipids and subsequently Na$^+$/K$^+$ ATPase activity. The latter further depresses myo-inositol uptake.

The key to this metabolic pathway is the enzyme, aldose reductase, which is responsible for the conversion of glucose to sorbitol (see Fig. 24.2). Animal experimentation has shown that the administration of inhibitors of this enzyme results in the complete reversal of all the metabolic abnormalities, including a return of reduced electrical conduction velocities towards normal. Hence sorbitol levels are maintained, myo-inositol levels increase and Na^+/K^+ ATPase activity is restored to normal, all of these features being totally independent of the blood glucose level.

So far, in human studies, administration of a variety of aldose reductase inhibitors has led to slight improvements in electrical conduction velocities and some improvements in clinical sensory symptoms. More detailed and extensive studies of these enzyme-inhibiting agents are awaited.

Vascular Hypothesis

For many years, small vessel disease has been demonstrated within the peripheral nerves of diabetic patients (Fig. 24.4). There are suggestions that peripheral nerves in diabetic animals are hypoxic and recent evidence in man has demonstrated *in vivo* the ischaemic nature of peripheral nerves from subjects with clinical neuropathy. In such subjects, the nerves were found to be hypoxic

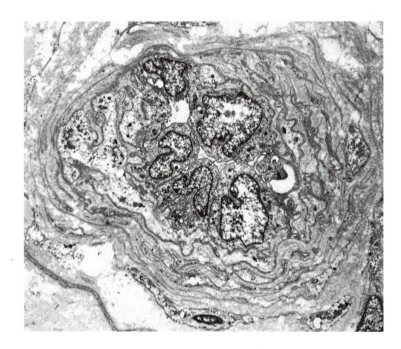

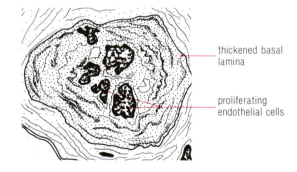

Fig. 24.4 Small vessel disease in the peripheral nerves. Intraneural capillary showing endothelial cell proliferation leading to total occlusion of the vessel lumen. EM × 7000.

INSERTION OF GLASS PLATINUM ELECTRODE INTO A PERIPHERAL NERVE

Fig. 24.5 Diagram of the insertion of a glass platinum microelectrode under direct vision using a dissecting microscope into a nerve fascicle. Use of the microscope confirms the exact site at which oxygen tension is being measured.

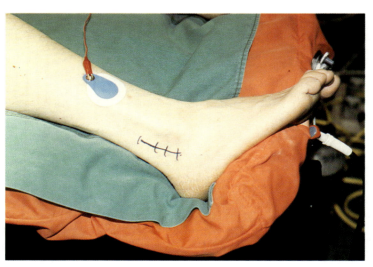

Fig. 24.6 Pen marking of site of sural nerve biopsy prior to incision and insertion of electrode under direct vision.

and the vessels within them occluded. Sorbitol levels were not elevated in many such studies and myo-inositol levels were not related to the severity of the nerve damage.

To measure nerve oxygenation, a glass platinum microelectrode may be inserted under direct microscopic control into a fascicle at the time of sural nerve biopsy (Figs 24.5 and 24.6).

Using this technique it has been shown that neuropathic nerves are hypoxic compared to normal and nerve oxygen tension significantly lower than that in venous blood taken from the foot at the time of the procedure. Moreover, the oxygen tension in venous blood from the neuropathic foot is higher than in the non-neuropathic foot (Fig. 24.7) in accordance with the clinical observation that gross distension of the veins in the neuropathic foot may result from arteriovenous shunting of blood (Fig. 24.8).

In the diseased vasa nervorum, the basal lamina may be grossly thickened (Fig. 24.9). Two mathematical parameters may be calculated: the capillary diffusion distance and the thickness of the basal lamina. The former correlates with myelinated nerve density, vibration perception threshold and oxygen gradient, while the latter correlates with both myelinated and unmyelinated fibre density and conduction velocity. Hence it is clear that there is a distinct relationship between the extent of vessel disease and the morphological abnormalities of peripheral nerve damage and its clinical features.

In more severe cases of neuropathy, endothelial cell number, basal lamina thickness and capillary diffusion distance are greater, but this finding is not apparent in vessels taken from muscle at the time of sural nerve biopsy, indicating that these specific features of diabetic neuropathy are not necessarily part of a diffuse, severe, small vessel disease of diabetes.

OXYGEN TENSIONS IN THE NEUROPATHIC AND NON-NEUROPATHIC FOOT			
	neuropathy (mmHg)	no neuropathy (mmHg)	p
nerve	38.8	53.6	<0.002
venous blood	52.3	37.8	<0.02

Fig. 24.7 Comparison of oxygen tensions in venous blood and nerves from a neuropathic and non-neuropathic foot.

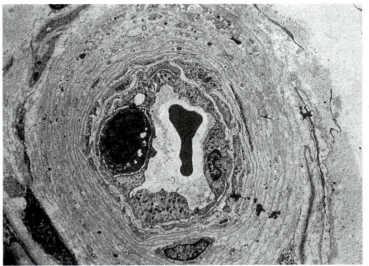

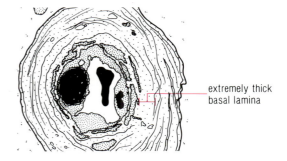

extremely thick basal lamina

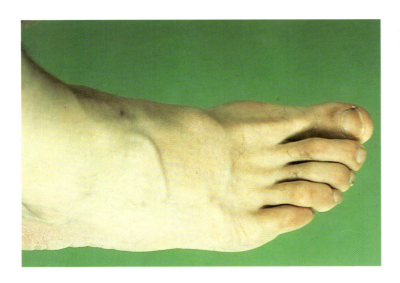

Fig. 24.8 Distension of veins on the dorsum of the foot. This may indicate arteriovenous shunting.

Fig. 24.9 Thickening of the basal lamina in a blood vessel within a peripheral nerve clearly showing the increased distance for diffusion from the centre of the lumen to tissues around the vessel. EM × 7000.

24.3

Development of Severe Clinical Neuropathy

Only a small number of diabetic subjects, in whom nerve chemistry is abnormal leading to functional and structural changes over a number of years, develop the clinical syndromes of severe neuropathy. Therefore it is essential to enquire what triggers the onset of these problems: is it the development of small vessel disease or some environmental or genetic factor? The presence of more severe vessel disease within peripheral nerve itself, when compared to skin and muscle, tends to suggest a specific neurovascular and chemical interaction.

Platelet abnormalities in diabetes may have some effect within the specific environment of the peripheral nerve and, as evidence of this, degranulating platelets may be seen in nerve capillaries (Fig. 24.10). The possible role of environmental poisons in the aetiology of neuropathy should not be forgotten. In clinical practice, either excessive alcohol consumption or drug therapy can be partly responsible for clinical neuropathy in a diabetic subject.

DEFINITIONS OF NEUROPATHY

It is important to establish satisfactory and accurate descriptions of clinical symptoms and signs, coupled with appropriate measurements of nerve function (Fig. 24.11).

Electrophysiology

There are many ways of measuring electrical nerve function (Fig. 24.12). It is important in all of these that the limb temperature should be constant and at 'body temperature'. There are major problems with the interpretation of most electrophysiological tests in peripheral nerves. For example, in a study of a group of newly diagnosed, Type II (non insulin-dependent) diabetic subjects in 1971, the patients were given simple dietary management resulting in a fall in blood glucose and an improvement in their motor conduction velocity of 3m/s. In 1982, a group of ten diabetic subjects with severe, unremitting, painful neuropathy was treated with continuous subcutaneous insulin infusion with marked improvement in their symptoms. These subjects also demonstrated an improvement in conduction velocity of 3m/s.

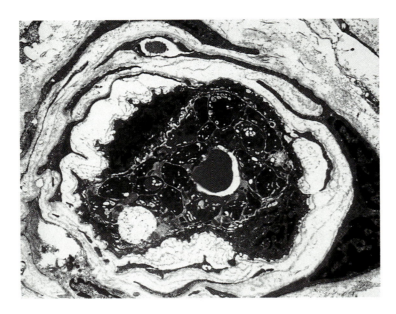

Fig. 24.10 Plug of degranulating platelets within a capillary of a peripheral nerve from a diabetic patient with neuropathy. EM × 7000.

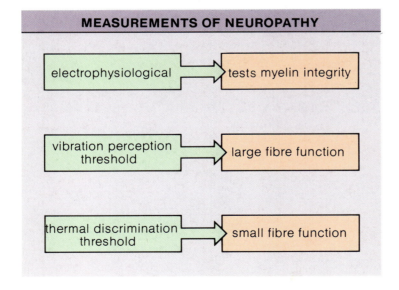

Fig. 24.11 Methods of measurement of neuropathy and their uses.

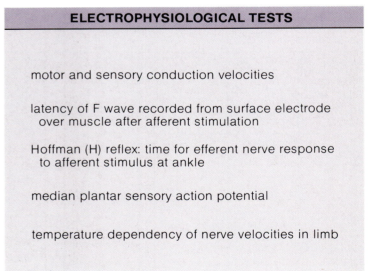

Fig. 24.12 Electrophysiological tests of nerve function.

This observation of two totally different groups of patients, one without and one with severe neuropathy, in whom improvement in glycaemic control led to exactly the same improvement in conduction velocity could suggest the possibility that conduction velocities merely reflect the fluid and electrolyte status of peripheral nerves. The improvement in glycaemic control may have led to the more satisfactory passage of the applied electrical stimulus.

Vibration Perception Threshold

The measure of large fibre function may be made by either the biothesiometer (Fig. 24.13) or the vibrameter (Fig. 24.14), the latter instrument incorporating a mechanism whereby the pressure of the stylus applied to the limb is standardized. Measurements of vibration perception threshold are abnormal in subjects with advanced neuropathy, are reproducible with some degree of accuracy and, in some studies, have been shown to improve with better glycaemic control.

Temperature Discrimination Threshold

Improved methods of measuring temperature discrimination (Fig. 24.15) provide a more sensitive index of peripheral nerve function by assessing the function of small nerves. These fibres seem to be damaged at a very early stage in diabetes, even before the development of overt clinical neuropathy, and in the future may prove a more sensitive and early measure of nerve dysfunction.

It is noteworthy that occasionally there are discrepancies between the abnormalities of the various electrophysiological, vibration sensation and thermal discrimination tests, although generally there is a reasonable correlation between the diagnosis of established neuropathy and abnormalities of these three tests.

It must also be stressed that in most studies the coefficients of variation in all of these tests are large. Reproducibility is often poor and at present no entirely satisfactory and accurate measurements of peripheral nerve function in diabetes are available. However, in all clinical studies, electrophysiological measurements, vibration perception and thermal sensation should be assessed in an attempt to give a general picture of nerve function.

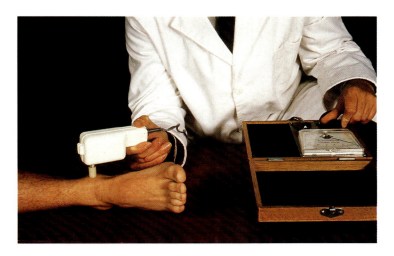

Fig. 24.13 Biothesiometer used to measure vibration perception threshold. The vibrating amplitude of the stylus applied to the skin is directly related to the square root of the voltage applied and is converted to a simple 0–50 unit scale.

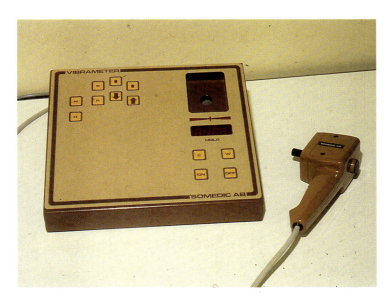

Fig. 24.14 Vibrameter used to measure vibration perception threshold. It operates on a similar principle to the biothesiometer, but within the head of the instrument the fulcrum is adjusted so that a constant pressure is applied at the site of measurement.

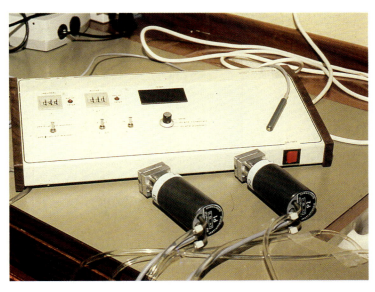

Fig. 24.15 Thermoaesthesiometer for the determination of warm and cold thermal thresholds using the forced choice principle. The patient is offered a standard temperature and a test temperature which is randomly hotter or colder than the standard. The patient is forced to choose whether the test is hotter or colder without the need to decide in which direction the temperature is changing.

DIABETIC NEUROPATHIES

chronic sensory

proximal motor

diffuse motor

focal

acute painful

syndromes in newly diagnosed diabetes

Fig. 24.16 Diabetic neuropathies.

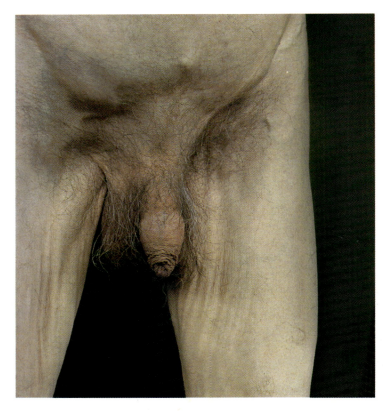

Fig. 24.17 Proximal muscle wasting.

Clinical Classification

Clinical observation has clearly shown that there are a number of different syndromes of diabetic neuropathy (Fig. 24.16). Chronic sensory neuropathy is diffuse and symmetrical, with typical symptoms of paraesthesiae, hyperaesthesia, cramps, or a burning sensation in the feet, which may be particularly troublesome at night. Proximal motor neuropathy may lead to wasting of specific groups of muscles and overlap with 'diabetic amyotrophy' (Fig. 24.17). Diffuse motor neuropathy has a subacute onset often in older Type II diabetic patients who may have reasonable glycaemic control and affects both proximal and distal muscles. Commonly in asymptomatic patients, small muscle wasting of the hands may be prominent (Fig. 24.18). Focal neuropathies may have a vascular origin and often affect the cranial or intercostal nerves, or result from pressure effects, producing a carpal tunnel syndrome or foot drop. An isolated third cranial nerve lesion is often due to diabetes (Fig. 24.19). Patients with newly diagnosed diabetes may have neurological symptoms and signs which resolve with treatment.

The differing clinical syndromes would deny the possibility of one simple aetiological mechanism and it is likely that in each of these an interaction of vascular and metabolic factors is at play. For example, diffuse sensory neuropathy could be due to diffuse metabolic dysfunction, although diffuse small vessel disease could also lead to a similar picture. In the syndrome of proximal motor neuropathy, the focal features on the background of generalized neuropathy suggest a metabolic disorder with focal vascular features. Diffuse motor neuropathy in older subjects, often with Type II diabetes, introduces the important possibility of an ageing factor. The focal neuropathies, on the other hand, strongly suggest that either pressure or local vascular factors are involved.

It is possible that more detailed study of newly diagnosed patients with diabetes, twenty per cent of whom demonstrate symptoms and clinical features of neuropathy, will provide the answer to the mechanisms underlying early nerve damage which are clearly reversible with improved glycaemic control.

MAJOR PROBLEMS IN DIABETIC NEUROPATHY
The Diabetic Foot

Ulceration in the diabetic foot results in such a degree of clinical morbidity and hospital bed usage that it should be regarded as the most important feature of diabetic peripheral nerve damage. The aetiology of foot ulceration involves a combination of the effects of

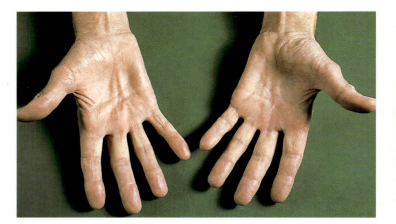

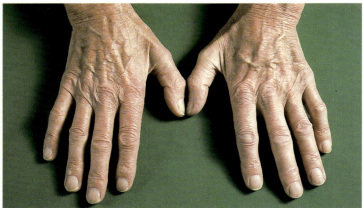

Fig. 24.18 Small muscle wasting in the first dorsal interosseous. There is contracture and thickening of the palmar fascia correlating with the presence of diabetic neuropathy.

deformity, local pressure, trauma, infection and abnormalities of blood flow and supply.

In the feet, a point may experience up to 50kg/cm^2 of pressure (Fig. 24.20). Fig. 24.21 illustrates the presence of a visible pulse within inches of gangrenous toes.

Infection in the neuropathic foot is not a major aetiological factor, but once such infection takes hold, it is the major reason for massive tissue destruction and loss of part of a foot, or even major amputation (Fig. 24.22). Amputation of a limb for purely neuropathic reasons should be totally preventable. To achieve this, there needs to be a strategy which will identify patients at risk and there should be education of patients and professionals about foot care. This will allow proper screening programmes.

Impotence

This common and tragic problem, possibly afflicting nearly half of men with diabetes over the age of forty-five years, is related to a combination of neurological, vascular and psychological problems. Detailed assessment of subjects from all these three aspects should be undertaken and appropriate advice and therapy offered. Attempts have been made at revascularization and there are various methods of surgical implantation to assist with penile erection. Glycaemic control should be improved at all times, although this alone does not lead to any significant improvement in most cases of chronic impotence. Very often the best that can be offered is a humane and sympathetic approach to a condition which can lead to unhappiness, depression and marital breakdown.

TREATMENT

Before attempting to treat diabetic neuropathy, other causes of neuropathy such as alcohol, drugs and vitamin B$_{12}$ deficiency should be sought and treated. Glycaemic control must be optimized as most studies have related the blood glucose level to the development of clinical neuropathy. This alone may improve functional tests and the pain threshold.

Two double-blind controlled studies have shown the benefits of tricyclic antidepressant drugs, which probably work through interference with α-receptor activity. Imipramine, amitriptyline and mianserin have all been tried in neuropathy as well as the phenothiazine, fluphenazine. To assess accurately the efficiency of any new treatments for neuropathy, further trials should include accurate clinical definitions, measurements of symptoms and signs and also the neurophysiological indices discussed above.

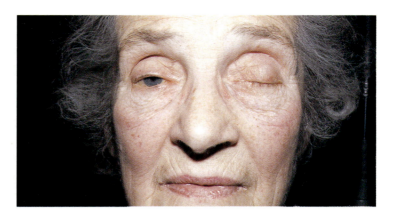

Fig. 24.19 Typical complete third cranial nerve palsy of sudden onset. It is accompanied by pain in the orbit and by high blood glucose.

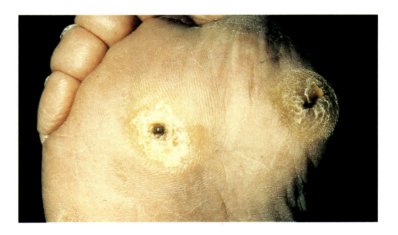

Fig. 24.20 Pressure points on the sole of the foot of a diabetic patient.

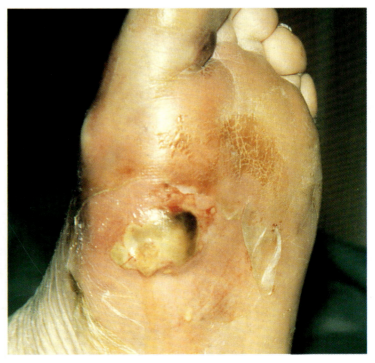

Fig. 24.22 Deep-seated foot infection. This is the major cause for loss of part of a foot, or even major amputation.

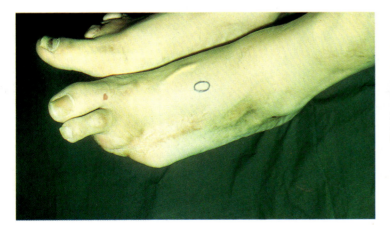

Fig. 24.21 The diabetic neuropathic foot. Despite recent loss of toes with gangrene and the presence on the plantar surface of this foot of two deep ulcers, the blue ring marks the site of an easily palpable and indeed visible bounding peripheral pulse. Near this pulse is a distended vein which suggests arteriovenous shunting.

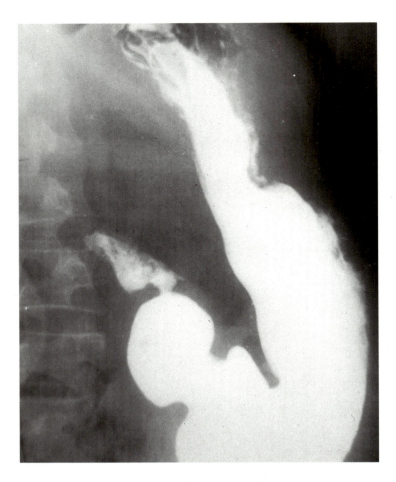

Fig. 24.23 Barium meal showing a distended stomach due to stasis from autonomic gastroparesis. The barium was taken two hours before this photograph.

Aldose reductase inhibitors, by reversing disordered metabolism in nerve tissue, have potential as therapeutic agents. However, it must be realized that subjects with diabetic neuropathy have axonal loss, segmental demyelination, often infarction of parts of the nerve and serious blockage of nutrient vessels (see Fig. 24.1). Clearly, to administer drugs at this stage with the hope of substantial recovery is demanding the impossible and it seems likely that demonstration of efficacy will depend upon longer term studies in which drugs are administered to subjects with either very early symptomatic neuropathy or, indeed, no neuropathy at all. With this in mind, it is important to realize that the severity of neuropathy does not necessarily relate closely to the severity of the pathological features seen on biopsy.

Moreover, in patients with neuropathy, although nerve glucose is high, sorbitol levels do not reach those found in diabetic animal models, such as the rat. Furthermore, there is no evidence, as yet, for significant depression of myo-inositol or for any relationship between myo-inositol depression and the severity of clinical neuropathy.

It seems likely that by the time a patient has severe clinical neuropathy the aetiological mechanisms initiating that problem have long since dissipated.

THE AUTONOMIC NEUROPATHIES

Interference with the autonomic nervous system leads to a wide variety of symptoms and signs. Autonomic neuropathy is unusual as a severe clinical syndrome, but when it does occur the features are very unpleasant. It is a serious development as studies have shown twenty per cent mortality within five years in those with

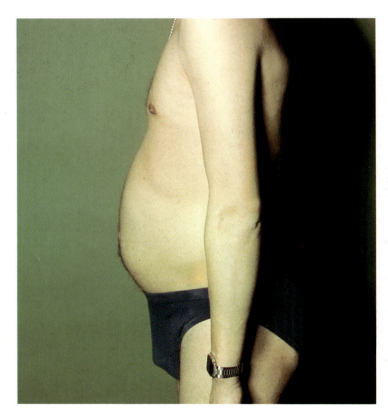

Fig. 24.24 Distended bladder due to autonomic neuropathy. This young man presented with painless swelling in the abdomen. He was not impotent indicating the highly selective damage which can occur in autonomic disease.

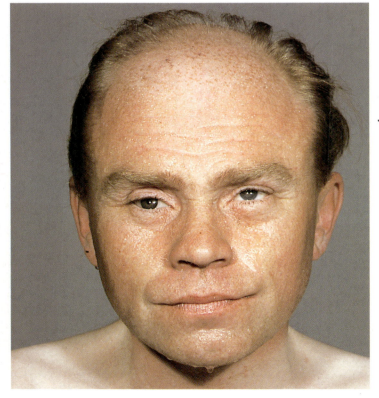

Fig. 24.25 Facial flushing and sweating after eating due to autonomic neuropathy. By courtesy of Dr P.J. Watkins.

24.8

established clinical autonomic neuropathy. The mixture of symptoms and signs due to autonomic dysfunction varies widely from patient to patient.

Cardiac denervation may be demonstrated by loss of beat-to-beat variation and postural hypotension, the latter sometimes occurring after insulin injection. It is possible that some abnormal sensations experienced by patients after injecting insulin may be due to low blood pressure rather than low blood glucose.

Gastrointestinal denervation may lead to disorders of oesophageal motility, gastric stasis (Fig. 24.23), diarrhoea or constipation. Genitourinary problems include impotence, incomplete bladder emptying or a neurogenic bladder (Fig. 24.24). Facial flushing or sweating may occur after eating, particularly savoury foods; the latter is termed 'gustatory sweating' (Fig. 24.25).

Autonomic Function Tests

A variety of autonomic function tests have been used to detect autonomic neuropathy. Following the Valsalva manoeuvre, there is a loss of the normal response of tachycardia followed by bradycardia (Fig. 24.26). On the resting ECG, there may be loss of the normal beat-to-beat variation of the heart rate (which may be accentuated by slow, deep respiration), loss of the normal rapid heartbeat increase on standing, or a simple demonstration of postural hypotension.

In patients with symptoms suggestive of autonomic neuropathy, it is likely that abnormal test results will be found and may help confirm the diagnosis. Many totally asymptomatic subjects with diabetes have a degree of abnormality of these tests and the exact significance of these abnormalities for future health, or the development of diabetic complications, is currently uncertain.

Treatment

Treatment of the symptoms of autonomic neuropathy is difficult. For those with cardiac problems an awareness of the potential danger is helpful, particularly if a general anaesthetic is required.

Metoclopramide may be of some benefit for gastric stasis and in extreme cases gastroenterostomy may be necessary. Tetracycline has been tried for diarrhoea on the basis that there may be an element of bacterial overgrowth. Fludrocortisone may help postural hypotension.

A paralysed bladder usually responds to bladder drill with regular emptying, although bladder neck resection may occasionally be required.

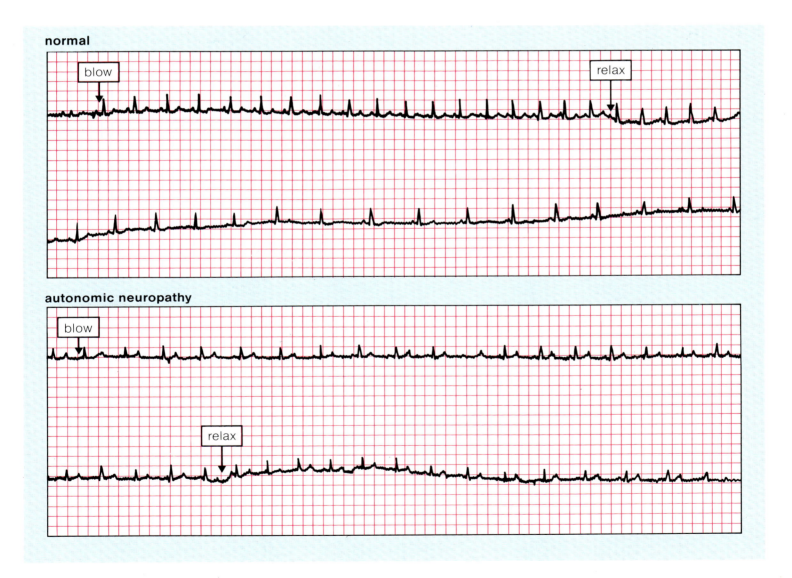

Fig. 24.26 ECG demonstrating impaired response to the Valsalva manoeuvre in autonomic neuropathy. The points where the subjects were asked to blow and relax are indicated. In the normal subject, there is an increase in heart rate with forced breathing followed by slowing on relaxation. In autonomic neuropathy, there is a fixed heart rate.

REFERENCES

Connor H, Boulton AJM & Ward JD (1987) *The Foot in Diabetes.* Chichester: John Wiley & Sons.

Dyck PJ, Thomas PK, Asbury AK, Winegard AI & Porte D (eds) (1987) *Diabetic Neuropathy.* Philadelphia: WB Saunders Company.

Ward JD (1985) Diabetic neuropathy. In *The Diabetes Annual, Volume 1.* Edited by Alberti KGMM & Krall LP. pp.288–309. Amsterdam: Elsevier Science Publishers B.V.

Ward JD (1986) Diabetic neuropathy. In *The Diabetes Annual, Volume 2.* Edited by Alberti KGMM & Krall LP. pp.197–208. Amsterdam: Elsevier Science Publishers B.V.

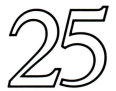

Diabetic Nephropathy

John T Ireland MD MB ChB FRCPEd ● **Anasuya Grenfell** MA MRCP

Diabetic nephropathy is a common and ultimately lethal complication of diabetes mellitus. It is a major cause of renal failure and twenty-five per cent of patients currently entering dialysis programmes in the U.S.A. are diabetic. The natural history is best documented in Type I (insulin-dependent) diabetic patients of whom approximately forty-five per cent develop nephropathy, with a peak incidence sixteen years after diagnosis. Death from renal failure or associated vascular disease occurs in half of these patients.

In 1936, Kimmelstiel and Wilson first described characteristic spherical hyaline masses in the lobules of glomeruli from eight diabetic patients who died of renal failure (Fig. 25.1). This followed illnesses characterized by albuminuria, nephrotic oedema and hypertension. Although these observations were initially received with scepticism, they led to the identification of other glomerular and renal arteriolar lesions which established the concept of a specific small blood vessel disease in diabetes. Thus, in 1954 Lundbaek proposed the idea of diabetic 'microangiopathy' based on the common finding of small vessel disease in both retinopathy and renal lesions of patients with diabetes of long duration.

Although the Kimmelstiel–Wilson nodule has remained the hallmark of diabetic renal disease, confusion has surrounded the pathogenesis of diabetic nephropathy. Using electron microscopy to view renal tissue obtained by percutaneous biopsy, it became apparent that there was a fundamental change diffusely affecting the glomerular capillary wall in diabetes; this was basement membrane thickening (Fig. 25.2). Successful attempts were made to relate this basement membrane lesion to the metabolic abnormalities of diabetes and it was found that chronic hyperglycaemia tended to lead to an increase in the glycoprotein structure of the membrane. It was difficult, however, to relate this widespread lesion to the development of the clinical features of albuminuria and progressive renal failure.

Recent intensive studies of functional changes in the diabetic kidney have somewhat clarified a hitherto confusing subject. The natural history of diabetic nephropathy can be divided into three distinct and contrasting stages: (i) early phase — renal hypertrophy and hyperfiltration; (ii) transitional phase — glomerular lesions with varying glomerular permeability leading to the development of microalbuminuria and elevated blood pressure; and (iii) late phase — development of persistent proteinuria and hypertension leading to uraemia and end-stage renal failure.

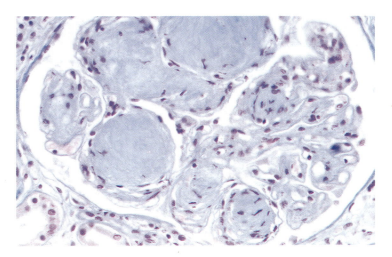

Fig. 25.1 A single glomerulus showing Kimmelstiel–Wilson nodules affecting the peripheral lobules. The nodules consist of spherical acellular hyaline masses seen in blue in this stain, toluidine blue.

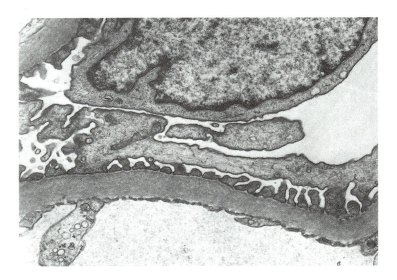

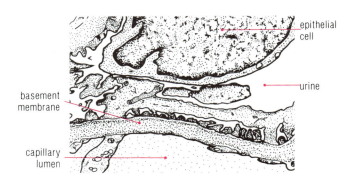

Fig. 25.2 Part of the glomerular capillary wall showing basement membrane thickening. EM × 10,000.

This chapter outlines two main aspects of diabetic nephropathy: structure and function. In both, the features are described according to the three stages in the natural history of diabetic renal disease, but with varying emphasis. Thus, the first phase of diabetic nephropathy, hypertrophy and hyperfiltration, is given greatest emphasis in the section on function. End-stage renal failure coincides with the best documented structural changes such as the Kimmelstiel–Wilson nodule and other glomerular lesions. It is in the second transitional phase, however, when glomerular lesions are developing and permeability is altering,

that the reader will find most interest in comparing the structural and functional changes.

STRUCTURE
Early Phase
Although reports in the early 1960's suggested that glomerular capillary basement membrane thickening might precede the onset of Type I diabetes, the detailed electron microscopy studies of Osterby–Hansen (1965) clearly showed that no structural abnormality was evident at the time of diagnosis. This was a

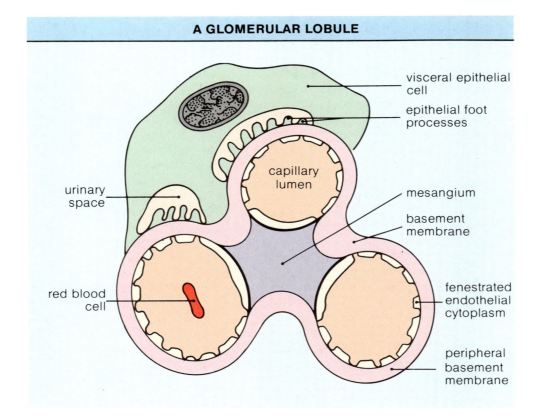

Fig. 25.3 Diagram of the glomerular lobule in cross-section showing how several capillaries are arranged around a centrilobular region called the mesangium.

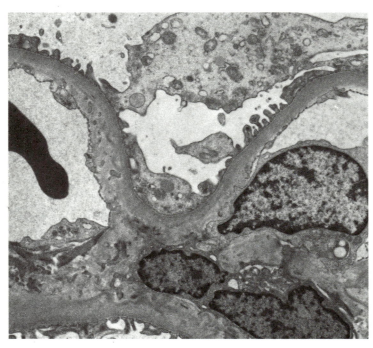

Fig. 25.4 Glomerular capillary wall and mesangial zone showing fenestrated endothelium, continuous basement membrane and foot processes of the epithelium. Also shown is the mesangial cell and matrix with some loose-textured basement membrane-like material. EM × 4500.

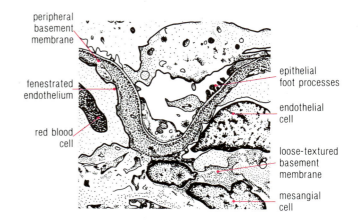

fundamental observation which helped to refute a widely held view that the glomerular changes might be genetically determined and therefore independent of the metabolic control of diabetes.

The normal anatomy of the glomerular lobule is shown in Fig. 25.3, which demonstrates how several capillaries are arranged around a centrilobular region, variously described as the axial zone, mesangium or intercapillary space. This central zone lies closest to the origin of the capillaries from the afferent arteriole and provides a core of supporting tissue from the centre of each lobule. The central mesangial cells are separated from the endothelial cells by loose-textured basement membrane material (Fig. 25.4) and have been likened to the pericytes in the retinal capillaries.

The peripheral parts of the capillary loops have only three distinct components: the endothelium, basement membrane and epithelium (Fig. 25.5). Of these, the basement membrane is the only continuous layer. The endothelium is composed of the attenuated periphery of the endothelial cells and is perforated by large pores or 'fenestrae' 50–100nm in diameter. The epithelium lies over the free surface of the capillaries and is attached to the basement membrane by foot processes, usually separated by a gap of about 25nm, bridged by a thin line called the slit membrane

(Fig. 25.5). These unique glomerular features allow assessment of basement membrane thickness, because when clearly seen the examiner can be confident of having obtained a true cross-section.

Transitional Phase: Glomerular Lesions

Basement membrane thickening

A gradual increase in basement membrane thickness becomes evident on renal biopsy after two to five years of Type I diabetes. This increase progresses slowly and relatively uniformly until after ten to twenty years the membrane is double its normal thickness. Simultaneously, basement membrane material accumulates in the mesangial zone (Fig. 25.6), so that the vascular and urinary spaces become compromised (Fig. 25.7).

Work on experimentally diabetic rats has confirmed that basement membrane thickening is a function of hyperglycaemia and time. Biochemical studies have shown that hyperglycaemia is associated with an absolute increase in basement membrane glycoprotein. In hyperglycaemia (or insulin deficiency), there is increased incorporation of carbohydrate into the membrane structure along non insulin-dependent pathways. This carbohydrate, in the form of polysaccharide units, tends to increase

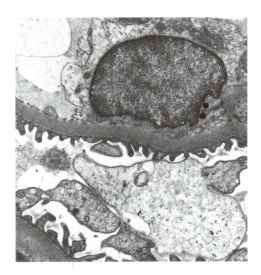
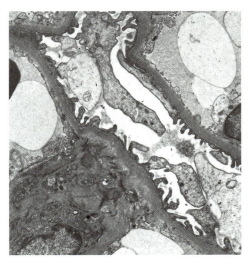
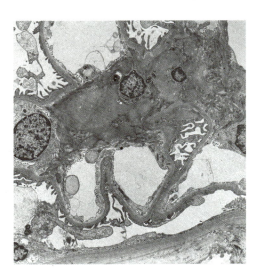

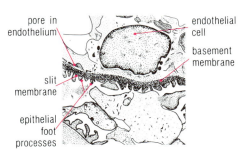
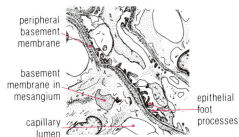
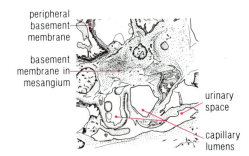

Fig. 25.5 Peripheral capillary wall made up of fenestrated endothelium, basement membrane and epithelium with foot processes. EM × 7000.

Fig. 25.6 Accumulation of basement membrane-like material in the mesangium causing mesangial expansion. EM × 4500.

Fig. 25.7 Accumulation of basement membrane-like material in the mesangium with mesangial expansion and compromise of the vascular and urinary spaces. EM × 3000.

with a concomitant loss of protein cross-linkages, with the result that, although the membrane is thickened, it may also become more permeable to protein and other macromolecules (Fig. 25.8). Increased non-enzymatic glycosylation of basement membrane protein and increased accumulation of glucose via the sorbitol pathway are other abnormalities of basement membrane biochemistry which have been identified in the diabetic state and which may lead to both the accumulation of basement membrane and its altered properties.

Fibrin deposition
Both the altered vascular permeability and the potential state of hypercoagulation in diabetes could influence fibrin deposition

(Fig. 25.9). Fibrin-derived macromolecules and fibrillar fibrin play a significant part in converting the early basement membrane lesions into the more dramatic and damaging features seen on light microscopy (see below). Other non-immunological circulating aggregates, apart from fibrin, may further stimulate mesangial matrix formation.

Glomerular Occlusion: End-stage Renal Failure
Diabetic glomerulosclerosis is the general term used to describe the various lesions which may be identified in the later stages of diabetic nephropathy, usually occurring after several years of gradual basement membrane accumulation. The various lesions described below often coexist and are probably variations on

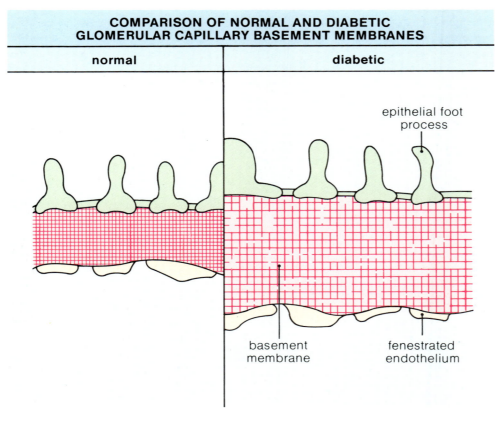

COMPARISON OF NORMAL AND DIABETIC GLOMERULAR CAPILLARY BASEMENT MEMBRANES

normal | diabetic

epithelial foot process

basement membrane

fenestrated endothelium

Fig. 25.8 Schematic diagram showing the contrast between normal and diabetic glomerular capillary basement membranes. The diabetic basement membrane is not only thickened but has an altered structure with loss of negative charge and protein cross-linking and an increase in polysaccharide content. As a result there is increased permeability to proteins and other macromolecules.

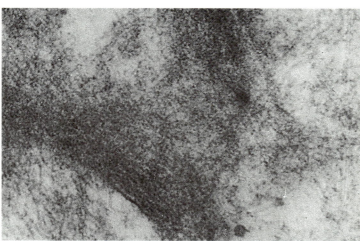

Fig. 25.9 Linear bundles of early fibrin in the capillary basement membrane. EM × 40,000.

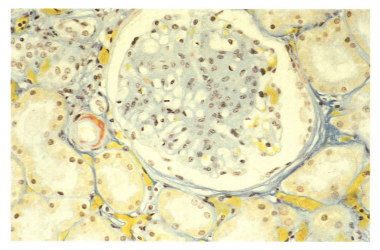

Fig. 25.10 Glomerulus showing diffuse basement membrane thickening and nodular glomerular change. Some red-staining fibrin can be seen in the wall of the afferent arteriole. Martius scarlet-blue stain.

several pathological processes secondary to basement membrane increase. The common histological end point is glomerular hyalinization.

Diffuse glomerular lesion

The degrees of renal failure and nephrotic syndrome correlate best with this lesion which begins with thickening of the whole circumference of the wall of peripheral capillaries in the glomerular tuft. These lesions become diffuse within the glomerulus and generalized throughout the kidney with increasing severity (Fig. 25.10). Further progression leads to narrowing of the capillary lumens and eventually to complete glomerular hyalinization.

Nodular glomerular lesion

Identifying a nodular lesion is the most reliable way of diagnosing diabetic nephropathy by light microscopy. Within an affected glomerulus, which may be normal in size or only slightly enlarged, nodules occupy the centres of single or multiple peripheral lobules. The fully developed lesion may be an almost spherical, homogeneous, vacuolated fibrillar or lamellar mass often having a patent or distended capillary running over its surface. The main diagnostic features are that the nodule is focal, peripheral, centrilobular and acellular (Fig. 25.11).

Exudative glomerular lesion

The exudative lesion is the least specific of the glomerular changes in diabetes. It also occurs in various non-diabetic disorders associated with renal failure. The lesion usually consists of rounded or crescentic deposits of either homogeneous or vacuolated, intensely acidophilic, material without nuclei, representing various proteins and fibrinoid matter which have leaked into the glomerular lumen (Fig. 25.12).

Glomerular hyalinization

As a consequence of the above lesions, increasing numbers of glomeruli become completely hyalinized in advanced cases of diabetes. There may be shrinkage of the glomerular tuft or periglomerular fibrosis with thickening of the Bowman's capsule by connective tissue fibrils (Fig. 25.13).

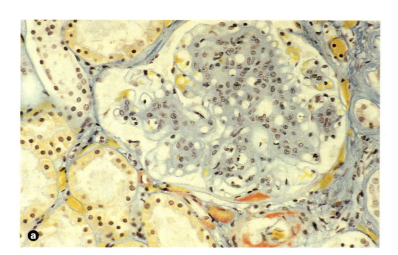

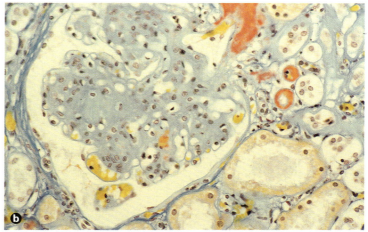

Fig. 25.11 Nodular glomerulosclerosis. Glomerular lesions (a) show a marked increase in the mesangial cell population. At the periphery of the nodules, a small fleck of red-staining fibrin can be seen at one point of the Bowman's capsule. In (b) the fibrillary nature of the nodular deposits can be seen as well as a dilated capillary loop passing over the surface of one of the nodules. Red-staining fibrin is present in the hyalinized extraglomerular vessels. Martius scarlet-blue stain.

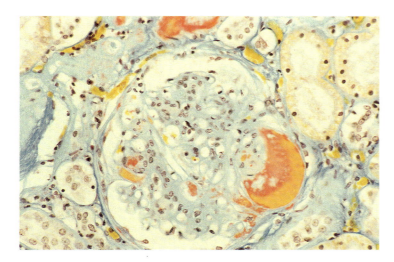

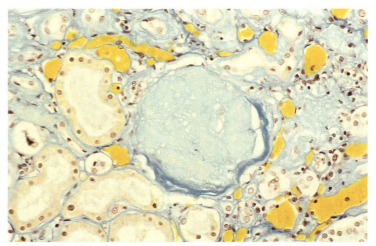

Fig. 25.12 Glomerulus showing crescentic exudative lesions. In addition to basement membrane thickening, one of the capillary loops shows a fibrin deposit staining red. This represents the so-called exudative type of capillary lesion in which there is thought to be marked inflow of plasma proteins into the abnormal capillary wall. Martius scarlet-blue stain.

Fig. 25.13 Complete hyalinization of a glomerulus in advanced diabetic nephropathy. The glomerulus is completely replaced by acellular hyaline. Tubular and interstitial changes of chronic pyelonephritis can also be seen. Martius scarlet-blue stain.

Arterial and arteriolar lesions

Although atheroma is considered to be more common in diabetes, there is no accurate documentation of any increase in its incidence in the larger renal vessels of diabetic patients at autopsy. Conversely, diffuse intimal fibrosis in these vessels, which is believed to be almost universal after the age of fifty years, has been found to be more frequent and advanced at autopsy in diabetic patients.

Bell (1942) established the importance of hyaline arteriolar lesions in diabetes. He emphasized that there was efferent arteriolar involvement, in addition to afferent arteriolosclerosis and showed that, although hypertension had been common in the 1465 diabetic patients he examined at autopsy, a large percentage without hypertension also had these lesions. Indeed, efferent arteriolar involvement is sufficiently characteristic of diabetes to be of aid to the light microscopist when concluding that associated glomerular disease is diabetic in origin (Fig. 25.14).

Bell originally stressed the parallel association between the severity of arteriolosclerosis and diffuse and nodular glomerular involvement. This has led some to conclude that the diabetic glomerular lesions might be a consequence of the arteriolar disease. This seems unlikely, however, since arteriolosclerosis, in the absence of diabetes, usually leads to ischaemic atrophy of the glomerular tuft, with thickening of the capillary wall at the hilum and shrinkage of the remaining vessels, instead of the diffuse and nodular changes that are seen.

Tubular lesions

Although various lesions may be found in the tubules of diabetic patients, few are thought to be of significance and they are generally secondary to glomerulosclerosis, ischaemia, pyelonephritis or chronic electrolyte disturbances. The 'Armanni–Ebstein lesion', or 'glycogen nephrosis', consists of glycogen-laden vacuoles in the tubules of the corticomedullary region. It was a common post-mortem finding in the pre-insulin era and is still occasionally found in those who die following uncorrected hyperglycaemia, acidosis and dehydration. Severe electrolyte and circulatory disturbances in profound diabetic ketoacidosis may also cause acute tubular necrosis.

Urinary tract infections

Many believe that diabetic patients are more prone than non-diabetic subjects to infections in general and pyelonephritis in particular. In autopsies on diabetic patients, changes interpreted as chronic pyelonephritis were frequently reported in association with diabetic arteriosclerosis and glomerulosclerosis. Indeed, some observers were sufficiently impressed by the association to conclude that the diabetic lesions might be a consequence of chronic pyelonephritis. However, it is now understood that most of the changes in the interstitial tissue and tubules which resemble healed chronic pyelonephritis are secondary to the ischaemia and the glomerular lesions of diabetes (see Fig. 25.13).

Because of the difficulty in establishing what is chronic pyelonephritis and what is not, opinions inevitably vary. This is reflected in the wide discrepancies in the frequency of pyelonephritis in autopsy series. Thomsen (1965) best reflects the more cautious view by stressing that what is called 'chronic' or 'healed pyelonephritis' pathologically, may be due to the ischaemia of arteriosclerosis and glomerulosclerosis. Nonetheless, there are several factors which may predispose the diabetic patient to urinary tract infection. These include the effect of diabetic autonomic neuropathy on bladder function, thus favouring stasis, the practice of catheterization in the management of ketoacidosis

and the probability that infection is more likely in renal tissue affected by such vascular lesions as arteriosclerosis and glomerulosclerosis.

Renal papillary necrosis

Renal papillary necrosis usually results from acute infection in which the tips of medullary tissue become necrotic and is reported to be more common in diabetic patients. These lesions may be exacerbated by ischaemia due to disease of the long thin vasa recta, although compression of the submucosal vessels by infective oedema may further compromise papillary blood supply. Radiological examination may help diagnosis by demonstrating a 'moth-eaten' appearance of the calyces; the 'ring-shadow' appearance corresponding to necrotic papillae is thought to be pathognomonic. With improved antibiotic therapy, this condition has been reported less frequently in diabetic subjects, although phenacetin abuse has been recognized as an alternative cause in non-diabetic subjects.

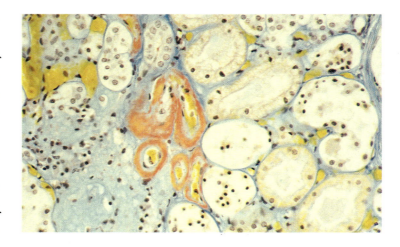

Fig. 25.14 Typical hyalinization of both efferent and afferent arterioles. Such arteriolosclerosis is said to be characteristic of diabetic small vessel disease in the kidney. Fibrin is again present in the walls of these vessels. Martius scarlet-blue stain.

FUNCTIONAL CHANGES IN DIABETIC NEPHROPATHY

Established diabetic nephropathy, which may be defined as persistent proteinuria of more than 0.5g/24 hours, usually develops after 12–20 years of diabetes. It is preceded by a long 'silent phase' during which both structural and functional changes can be detected in the kidney, often from very early in the course of diabetes. These functional changes can be considered in terms of the three main phases in the natural history of diabetic nephropathy (Fig. 25.15) outlined earlier: (i) the early phase; (ii) the transitional phase; and (iii) the late phase.

Early Phase

Glomerular filtration rate

At the onset of Type I (insulin-dependent) diabetes, functional changes occur in the kidney which appear to be related to structural changes that occur at the same time. The glomerular filtration rate (GFR) may be elevated and this is associated with an increase in renal size (Fig. 25.16). Glomerular hypertrophy accompanies these changes and there is an increase in the capillary filtration surface area which correlates with the elevated GFR. The contribution of these early functional and structural changes to the future development of diabetic glomerulosclerosis is unknown, but renal size and GFR remain elevated in between twenty-five and forty per cent of patients for several years after the diagnosis of diabetes.

Albumin excretion

Albuminuria above the normal range, but well below the usual clinical levels of detection (Albustix-negative) may be found at the time of diagnosis or in short-duration Type I diabetic patients after the withdrawal of insulin for several days. At this early stage it appears to have little significance in terms of future diabetic nephropathy in contrast to its importance at later stages.

NATURAL HISTORY OF DIABETIC NEPHROPATHY		
early phase	**transitional phase**	**late phase**
GFR increased	GFR increased	GFR decreased
renal size increased	renal size increased	renal size normal or increased
AER increased (poor control)	AER increased (micro-albuminuria)	AER greatly increased (persistent proteinuria)
blood pressure normal	blood pressure increased	blood pressure greatly increased
reversible	?reversible	irreversible

Fig. 25.15 Natural history of diabetic nephropathy. GFR = glomerular filtration rate; AER = albumin excretion rate.

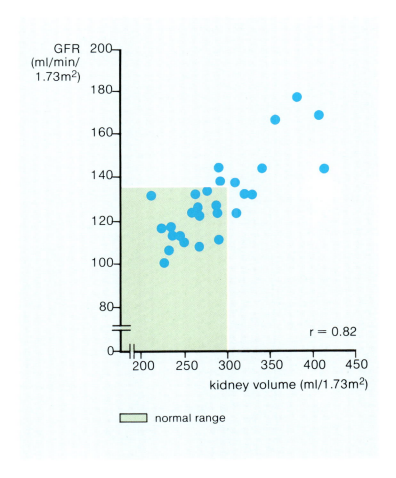

Fig. 25.16 Relationship between glomerular filtration rate (GFR) and kidney volume in diabetic patients. The relationship is statistically highly significant.

Transitional Phase

Microalbuminuria

Elevation of albumin excretion above normal but below that detected by Albustix (a reagent strip for proteinuria detection) has been demonstrated in thirty to forty-five per cent of patients with diabetes of ten to twenty years duration (Fig. 25.17). This mild elevation of urinary albumin excretion has been termed 'micro-albuminuria'. The upper limit of the normal albumin excretion rate (AER) is approximately 30mg/24 hours, while urine is usually positive with Albustix testing at rates above 250mg/24 hours. Microalbuminuria thus refers to a wide subclinical range of albumin hyperexcretion of between 30–250mg/24 hours (Fig. 25.18). These values are not absolute and common sense should be used in assigning a borderline value to one or other category, especially at the lower end. The day-to-day variation in AER may be between forty and fifty per cent and partly reflects the influence of plasma concentration, urine flow and exercise.

Microalbuminuria carries the risk of progression to diabetic nephropathy, although the AER which is thought to be predictive varies over a wide range from 15–70µg/min. This range may be explained by differences in methods, timing of urine collection and length of follow-up (Fig. 25.19). Despite these differences, most studies have similar findings. Diabetic patients with overnight or twenty-four-hour urinary AERs of 50–250mg/24 hours show a twenty-fold increase in the risk of developing clinical nephropathy compared to patients whose AERs are below this.

The structural basis for the increased AER remains obscure. Mauer and colleagues (1984) have shown that the AER correlates

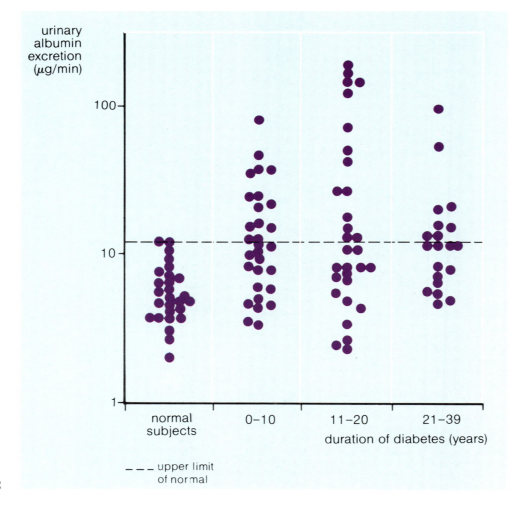

Fig. 25.17 Albumin excretion in patients who have had diabetes for differing durations. There is an increase in those patients who have had the disease for ten or twenty years.

with the mesangial volume, but not the basement membrane width, whereas Osterby (1986) has shown a correlation with basement membrane thickening as well. Patients with an increased AER may also show some glomerular occlusion, but this occurs in only a small proportion of glomeruli.

The glomerular capillary blood–urine barrier may be considered functionally as a membrane perforated by negatively-charged pores, 55 Å in diameter. The factors which determine the passage of proteins across this barrier therefore include the size and charge of the molecules as well as the transglomerular pressure gradient. As microalbuminuria develops, the selectivity of the glomerular barrier alters. Normally, the albumin/total protein ratio is approximately eleven per cent, but with the development of microalbuminuria this increases to approximately twenty-two

per cent due to an increase in the relative amount of filtered albumin. It has been suggested this alteration in selectivity is due to loss of negative charge from the basement membrane such that the filtration of albumin, a polyanionic molecule (molecular weight 69,000 daltons, Stokes' radius 36 Å) is increased compared with an electrically neutral molecule such as IgG (molecular weight 160,000 daltons, Stokes' radius 55 Å). There is considerable experimental evidence and some evidence from *in vivo* renal conditions other than diabetes to support this hypothesis. It has been postulated that the loss of negative charge is due to reduction in the heparan sulphate anionic sites within the glycosamino-glycans of the basement membrane. The mechanism by which this loss of negative charge occurs remains uncertain.

ALBUMIN EXCRETION DURING DIFFERENT PHASES OF DIABETIC NEPHROPATHY			
	normo-albuminuria	micro-albuminuria	clinical proteinuria
albumin excretion (per 24 hours)	<26mg	26–250mg	>250mg
albumin/total protein ratio	11%	22%	50%

Fig. 25.18 Albumin excretion during different phases of diabetic nephropathy.

LEVELS OF MICROALBUMINURIA PREDICTING CLINICAL NEPHROPATHY			
group	follow-up (years)	urine collection	predictive AER (μg/min)
London, U.K.	14	overnight	30
Copenhagen, Denmark	6	24 hours	70
Åarhus, Denmark	6–14	1–2 hours	15

Fig. 25.19 Levels of microalbuminuria which predict clinical nephropathy. The variation in predictive values may be due to differences in method, timing of urine collection and length of follow-up.

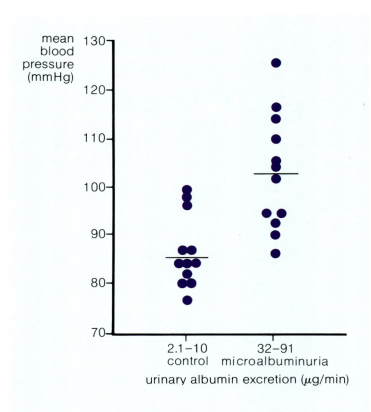

Glomerular filtration rate

It has been suggested that an elevated GFR of greater than 150ml/min/1.73m^2 may be important in the pathogenesis and progression of diabetic nephropathy. In association with microalbuminuria, it could be a marker for those at increased risk. However, the prognostic significance of a high GFR in the absence of microalbuminuria is uncertain. This raised GFR has been shown to correlate well with an increase in the filtration surface area of the glomeruli.

Hypertension

Patients with microalbuminuria have been shown to have higher blood pressure than those without it, although their blood pressure is still within the normal range (Fig. 25.20). In addition, it has been shown that there is a positive correlation between albumin excretion rate and blood pressure. The significance of this raised blood pressure to the progression of the underlying renal disease at this early stage is uncertain.

Fig. 25.20 Blood pressure in diabetic patients with either microalbuminuria or normal protein excretion (controls). Those patients with microalbuminuria have higher blood pressure. The mean value is indicated in each case.

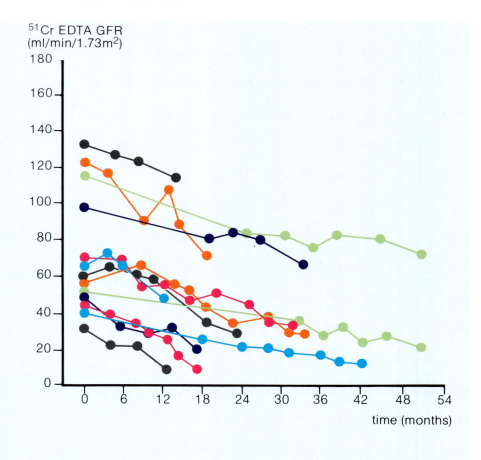

Fig. 25.21 Decline in renal function with time in diabetic patients with proteinuria. Renal function was assessed by measuring the excretion rate of radiolabelled EDTA (^{51}Cr EDTA).

Late Phases: Established Diabetic Nephropathy

Intermittent proteinuria is usually the first manifestation of overt diabetic nephropathy and it may continue for several years before the development of persistent proteinuria. The appearance of persistent proteinuria heralds the onset of a gradual and progressive decline in renal function (Fig. 25.21). The interval between the onset of persistent proteinuria and death from uraemia can range from between a few to twenty years. The factors responsible for this highly variable decline in renal function are unknown, but patients with heavy proteinuria and hypertension seem to have the worst prognosis.

Glomerular filtration rate

The glomerular filtration rate, while initially normal or elevated, gradually declines with time. It has been shown to correlate with the degree of glomerular capillary occlusion and the resultant reduction in filtration surface area. A correlation has also been shown between declining GFR and an increase in basement membrane thickening. The deterioration in GFR varies considerably from one patient to another, with rates ranging from 0.1–2.4ml/min/month, but it is strikingly linear with time for each individual. Age, sex, onset or duration of diabetes, albumin clearance rate, initial GFR and blood glucose control are all unrelated to the rate of decline of GFR.

Monitoring renal function in patients with diabetic nephropathy is important because the time course of events can be predicted. In the early stages, GFR should be measured, as serum creatinine does not rise until the GFR is reduced by between fifty and seventy-five per cent. Once the serum creatinine level has risen above 200μmol/l, it correlates closely with the stage of renal impairment and this can then be estimated by plotting the reciprocal of the serum creatinine against time (Fig. 25.22).

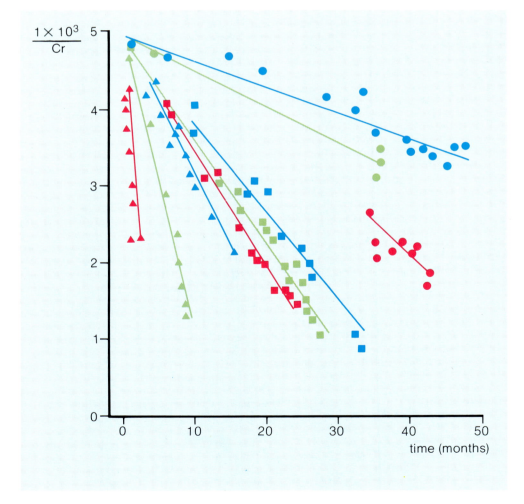

Fig. 25.22 Progression of renal failure in nine diabetic patients. Serum creatinine (Cr) was only recorded above levels of 200μmol/l. Its measurement can lead to an estimate of the state of renal impairment. From Jones *et al.* (1979), by courtesy of the *Lancet*.

Hypertension

Hypertension is common in patients with established diabetic nephropathy and may occur early in its course (Fig. 25.23); blood pressure rises as GFR falls (Fig. 25.24). The rate of decline in the GFR does not appear to be related to blood pressure although antihypertensive treatment appears to retard the rate of decline.

Proteinuria

Proteinuria increases as diabetic nephropathy progresses. The daily excretion of proteins varies considerably between individuals, although urinary excretion increases as GFR falls. Not only does urinary protein excretion increase, but the selectivity of the glomerular barrier also continues to change. The albumin/total protein ratio, which is increased to approximately twenty per cent in patients with microalbuminuria, increases even further up to fifty per cent in those with established nephropathy. The high relative selectivity for albumin remains until the GFR falls below 20ml/min/1.73m², when the filtration of IgG relative to albumin increases. Once the GFR declines to approximately 10ml/min/1.73m², there is a low selectivity proteinuria with increased filtration of both albumin and IgG. The loss of selectivity late in the course of diabetic nephropathy is thought to be due to the development of a small population of large pores, or membrane defects, within the glomerular basement membrane.

End-stage renal failure

End-stage renal failure usually develops approximately seven years after the onset of persistent proteinuria with a range of between five and twenty years. During this time, other diabetic complications develop and progress. By the time treatment is required for end-stage renal failure, the patient is usually thirty to forty years of age, with diabetes of between twenty and twenty-five years duration, and is troubled by severe retinopathy, neuropathy and cardiovascular disease (Fig. 25.25).

INTERVENTION
Glycaemic Control

The metabolic abnormalities of diabetes are believed to be important in the pathogenesis of the renal functional abnormalities of hyperfiltration, raised albumin excretion rate and renal hypertrophy. Attempts have therefore been made to prevent or correct these abnormalities with tight glycaemic control.

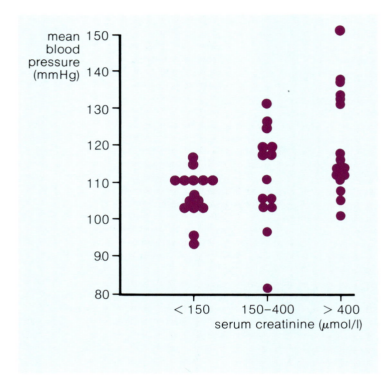

Fig. 25.23 Mean blood pressure in diabetic patients with nephropathy who have different serum creatinine levels. Increased serum creatinine is associated with decreased GFR.

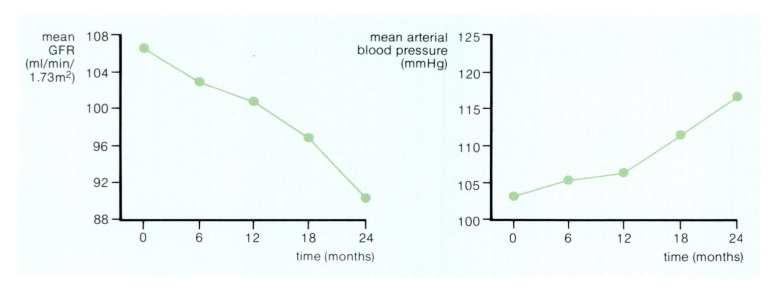

Fig. 25.24 Rise in mean blood pressure as GFR declines in diabetic patients with proteinuria.

Early phase

Primary prevention studies in experimental animals with diabetes have shown that those animals with poor glycaemic control develop hyperfiltration, albuminuria, nephromegaly and renal histological lesions, whereas those with tight control fail to develop these abnormalities. Attempts to reverse such abnormalities, once established, with strict control have also been successful. In diabetic patients at the time of diagnosis, strict glycaemic control will reduce, and in many cases normalize, both the GFR and the raised albumin excretion rate. The effects on renal size are controversial and, as yet, it remains uncertain whether renal size can be reduced by tight metabolic control.

Transitional phase

Initial studies suggest that tight control may reduce or prevent the progression of microalbuminuria, but these results remain tentative as they involve only small numbers of patients followed for short periods of time. So far no one has shown that histological lesions can be reversed or that the progression to diabetic nephropathy can be prevented.

Late phase

Once persistent proteinuria has developed and diabetic nephropathy is established, tight metabolic control does not appear to have any effect. Proteinuria is not altered and there is little effect on the rate of decline in GFR. Even at the earlier stage of intermittent proteinuria, tight glycaemic control does not appear to have any effect.

The failure of metabolic control to influence the decline in renal function suggests that the destructive process in the kidney has become self-perpetuating and independent of the underlying metabolic abnormality that initiated it. The inevitable progression, once renal disease has advanced to a certain point, is common to many nephropathic processes and it has been suggested that the compensatory hyperfiltration in surviving nephrons may be self-destructive.

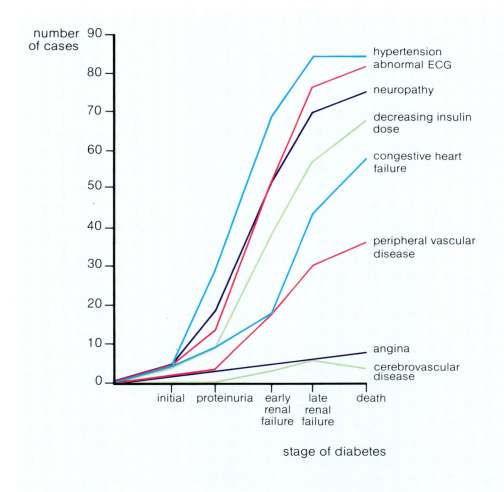

Fig. 25.25 Frequency of diabetic complications in various stages of nephropathy. From Goldstein (1974), by courtesy of Springer Verlag.

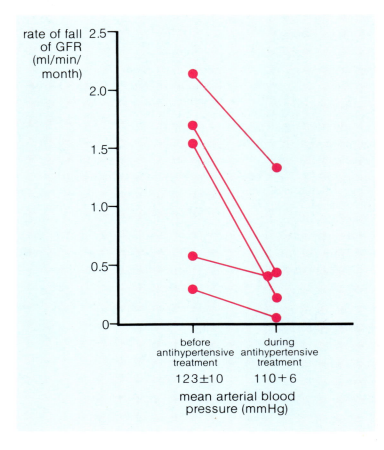

rate of fall
of GFR
(ml/min/
month)

before
antihypertensive
treatment
123±10

during
antihypertensive
treatment
110+6

mean arterial blood
pressure (mmHg)

Fig. 25.26 Effect of antihypertensive treatment on rate of decline of GFR in patients with diabetic nephropathy. Treatment greatly decreases the rate of decline of GFR. From Mogensen (1982), by courtesy of the *British Medical Journal*.

Blood Pressure

In established diabetic nephropathy, reducing the blood pressure has been shown to slow the rate of decline in GFR (Fig. 25.26). The finding that blood pressure is already elevated in micro-albuminuria and that albumin excretion rate correlates with blood pressure suggests that hypotensive treatment at this stage may be important in retarding the progression of the disease. Both acute and long-term studies of blood pressure treatment in patients with microalbuminuria have shown a reduction in albumin excretion rate.

Protein Restriction

Both in animals and in man, acute and chronic protein ingestion lead to an increase in GFR and in some cases renal enlargement. Restriction of protein intake in diabetic animals results in a decrease in intraglomerular pressure and reduces renal damage

Fig. 25.27 Effect on kidney function of intervention at different stages of diabetic nephropathy.

		manoeuvre		
phase	variable	decreased blood pressure	decreased blood glucose	decreased protein intake
early	GFR	?	↓	↓
	AER	↓	↓	↓
	kidney size	?	?	?
transitional	GFR	↓→	↓	↓
	AER	↓	?↓	↓
	kidney size	?	?	?
late	GFR	↓ rate of decline	→	?↓ rate of decline
	AER	↓	→↑	?↓
	kidney size	?	?	?

INTERVENTION AT DIFFERENT STAGES OF DIABETIC NEPHROPATHY

↓ decreased
↑ increased
? uncertain
→ unchanged

independent of glycaemic control, while high protein intake results in severe glomerular lesions and heavy albuminuria. Studies on protein restriction in man are still very preliminary, but short-term protein restriction reduces supranormal GFR and decreases the albumin excretion rate in diabetic patients with microalbuminuria. Whether these effects prevent future kidney damage remains to be established.

A summary of the effects of intervention at the different stages of diabetic nephropathy is shown in Fig. 25.27.

Conclusions

A sequence of events in the transition from early renal abnormalities to glomerulosclerosis and renal failure is suggested in Fig. 25.28. Diabetes mellitus in some patients results in an elevation in GFR and an increase in the glomerular filtration of proteins (microproteinuria). These changes lead to basement membrane thickening, mesangial expansion and Albustix-positive proteinuria (clinical proteinuria). This, in turn, causes further mesangial expansion leading to glomerulosclerosis and glomerular occlusion. This then produces compensatory hyperfiltration in the surviving glomeruli which, in turn, causes further destruction of glomeruli, so initiating a vicious cycle. Loss of glomeruli leads to a decline in function of the whole kidney and end-stage renal failure.

Renal functional changes are present from very early in the course of diabetic nephropathy and show some correlation with early structural changes in the kidney. These functional changes allow the identification of patients at risk of future clinical nephropathy and signal the need for intervention. Tight glycaemic control, the treatment of hypertension and dietary protein restriction have all been shown to be effective in reducing some of these functional abnormalities. Their use together may be even more effective.

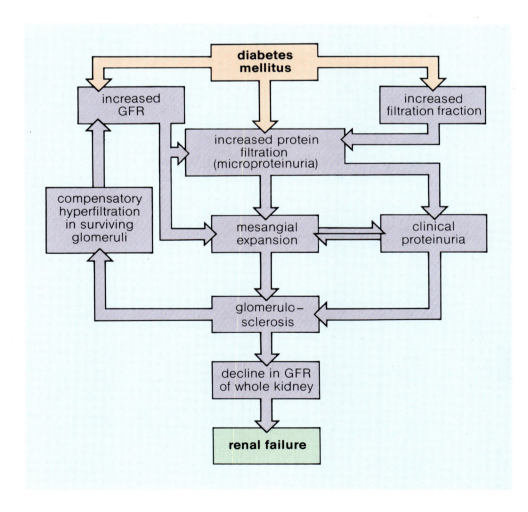

Fig. 25.28 Possible sequence of events in the transition from early renal abnormalities to glomerulosclerosis and renal failure.

MANAGEMENT OF RENAL FAILURE IN DIABETES
Assessment of Other Diabetic Complications

Renal disease is not an isolated complication of diabetes. The majority of patients also have widespread vascular disease, severe retinopathy and neuropathy by the time they reach end-stage renal failure. These complications are often overwhelming and may limit the success of renal replacement therapy. Thorough assessment of complications early in the course of diabetic nephropathy with appropriate intervention and follow-up may help minimize the problems and improve the outcome of these patients.

Cardiovascular disease

Cardiovascular disease is common in diabetic patients with advanced nephropathy, even those who are in their twenties and thirties. Approximately one third of Type I diabetic patients with diabetic nephropathy will die of cardiovascular disease before they even reach end-stage renal failure. Asymptomatic ischaemic heart disease is common. Abnormal electrocardiograms are present in fifty to seventy per cent of patients with end-stage renal failure while approximately fifty per cent have cardiomegaly (CT ratio >0.5) on chest radiography.

The cardiovascular system should be assessed early in the course of diabetic nephropathy and patients should be followed carefully as renal failure progresses. All have left ventricular hypertrophy on echocardiography (Fig. 25.29) and this is thought to reflect chronic hypertension. Blood pressure should be measured regularly and treated aggressively at an early stage.

Coronary angiography provides the best method of assessment and should be performed in younger patients and those being considered for renal transplantation. Several studies have shown the presence of significant coronary occlusive disease in between twenty and one hundred per cent of patients, depending upon the selection criteria and definition of coronary occlusion. Bypass surgery or angioplasty should be offered where feasible before renal replacement therapy. Neither those with coronary artery disease who are not suitable for intervention nor those with severe left ventricular dysfunction should be considered for transplantation. In addition, those with fifty per cent coronary artery stenosis should be re-studied within six months because of the rapid progression of lesions in some patients.

Peripheral vascular disease

Peripheral vascular disease is an important cause of morbidity and occasionally mortality in patients with diabetic nephropathy. All patients with symptoms (claudication and rest pain) and those with foot lesions and absent foot pulses should be investigated as prompt treatment may salvage a limb. Non-invasive investigations include: measurement of systolic ankle and toe pressures, although these may be difficult to interpret as vascular calcification (Fig. 25.30) results in rigid arterial walls and so an artificially raised blood pressure; Doppler ultrasound to determine blood velocity wave forms; and transcutaneous oxygen tension measurements. These investigations together with arteriography help to locate the site of arterial disease and to predict whether conservative management will be successful or whether amputation

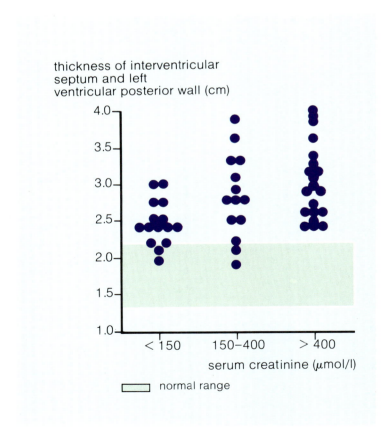

Fig. 25.29 Left ventricular dimensions on echocardiography in diabetic patients. The patients had proteinuria and different levels of serum creatinine.

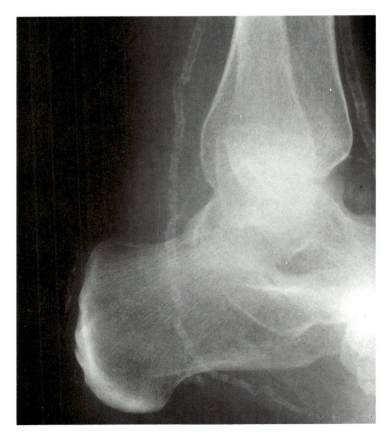

Fig. 25.30 Vascular calcification in the lower limb and ankle of a patient with diabetic nephropathy.

is required. Those suitable for intervention should be treated with angioplasty or bypass surgery. This is particularly important if an ischaemic ulcer is present, as all efforts should be made to heal the lesion before transplantation. The correct management of such lesions can result in healing in the majority of cases which limits the amputation rate.

Neuropathy
Neuropathy is present in almost all patients with advanced diabetic nephropathy, but its clinical manifestations are very variable. Some patients are completely asymptomatic, while others are troubled by severe features of somatic and autonomic neuropathy. Formal tests of thermal and vibration sensation (see *Chapter 24*) as well as autonomic function should be performed to identify those patients at risk.

Autonomic neuropathy may lead to urinary retention due to a neurogenic bladder and this partly explains the susceptibility of these patients to recurrent urinary tract infections. A neurogenic bladder is a relative contraindication to transplantation and a micturating cystogram to assess bladder size and emptying should be performed routinely before transplantation.

Vomiting due to gastroparesis is rare and difficult to assess in the presence of uraemia. A barium meal is of little help in its assessment and more sophisticated tests of stomach emptying are required. It can be very difficult to manage complications successfully.

Respiratory arrest in association with sedative drugs or anaesthesia occasionally occurs in patients with autonomic neuropathy and anaesthetists should be aware of this possibility.

Retinopathy
Retinopathy is almost always present in patients with advanced nephropathy and tends to deteriorate as renal failure progresses, due to a combination of hypertension and fluid overload. Severe deterioration occurs in those who have had no treatment prior to the development of renal failure and there is an increased risk of blindness once clinical uraemia has developed. Early examination and photocoagulation are essential.

Rehabilitation of patients with nephropathy may be affected by the presence of severe visual impairment or blindness, but there is no evidence that the outcome of renal failure treatment is adversely affected. Thus proliferative retinopathy and blindness do not constitute a contraindication to the treatment of diabetic nephropathy.

Treatment of Diabetic Patients with End-stage Renal Failure
Treatment of diabetic patients with end-stage renal failure needs careful planning and should be tailored to the severity of the illness and the situation of the patient. Early treatment probably improves the chances of a successful outcome as diabetic patients exhibit the symptoms of uraemia at lower levels of creatinine than non-diabetic subjects. In addition, there appears to be an acceleration in the progression of other diabetic complications as end-stage renal failure develops. Thus, patients should be considered for treatment when their creatinine levels reach $400-500 \mu mol/l$.

Transplantation
Transplantation is the treatment of choice for the diabetic patient with renal failure and should be performed before the need for dialysis to give the best results. However, some degree of chronic uraemia has a useful immunosuppressant effect and patients should not be given a transplant too early. Contraindications to transplantation vary from one renal unit to another, but usually include age over seventy years, severe cardiac disease which is not amenable to surgery and chronic sepsis.

Dialysis
Although transplantation is the best treatment for the diabetic patient with renal failure, some patients may be unsuitable and others may need dialysis either while awaiting transplantation or after graft failure.

The early results of haemodialysis in diabetic patients were very poor with one year survival rates of only twenty-two to thirty-three per cent and a high morbidity rate which discouraged the treatment of these patients. This was due to particular problems that complicated haemodialysis in diabetic patients (Fig. 25.31). Vascular access in such patients has always been a problem and frequent revision of the access site may be necessary. Ischaemic pain and gangrene of the operated limb may occur. The rapid fluid shifts associated with haemodialysis are not well tolerated and severe hypotension may develop. This is particularly the case in the presence of autonomic neuropathy. Progression of retinopathy often to blindess was a common problem and rehabilitation was very poor.

Results have improved considerably with experience and increasing numbers of patients have been treated by haemodialysis over the past decade with one year survival rates of over seventy

PROBLEMS OF HAEMODIALYSIS IN DIABETIC PATIENTS
vascular access
haemodynamic instability
progression of retinopathy
poor rehabilitation

Fig. 25.31 Problems of haemodialysis in diabetic patients.

CONTINUOUS AMBULATORY PERITONEAL DIALYSIS
vascular access not required
haemodynamic instability rare
good metabolic control
less risk of deterioration in retinopathy
rehabilitation better

Fig. 25.32 Advantages of continuous ambulatory peritoneal dialysis.

per cent. Although mortality and morbidity are still greater than in non-diabetic patients, the complications associated with haemodialysis are far fewer due to the better management of retinopathy, blood pressure and fluid balance.

Glycaemic control on dialysis is important and may be hard to achieve. Fluid restriction may be difficult to impose on patients who are thirsty due to hyperglycaemia. Insulin requirements will vary considerably depending upon activity, appetite and associated medical problems.

Blood pressure control may be difficult as the problems of hypotension during dialysis make it hard to achieve dry weight. Supine hypertension and postural hypotension may be a problem and careful fluid and salt restriction is needed between dialyses.

Continuous ambulatory peritoneal dialysis has become an increasingly popular form of treatment for diabetic patients with renal failure. It is particularly suitable for such patients and has certain advantages over haemodialysis (Fig. 25.32). There are no access problems and rapid fluid shifts do not occur. It is simple to use and offers the possibility of good metabolic control with the use of intraperitoneal insulin. Visual impairment and even blindness do not appear to be a contraindication and blind patients appear to do as well as those with normal vision. Peritonitis may be a problem and usually results in a marked rise

in blood glucose levels partly due to increased absorption of glucose from the peritoneal dialysis fluid. Intravenous insulin may be required during such episodes if they are severe. Long-term experience with continuous peritoneal dialysis is limited and it remains to be seen if this form of treatment will be suitable for chronic dialysis.

CONCLUSION

Diabetic nephropathy is a major cause of renal disease and may account for up to twenty-five per cent of new cases accepted for renal replacement therapy in some centres. Diabetic patients are no longer considered unsuitable candidates for treatment. Considerable improvements in the results of renal replacement therapy over the past few years mean that, in centres with considerable experience, results approach those in non-diabetic patients. Despite these advances, the presence of often overwhelming complications in diabetic patients with renal failure means that, in most cases, survival is poorer than in non-diabetic patients. Assessment and aggressive management of concomitant diabetic complications from an early stage in the natural history of nephropathy is important so that patients who reach end-stage renal failure are fitter and hence have a better chance of survival.

REFERENCES

Andersen AR, Christiansen JS, Andersen JK, Kreiner S & Deckert T (1983) Diabetic nephropathy in Type I (insulin-dependent) diabetes. An epidemiological study. *Diabetologia*, **25**, 496–501.

Bell ET (1942) Renal lesions in diabetes mellitus. *American Journal of Pathology*, **18**, 744–745.

Goldstein HH (1974) Discussion: The problem of end-stage diabetic nephropathy. *Kidney International*, **6** (Suppl. 1), 21–23.

Grenfell A & Watkins PJ (1986) Clinical diabetic nephropathy: natural history and complications. *Clinics in Endocrinology and Metabolism*, **15**, 783–805.

Jones RH, Hayakawa H, Mackay JD & Parsons V (1979) Progression of diabetic nephropathy. *Lancet*, **1**, 1105–1106.

Lundbaek K (1954) Diabetic angiopathy — a specific vascular disease. *Lancet*, **1**, 377.

Mauer SM, Steffes MW, Ellis EN, Sutherland DER, Brown DM & Goetz FC (1984) Structural–functional relationship in diabetic nephropathy. *Journal of Clinical Investigation*, **74**, 1143–1155.

Mogensen KE (1982) Long-term antihypertensive treatment inhibiting progression of diabetic nephropathy. *British Medical Journal*, **285**, 685–688.

Osterby-Hansen R (1965) A quantitative estimate of the peripheral glomerular basement membrane in recent juvenile diabetes. *Diabetologia*, **1**, 97–100.

Osterby R (1986) Structural changes in the diabetic kidney. *Clinics in Endocrinology and Metabolism*, **15**, 733–751.

Parving H-H, Andersen AR, Smidt UM & Svendsen PA (1983) Early aggressive antihypertensive treatment reduces rate of decline in kidney function in diabetic nephropathy. *Lancet*, **2**, 1175–1179.

Thomsen AC (1965) *The Kidney in Diabetes Mellitus*. Copenhagen: Munksgaard.

Viberti GC & Wiseman MJ (1986) The kidney in diabetes: significance of the early abnormalities. *Clinics in Endocrinology and Metabolism*, **15**, 753–782.

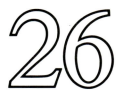

26 Dermatological Problems in Diabetes

Dowling D Munro MD FRCP

In diabetes mellitus, blood vessels become abnormal in all parts of the body. Histological examination shows endothelial proliferation and PAS-positive material deposited in the thickened basement membranes of arterioles, capillaries and venules causing luminal narrowing. The manifestations of skin disease in diabetes commonly result from these vascular abnormalities. In addition, diabetic patients are generally predisposed to infection with bacteria and fungi, including yeasts, and some develop skin lesions of obscure aetiology. These lesions are sufficiently common to make their association with diabetes more significant than might occur by chance alone.

DISEASES RELATED TO DIABETIC VASCULAR ABNORMALITIES
Diabetic Dermopathy

This dermatosis, which presents most commonly on the shins (Fig. 26.1), is a manifestation of small vessel disease. It is by far the most common dermatological presentation of diabetes. The lesions may be single or multiple and are seen not only on the front of the legs but also occasionally on the forearms, thighs and over bony prominences such as the knees.

The lesions may present in an acute phase with a 0.5–1.0cm diameter purplish-red macule, which becomes darker and haemorrhagic, forms a small scab and slowly heals leaving a tiny shiny scar comparable to the scar seen in chickenpox (Fig. 26.2). When the origin of such a lesion is discussed, the patient will commonly suggest that the site has been traumatized, but on closer questioning the patient may admit that no trauma was actually noticed at the site. If the lesions are multiple they are more readily commented upon by the patient. There may be twenty or more 0.5cm haemorrhagic scabs on the lower legs and around the ankles which give little in the way of symptoms and heal leaving scars. A biopsy of one of these lesions in the acute stage shows PAS-positive thickening of the vessel wall and proliferation of the small vessel endothelium. Commonly, the lumen is narrowed enough to occlude the vessel.

The presence of diabetic dermopathy is not closely correlated with either the severity or duration of the disease, but in patients with this manifestation of microangiopathy, clinical examination may reveal retinopathy or nephropathy.

Diabetic Erythema

Elderly diabetic patients may develop well-demarcated red areas on the lower legs and feet. Superficially, their appearance is similar to cellulitis or erysipelas, but these lesions are painless and the lower legs and feet are often oedematous. Elderly patients with these lesions often have a degree of cardiac decompensation and atherosclerosis of the lower limb vessels. Radiological examination may show evidence of underlying bony destruction due presumably to small vessel insufficiency.

One variant of diabetic erythema has been termed 'diabetic rubeosis'. It occurs in fair-skinned patients who have had diabetes for several years and who may present with redness of the face, and occasionally of the hands and feet, which is associated with local burning discomfort. The differential diagnosis includes rosacea, when it occurs on the face, and simple perniotic changes when the discoloration occurs on the limb periphery. Small vessel disease is again thought to be the cause of this condition which may also produce an exaggerated flushing response to alcohol or temperature change, or possibly due to decreased vascular tone.

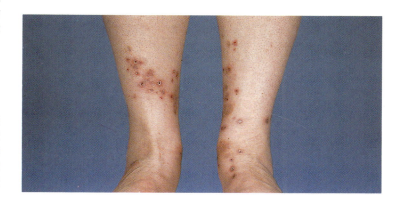

Fig. 26.1 Diabetic dermopathy. The usual distribution on the lower legs is shown. There are more lesions present here than in many patients.

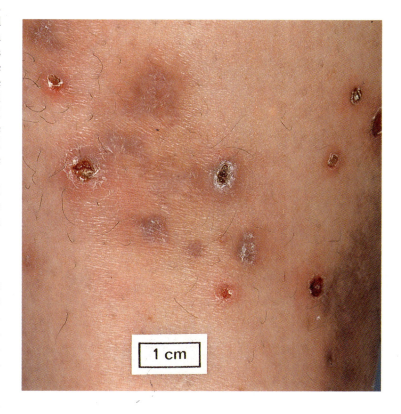

Fig. 26.2 Diabetic dermopathy: close-up view of the leg shown in Fig. 26.1. These lesions are typical of the relatively acute phase of the disease. Each of these circular lesions will form a small shiny, atrophic white scar.

26.1

Wet Gangrene

Ischaemic changes in the lower limbs of diabetic patients, especially in the toes and heels, may result from small vessel disease rather than the large vessel disease due to atherosclerosis. Such tissues readily become infected and the resultant 'wet gangrene' (Fig. 26.3) is often associated with marked pain.

Conventional management involves the use of antibiotics, including metronidazole for any anaerobes, angiography to establish the vascular status and an urgent surgical opinion. If wet gangrene is rapidly progressive, especially if malodorous due to anaerobes, urgent amputation is usually required.

Dry Gangrene

Ischaemic change resulting from dry gangrene (Fig. 26.4) usually occurs in the toes and is most commonly associated with occlusive macroangiopathy, although microangiopathy may also contribute. The digits often become thin and appear to be nourished poorly due to the ischaemic changes which have occurred over a long period. Hair loss on the toes may be an early sign. Gangrenous areas of the skin and toes may separate spontaneously if the dead tissue is kept free of secondary bacterial infection and dramatic surgical intervention should be avoided unless it is obvious that the digits will not survive.

Perforating Ulcers of the Feet

Diabetic ulcers of the feet usually result from mixed vascular and neuropathic damage and may be the presenting feature of diabetes (Fig. 26.5). Although a sensory abnormality may be detected, it sometimes requires remarkably careful assessment of superficial and deep sensation before the neurological abnormality can be determined. Nerve conduction studies may reveal early neuropathic changes; diabetic foot ulcers are seldom due to ischaemia alone.

DISEASES DUE TO INFECTIONS
Staphylococcal Folliculitis and Streptococcal Erysipelas

Although patients with poor glycaemic control are more prone to bacterial or fungal infections, the correlation between presentation with staphylococcal infection and diabetes is poor. Although nursing and junior medical staff commonly test the urine of a patient who presents to the Accident and Emergency Department with a large furuncle or carbuncle (Fig. 26.6), in practice, young adults with diabetes rarely present in this way. This group of patients usually present with typical diabetic symptoms before staphylococcal folliculitis becomes apparent. However, it is seen in diabetes, particularly in patients with poor glycaemic control, possibly because of abnormalities of neutrophil function. Migration of leucocytes through small vessel walls may be impeded because of the basement membrane thickening and, in experimental

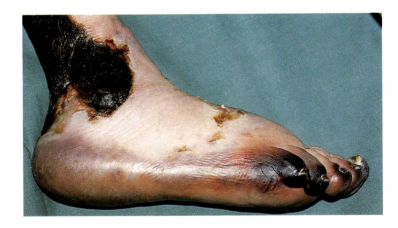

Fig. 26.3 Wet gangrene due to ischaemia of the extremities with superadded infection. This is often due to mixed bacterial growth. The presence of anaerobes produces a foul smell and is a bad prognostic feature. By courtesy of Dr D. Barnett.

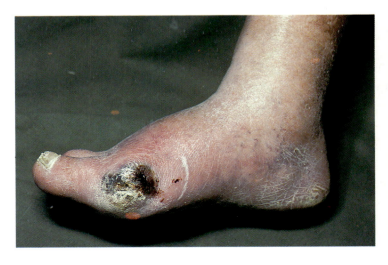

Fig. 26.4 Dry gangrene showing ischaemic areas without superadded infection.

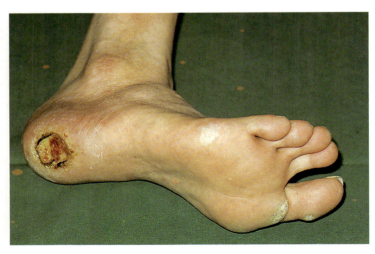

Fig. 26.5 Perforating ulcer on the sole of the foot. Patients who present with perforating ulcers must be assessed for diabetes and peripheral neuropathy.

situations, leucocyte function, including chemotaxis and phagocytosis, has been demonstrated to be deficient in diabetic patients.

Streptococcal erysipelas may also be seen in the lower legs of diabetic patients and may be associated with staphylococcal cellulitis. This dual infection requires appropriate and prolonged antibiotic therapy as the devitalized tissues of the lower legs, especially in elderly diabetic patients, may not respond to treatment as readily as those of younger healthier patients.

Chronic Candidal Paronychia

Finger-nail fold infection with *Candida* is an occupational disease of those, such as barmaids and nurses, who have their hands frequently in water. It is also a disease which is seen more commonly in diabetic patients than in the general population. At presentation, there is redness, tenderness and swelling of the nail fold. There is associated loss of the cuticle thus allowing secondary bacterial infection to become superimposed upon the candidal infection (Fig. 26.7). Middle-aged patients presenting to the dermatologist with candidal skin infections are often found to have previously unrecognized diabetes.

It should be emphasized that chronic candidal paronychia is not treated in the same way as acute bacterial paronychial infection and performing surgery on the condition only slows resolution. The correct therapy is to use antiseptic or antibiotic paints, such as fifteen per cent sulphacetamide in spirit. This is applied around the nail fold approximately five-times daily. Before retiring to sleep, an ointment containing an anticandidal chemical, such as nystatin, is applied around the nail fold to give treatment throughout the night. Treatment must be continued for many weeks or even months if the condition is to resolve, but optimal glycaemic control will speed resolution.

Candidal Vulvitis and Balanitis

Candidal vulvitis (Fig. 26.8) or balanitis (see *Chapter 6*) is a manifestation of candidal infection which is another common way that diabetes presents to the dermatologist. Middle-aged obese women and men who complain of itching of the vulva or penis, respectively, should be suspected of having undiagnosed diabetes. Treatment is best undertaken with combination creams containing a corticosteroid, nystatin and an antibiotic, as in these sites of the body inflamed areas sometimes become secondarily infected with bacteria in addition to the primary candidal disease.

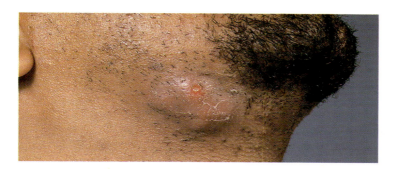

Fig. 26.6 Staphylococcal folliculitis occurring on the beard area. When several follicles are involved, the lesion is termed a carbuncle.

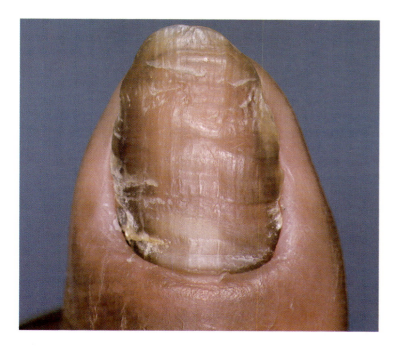

Fig. 26.7 Chronic candidal paronychia. There is loss of the nail cuticle and ridging of the nail secondary to the inflammation of the nail fold.

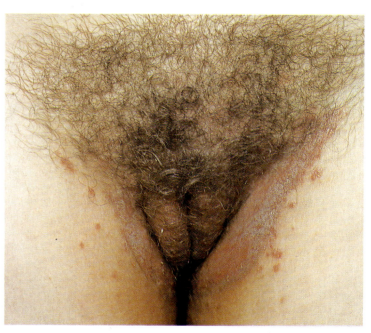

Fig. 26.8 Candidal vulvitis. This is a common way for diabetes to present to the dermatologist. The satellite lesions away from the edge of the main patch of dermatosis are a feature of *Candida*.

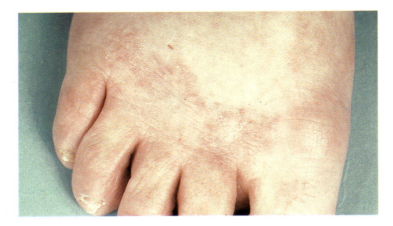

Fig. 26.9 Dermatophytosis: tinea pedis. This fungal infection commonly starts in the fourth toe web and then spreads on to the dorsum of the foot and into the nails.

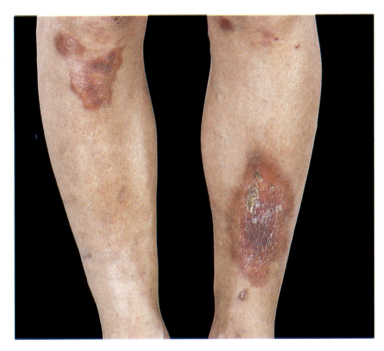

Fig. 26.10 Necrobiosis lipoidica diabeticorum. The characteristic plaques on the front of both shins are shown.

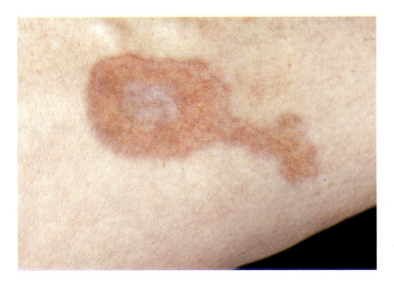

Fig. 26.11 Necrobiosis lipoidica diabeticorum. A close-up of a lesion shows atrophy in the centre with a yellow discoloration and dilated capillaries coursing over the surface of the plaque.

Dermatophytosis

Chronic fungal infection of the toe clefts, toe nails and feet, due to the ringworm group of fungi, causing tinea pedis (Fig. 26.9) is seen more commonly in diabetic adults than in the general population. The commonest fungal infection to cause this problem is *Trichophyton rubrum*. It is unclear whether this predisposition to fungal infection in diabetic patients is due to chronic hyperglycaemia or is secondary to the peripheral vascular disease which often accompanies the diabetic state. In a comparative study of patients attending a dermatology department, the greatest incidence of tinea pedis was in patients with peripheral vascular disease without diabetes, although diabetic patients more often had this disease than a control group matched for age and sex. Treatment is with systemic anti-fungal agents, such as griseofulvin, together with topical anti-fungal creams of the miconazole type.

DISEASES OF OBSCURE CAUSE OR RELATED TO DIABETIC METABOLIC DISORDERS

Necrobiosis Lipoidica Diabeticorum (Diabetic Necrobiosis)

The aetiology of diabetic necrobiosis is unclear and its association with diabetes is also a matter of controversy. Fifty per cent of patients who present with this condition do not have clinical diabetes, but a significant proportion show glucose intolerance if their carbohydrate metabolism is stressed with glucocortico-steroids. However, subjects may have identical lesions to those of diabetic patients, yet have no evidence of a diabetic state, either by testing with a glucose load or in their family history.

The disease is three times more common in women than in men. It appears in young adults or early middle-aged individuals and the incidence in patients who have diabetes is about 0.3%.

The lesions present as oval or irregularly indurated plaques most commonly on the shins (Fig. 26.10) but also on the thighs, arms and even occasionally the face. The dull red plaques gradually increase in size, the edges become yellowish-brown, the centres take on a yellow atrophic smooth appearance and the surface of the skin is covered with tiny dilated capillaries (Fig. 26.11). The lesions are very easily traumatized and when they ulcerate they are slow to heal.

Histologically, the basic lesion is an area of dermal collagen necrosis with a palisade of chronic inflammatory cells and later, macrophages appear filled with lipid. It is this fat, contained in foamy macrophages, which gives the lesion its xanthomatous appearance. Microangiopathy is much more obvious in diabetic than in non-diabetic patients, but it is clearly not a prerequisite for the development of these lesions.

Present treatment is very unsatisfactory. Glycaemic control is not thought to be particularly relevant to the healing of the lesions. Intra-lesional injections with corticosteroids sometimes help to soften the plaques if they are hard, but this therapy may predispose to ulceration.

In the small proportion of patients who have a major continuing problem from ulceration, excision and skin grafting may be helpful. However, occasionally following skin grafting, the process continues around the edges of the skin graft and the resultant cosmetic appearance is unsatisfactory.

Granuloma Annulare

Necrobiosis lipoidica diabeticorum is commonly associated with diabetes but granuloma annulare is very uncommonly associated with it. However, approximately fifty per cent of patients with granuloma annulare show a diabetic curve on a steroid-stressed glucose tolerance test.

The clinical appearance of this disease is of flesh-coloured nodules and rings of dermal thickening, usually measuring 1–5cm in diameter (Fig. 26.12). They occur most commonly over the knuckles and around the ankles, but occasionally may be quite extensive on the backs of the hands, and on the feet and shins. In a small proportion of patients the condition becomes widespread.

The histology of granuloma annulare lesions is very similar to that of diabetic necrobiosis, although the degree of macrophage infiltration and fat-filled cells is much less. It is also similar to that of rheumatoid nodules and in some patients a clinical picture which overlaps the three histologically similar conditions seen.

Treatment of granuloma annulare is either with injection of corticosteroids or by the use of a potent topical steroid ointment which is covered with polyurethane film to aid absorption.

Many patients with granuloma annulare have the disease for one or two years and then it spontaneously resolves. This is not a pattern seen with diabetic necrobiosis.

Idiopathic Bullae

Blister formation occurs occasionally on the skin of middle-aged and elderly patients without obvious cause. It is, however, much more common in diabetic subjects. The lesions occur most commonly on the periphery of limbs and arise without known trauma (Fig. 26.13). The blisters resolve over a few days and histological examination commonly shows that they arise within the thickness of the epidermis. Biopsies from early lesions indicate that the split occurs at the epidermal–dermal junction. Early re-epithelialization explains why a late biopsy reveals epidermis above and below the fluid-containing bullae.

The differential diagnosis includes the more serious blistering diseases such as pemphigus vulgaris and pemphigoid, but there is no sinister significance to these bullae in diabetic patients.

Vitiligo

The spontaneous appearance of pure white patches of vitiligo, commonly of a symmetrical distribution and occurring in patients of any age, causes alarm, especially in patients with dark skin as the cosmetic implications in such patients can be great (Fig. 26.14).

Vitiligo is associated with a series of autoimmune diseases such as alopecia areata, autoimmune thyroid disease, pernicious anaemia and adrenalitis. In children with diabetes and vitiligo, there is an increased incidence of autoantibodies to other endocrine organs such as the thyroid. In late onset (Type II) diabetes, twenty per cent of patients have vitiligo but endocrine autoimmunity is not increased in this group. There is no satisfactory treatment for this condition.

Pruritus

Idiopathic itching of the skin without any obvious rash was formerly considered to be associated commonly with diabetes, but this view is no longer held. Itching is not uncommon in the elderly due to degreasing of the skin by excessive use of water and detergents. The association with diabetes is very tenuous apart from irritation of the groin, genitals and perianal skin in those who have candidal or bacterial infection at these sites.

If a diabetic patient presents with pruritus without a rash, evidence of coincidental liver disease, uraemia, or some occult lymphoma or malignancy should be sought. Some elderly patients develop pruritus as a manifestation of chronic iron deficiency and a serum iron or ferritin estimation should be undertaken even in patients who have a normal haemoglobin. If these investigations all prove negative, then the pruritus should be treated with emollient creams and bath oils.

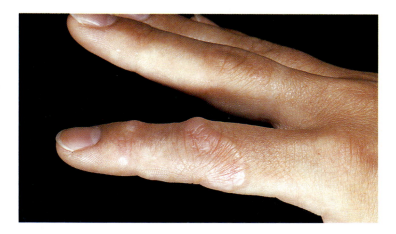

Fig. 26.12 Granuloma annulare. The lesions are seen as flesh-coloured, slightly shiny, rings and nodules on the fingers.

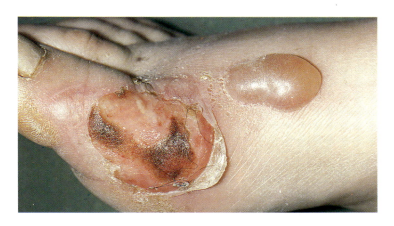

Fig. 26.13 Idiopathic diabetic bullae. A lesion that has burst and one that is intact are shown.

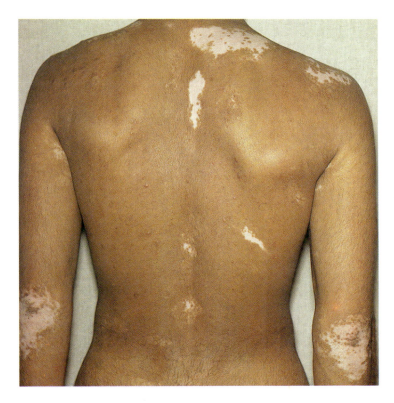

Fig. 26.14 Vitiligo. The symmetrical nature of the disease is shown by the lesions on both elbows. Vitiligo is pure white as opposed to the hypopigmented changes seen in diseases such as leprosy.

Xanthomata

Hyperlipidaemia is common in diabetic patients and involves raised triglyceride and cholesterol levels more than phospholipids. This type of hyperlipidaemia is characterized by chylomicrons and the cutaneous manifestation of chylomicronaemia is the presence of eruptive xanthomata (Fig. 26.15). These lesions present as small reddish-yellow nodules up to 5mm in diameter arising particularly on the buttocks and extensor surfaces of the limbs. They are usually asymptomatic but occasionally may be intensely pruritic when they first erupt. Eruptive xanthomata on histological examination show histiocytes and macrophages laden with neutral lipids.

The cutaneous xanthomata associated with elevated levels of cholesterol alone are usually non-pruritic and the lesions are much larger nodules.

Xanthelasma are sometimes seen on the eyelids of diabetic patients even without demonstrable hyperlipidaemia. In a small proportion of patients, the palms may be yellow due to deposition of carotene which is selectively retained within the horny layer of the skin.

Treatment of eruptive xanthomata is by control of the underlying lipid disorder. Xanthelasma may be treated by cautery of the lesions either with trichloracetic acid or diathermy, or by local surgery.

Lipodystrophy and Lipohypertrophy

Atrophy of the subcutaneous fat may occur in areas where insulin injections have been given (Fig. 26.16). The lesions are more commonly seen in female than in male patients and are thought to result from an immune-mediated reaction to impure insulin. With the use of very highly purified insulin, their frequency should diminish (see *Chapter 16*). Treatment is difficult but it has been suggested that injecting around the edge of the lesions to cause local hypertrophy may be helpful.

Lipohypertrophy probably reflects the anabolic effect of insulin on fat metabolism and this results in fatty lumps occurring in the subcutaneous tissue at the site of repeated injection (Fig. 26.17). It should not occur if the injection sites are regularly rotated.

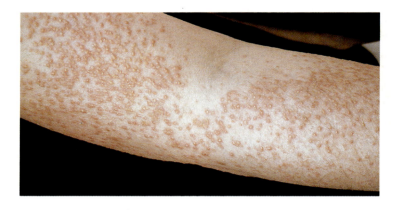

Fig. 26.15 Eruptive xanthomata. Showers of reddish-yellow nodules occur especially on the extensor surfaces of the limbs.

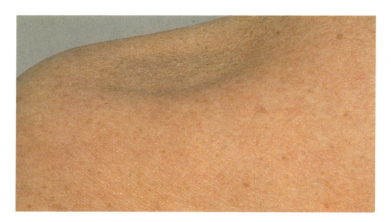

Fig. 26.16 Lipodystrophy at the site of injection of insulin.

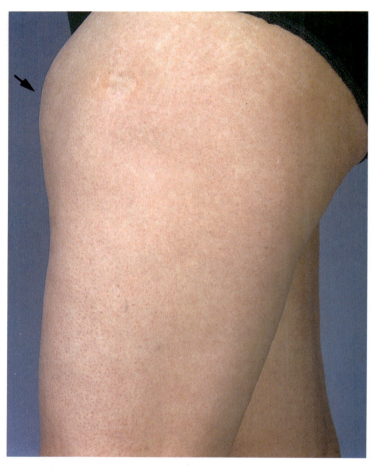

Fig. 26.17 Lipohypertrophy on the front of the thigh. Fatty lumps (arrowed) occur at the sites of repeated insulin injections.

REFERENCES

Bauer M & Levan NE (1970) Diabetic dermangiopathy. A spectrum including pigmented pretibial patches and necrobiosis lipoidica diabeticorum. *British Journal of Dermatology*, **83**, 528–535.

Danowski TS, Sabeh G, Sarver ME, Shelkrot J & Fisher ER (1966) Shin spots and diabetes mellitus. *American Journal of Medical Sciences*, **251**, 570–575.

Feingold KR & Elias PM (1987) Endocrine–skin interactions. *Journal of the American Academy of Dermatology*, **17**, 921–940.

Huntley AC (1982) The cutaneous manifestations of diabetes mellitus. *Journal of the American Academy of Dermatology*, **7**, 427–455.

Jelinek JE (Ed) (1986) *The Skin in Diabetes*. Philadelphia: Lea & Febiger.

Vallanca-Owen J (1969) Diabetes mellitus. *British Journal of Dermatology*, **81**, 9–13.

27 Paediatric Diabetes

Martin O Savage MA MD FRCP

Diabetes mellitus is the commonest endocrine disorder of childhood. Over ninety-five per cent of children and adolescents developing diabetes in the Western World have the insulin-dependent form (Type I diabetes mellitus). These patients require insulin therapy on a permanent basis to prevent progressive deterioration. Maturity onset diabetes in youth (MODY) is an uncommon disorder which appears to result from an autosomal dominant defect. Approximately fifty per cent of patients with Type I diabetes will present before the age of twenty years.

It is the dependence on insulin therapy, the requirement of a controlled carbohydrate diet and the need for regular monitoring which place the child with diabetes under considerable psychological and physical strain. The maintenance of acceptable glycaemic control poses a challenge to the family and to the paediatrician to a degree equalled by very few other childhood disorders.

EPIDEMIOLOGY

Epidemiological studies of childhood diabetes have only been performed recently. The prevalence was calculated in Pittsburgh, U.S.A., to be 1.7 per thousand subjects aged from five to seventeen years. Other studies in the U.S.A. have given figures ranging from 0.6 to 2.5 cases per thousand. The incidence of diabetes which may be expressed as the number of new cases in one year per hundred thousand subjects in the general population shows considerable geographical variation ranging from 0.8 in Japan to nearly thirty in Finland (Fig. 27.1).

The incidence of childhood diabetes increases with age, peaking in adolescence. This peak occurs two years earlier in females and relates to the earlier pubertal development in girls.

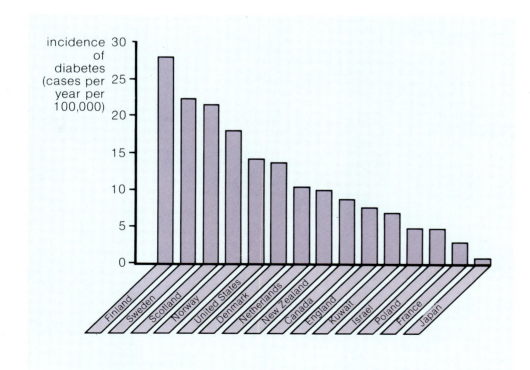

Fig. 27.1 Incidence of Type I diabetes by country. There is considerable geographical variation. From Diabetes Epidemiology Research International (1987), by courtesy of the *British Medical Journal*.

CLINICAL PRESENTATION

The presentation of diabetes in childhood is characterized by a short history compared to that seen in adults (Fig. 27.2). Almost all children have symptoms for less than eight weeks and the majority for less than two weeks. Presenting features can be divided into those associated with hyperglycaemia (Fig. 27.3) and those with ketosis.

Hyperglycaemia

Hyperglycaemia causes polyuria and nocturia which may present as enuresis. There is increasing thirst with weight loss (Fig. 27.4), fatigue and often increased appetite. The patient may, however, remain well despite these symptoms. Infection is unusual at presentation, being commonest in the form of monilial vulvovaginitis in adolescent girls. Transient visual disturbance due to osmotic changes in the lens is a rare but recognized symptom.

Ketosis

The clinical features of ketosis (Fig. 27.5) are, in contrast, more severe and are associated with rapid deterioration of the child's condition leading to hospitalization. Ketosis causes central nervous system depression with drowsiness and may lead ultimately to coma. The accompanying metabolic acidosis results in abdominal pain, vomiting, dehydration, hyperventilation and tachycardia. The combination of hyperosmolality due to progressive hyperglycaemia and dehydration may result in circulatory collapse.

Prediabetes

Prediabetes is a rather ill-defined state in which immunological risk factors for diabetes, for example, islet cell antibodies, are present. In some patients, evidence of early metabolic abnormalities of islet B cell function may be seen, such as diminution of the first phase of insulin release in response to intravenous glucose. The patient, however, remains clinically well. It is likely that a child can remain symptom-free with less than ten per cent of functional endocrine pancreatic tissue remaining. This implies that childhood diabetes may have a long latent period, during

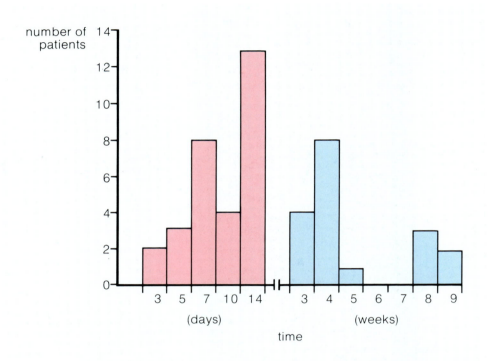

Fig. 27.2 Duration of symptoms in children presenting with Type I diabetes. Sixty-two percent presented within fourteen days of the onset of symptoms.

PRESENTING SYMPTOMS OF HYPERGLYCAEMIA IN CHILDHOOD DIABETES	
polyuria	weight loss
nocturia	fatigue
enuresis	increased appetite
thirst	monilial infection

Fig. 27.3 Presenting features of diabetes in childhood that are associated with hyperglycaemia.

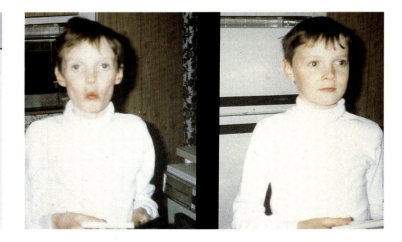

Fig. 27.4 Child with diabetes, at presentation and on insulin therapy. There is wasting and dehydration prior to therapy. By courtesy of Dr A.C. Tarn.

which there is progressive loss of islet B cells leading eventually to metabolic decompensation and the typical 'acute' presentation. Such a case history is shown in Fig. 27.6.

THE FIRST HOSPITAL ADMISSION

Most children with newly presenting diabetes are admitted to hospital. This is not mandatory and home management is successfully practised in some areas where skilled community nurses who are specialists in diabetes can perform regular home visits. Whether at home or in hospital, the diagnosis of diabetes is a shattering experience for both the child and the family. Approximately forty per cent of new cases have significant ketoacidosis. However, most children are well, which adds to their confusion at their sudden involvement in a new world of injections, monitoring, dietary restriction and parental anxiety.

The main aims of the first admission are for the family to become acquainted with the diabetes team; to learn the fundamentals of insulin injection, blood and urine testing, and dietary requirements; and to receive counselling about the significance of the diagnosis. Insulin therapy is started with an approximate dose of 0.5–0.6 units/kg per day. A controlled hypoglycaemic episode is arranged, the school is informed and assurance given to the family that regular appointments at the diabetic clinic will follow.

OUTPATIENT MANAGEMENT OF CHILDHOOD DIABETES
Paediatric Diabetic Clinic

Most paediatricians now agree that children with diabetes should be followed by a specialist in this field. The diabetic clinic provides the focus for the child's care where a team of doctors, nurses, a dietician and a psychologist, or child psychiatrist, can combine in a uniformed approach to management. Patients are seen frequently after the first admission with intervals between appointments lengthening to two, three or four months. A number of specific procedures are carried out at clinic visits (Fig. 27.7). Clinical examination includes measurement of height and weight and plotting of these on percentile charts.

PRESENTING SYMPTOMS OF KETOSIS IN CHILDHOOD DIABETES	
vomiting	dehydration
abdominal pain	drowsiness
hyperventilation	coma
tachycardia	

Fig. 27.5 Presenting symptoms of ketosis in childhood diabetes.

CASE HISTORY ILLUSTRATING PREDIABETES		
date	symptoms	post-prandial blood glucose measured retrospectively (mmol/l)
September 1982	none	3.3, 4.4
April 1983	none	29.4
September 1983	none	31.1
May 1984	none	25.7
January 1985	none	35.0
January 1986	tiredness, upper respiratory infection Type I diabetes diagnosed	32.4

Fig. 27.6 Sequential blood glucose values over a three-year period in a fifteen-year-old girl with asymptomatic prediabetes. From Tarn AC et al. (1987), by courtesy of the British Medical Journal.

PROCEDURES IN A PAEDIATRIC DIABETIC CLINIC	
clinical	**laboratory**

measure weight and height
stage pubertal development
measure blood pressure
examine:
    thyroid
    fundi
    teeth
    liver
    joint mobility
    infection sites
assess control from monitoring
    records
	urine analysis for:
	    glucose
	    ketones
	    albumin
	HbA$_{1c}$
	fructosamine
	thyroid function
	organ-specific antibodies
	urinary microalbumin excretion

Fig. 27.7 Procedures in a paediatric diabetic clinic.

Pubertal development should be staged. Examination of the thyroid, fundi, liver, teeth and injection sites is performed and the blood pressure is recorded. Urine analysis is performed for glucose, ketones and albumin, and blood taken for haemoglobin A1 (HbA_{1c}) every three to four months and for thyroid function if clinically indicated.

It is in the diabetic clinic that the insulin regimen is evaluated. The difficulties of the patients and families are discussed in a non-confrontational atmosphere and assessment of home urine and blood glucose monitoring is carried out. As the patient grows older and more confident with diabetes management, it is important for the child himself to gradually become responsible for his own management.

Insulin Therapy

The majority of newly diagnosed patients show some recovery of islet B cell function during the first few months after diagnosis.

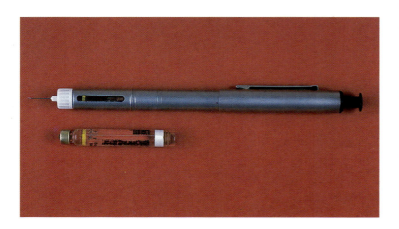

This remission or 'honeymoon period' is variable and is less common in very young patients. The choice of insulin regimen depends upon the preference and practice of the individual paediatrician. One regimen uses a combination of intermediate- and short-acting insulins from the time of diagnosis. Most children under the age of six years have a single morning injection with a ratio of two-thirds intermediate- and one-third short-acting insulin. After this age, depending upon the level of glycaemic control, an evening injection is started, initially with short-acting insulin and then intermediate-acting insulin is added in a similar ratio to the morning. Approximately two-thirds of the total dose is given in the morning and one-third in the evening.

Prepubertal children usually need 0.5–1.0 units/kg per day. During puberty, requirements increase and girls may need marginally more insulin than boys. Human insulin may act more rapidly than monocomponent porcine insulin, hence predisposing to hypoglycaemia in young children.

A regimen involving the use of multiple-injection pens (Fig. 27.8) is gaining popularity. Its principle is that a background concentration of long-acting insulin, for example, Ultratard, is present over the twenty-four-hour period with boosts of short-acting insulin, such as Actrapid, given thrice daily before meals. The proportion of the two insulins is about 1:1 and better glycaemic control has been found in the mornings when Ultratard is given at 2000h. A modification of this regimen involves the use of an intermediate-acting insulin, such as Insulatard, at bedtime in place of the evening injection of long-acting insulin. Multiple injection therapy is popular with adolescents giving more flexibility for meal-times.

Diet

The nutritional requirements of a diabetic child are similar to those of a healthy non-diabetic child of comparable age, sex,

Fig. 27.8 Multiple-dose insulin injection pen, the 'Novopen'.

Fig. 27.9 Mean twelve-month HbA_{1c} values in forty-nine children attending a paediatric diabetic clinic. The overall mean value is 10.9%.

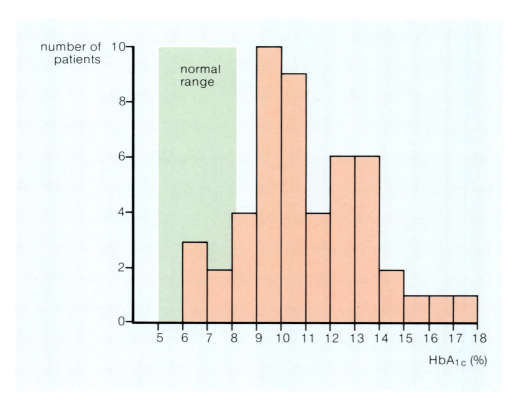

weight and activity. Carbohydrate intake should be relatively constant to complement the usual daily insulin dosage. Carbohydrates should not, however, be rigidly restricted as this energy source is important for normal growth and development. It is suggested that the calorie intake be divided as follows: carbohydrate 55%, fat 30% and protein 15%. Approximately 70% of the carbohydrate should be derived from complex sources, with particular emphasis on high-fibre foods to delay absorption. Glucose and highly refined sugars should generally be avoided as their ingestion results in marked increases in blood glucose causing swings in metabolic control.

Monitoring of Diabetic Control

During the first hospital admission, the purpose and practice of regular urine and blood testing for glucose is explained. The successful practice of home monitoring requires considerable motivation from both patient and family and the paediatrician must take a flexible attitude towards this. Twice-daily urine testing should be encouraged as should thrice-daily blood testing for glucose, that is, before each insulin injection and before bed. Some children may not be able to manage this and the regimen can be modified in line with the child's capabilities. The aim of home blood glucose monitoring is for the child to be sufficiently aware of his or her blood glucose levels for changes in the insulin regimen to be made at home. A record of glucose values is made and discussed with the doctor at the diabetic clinic. Too much pressure on the child will result in falsification of records. Home blood glucose monitoring can improve glycaemic control in a proportion, albeit rather small, of diabetic children.

The HbA_{1c} concentration is not open to manipulation and represents a mean level of blood glucose values over approximately the preceding three months. These values are educative for both patient and doctor. Only a small percentage of patients in the clinic will have values in the normal range (Fig. 27.9). Plasma fructosamine is gaining popularity as a means of assessing control over the preceding four-week period.

MANAGEMENT OF DIABETIC KETOACIDOSIS

The principles and practice are similar to those in the adult (see *Chapter 21*).

Management Related to the Child Patient

Guidelines for the management of ketoacidosis in childhood are shown in Fig. 27.10.

Resuscitation

Even more than in the adult, the first priority is to ensure a patent airway followed by nasogastric suction of stomach contents to avoid aspiration. Peripheral circulation is established by repletion of circulating blood volume using an intravenous infusion of an isotonic solution, for example, normal saline. This is given at a rate of 10–20ml/kg/h for the first one to two hours. The bladder is catheterized if the child is unconscious, and the heart monitored. Urea and electrolyte concentrations are recorded frequently to avoid initial hyperkalaemia or subsequent hypokalaemia.

Insulin therapy

Short-acting insulin is given by an intravenous infusion pump initially in a dose of 0.1 units/kg per hour. This rate may be halved when the blood glucose level falls to 10–15mmol/l.

Fluid and electrolyte therapy

The child is usually ten per cent dehydrated, that is, 100ml/kg body weight. Fluid loss is replaced on the basis of deficit plus estimated urine losses plus maintenance requirements and should be corrected over twenty-four to thirty-six hours. Following establishment of peripheral circulation, 0.45% saline can be used as the principal rehydrating fluid, to which dextrose is added when the blood sugar level falls to 10mmol/l. Hypokalaemia is an extremely important complication of the management of diabetic ketoacidosis and must be identified and treated with intravenous potassium chloride in a dose of 40mmol/l. A bicarbonate supplement is not needed.

MANAGEMENT OF KETOACIDOSIS IN CHILDHOOD

1. confirm clinical diagnosis
  cardinal features:
    hyperventilation
    lethargy
    polyuria

2. resuscitation
  ensure patent airway; nasogastric suction
  i.v. normal saline 10–20ml/kg/h
  if unconscious, nurse in intensive care unit

3. monitoring of clinical and biochemical status
  cardiac monitor for hyper- or hypokalaemia
  plasma glucose and electrolyte estimations
    2–4 hourly
  hourly bed-side glucose estimations

4. insulin therapy
  i.v. soluble insulin in dose of 0.1 units/kg/h
    by infusion pump

5. fluid and electrolyte therapy
  assume 10% dehydration (100ml/kg body weight)
  correct over 24–36 hours
  following resuscitation give 0.45% saline
    (± dextrose) and KCl, 40mmol/l

Fig. 27.10 Guidelines for the management of ketoacidosis in childhood.

COMPLICATIONS

The complications of diabetes mellitus in childhood (Fig. 27.11) can be divided into two categories: (i) metabolic disturbances or inadequacies of management; and (ii) chronic abnormalities possibly related to the quality of long-term glycaemic control.

Metabolic Disturbances

Diabetic ketoacidosis is the commonest cause of rehospitalization, but it is becoming less frequent as outpatient management improves. Hypoglycaemia is caused by excessive insulin action, inadequate food intake, or increased exercise. All three factors may occur in combination. The features of hypoglycaemia in childhood are shown in Fig. 27.12. Young children may suffer intellectual impairment from recurrent hypoglycaemic episodes. Iatrogenic over-treatment, particularly with short-acting insulin, must be avoided in young patients.

Chronic Abnormalities

Psychological disturbances are common, understandable and important. These will not be discussed in detail as a brief review would be simplistic. Childhood diabetes, however, must affect or modify emotional development (Fig. 27.13). Parental over-protection and adolescent denial are common features.

Microvascular disease is seldom seen in childhood or adolescence but the paediatrician must be aware of potential changes and early abnormalities can be detected by techniques such as the urinary microalbumin excretion rate and fluorescein angiography.

Delayed linear growth and pubertal development is probably only seen with very poor control. Limited joint mobility (the diabetic hand syndrome) is another feature which may be related to chronic hyperglycaemia and has been correlated with early microvascular abnormalities. Its presence is an indication for critical appraisal of glycaemic control.

COMPLICATIONS OF DIABETES IN CHILDHOOD

metabolic disturbance	chronic abnormalities
ketoacidosis	psychological disturbances
hypoglycaemia	microvascular disease
	delay of growth and puberty
	limited joint mobility

Fig. 27.11 Complications of diabetes in childhood.

FEATURES OF HYPOGLYCAEMIA IN CHILDHOOD

pallor	headache
weakness	confusion
irritability	drowsiness
sweating	coma
hunger	convulsions
blurring of vision	circumoral tingling

Fig. 27.12 Features of hypoglycaemia in childhood.

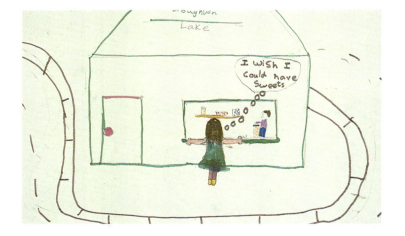

Fig. 27.13 Drawing by a diabetic child which emphasizes the stress of dietary restriction. This may be worse than the trauma of daily injections. By courtesy of Dr E.A.M. Gale.

REFERENCES

Diabetes Epidemiology Research International (1987) Preventing insulin dependent diabetes mellitus: the environmental challenge. *British Medical Journal*, **295**, 479–481.

Drash AL (1986) Diabetes mellitus in the child and adolescent: parts I & II. *Current Problems in Pediatrics*, **16**, 413–466 & 469–542.

Krane EJ (1987) Diabetic ketoacidosis: biochemistry, physiology, treatment and prevention. *Pediatric Clinics of North America*, **34**, 935–960.

Rosenbloom AL (1983) Long-term complications of Type I (insulin-dependent) diabetes mellitus. *Pediatric Annals*, **12**, 665–685.

Ryan C, Vega A & Drash A (1985) Cognitive deficits in adolescents who develop diabetes early in life. *Pediatrics*, **75**, 921–927.

Sperling MA (1987) Outpatient management of diabetes mellitus. *Pediatric Clinics of North America*, **34**, 919–934.

Tarn AC, Smith CP, Spencer K, Bottazzo GF & Gale EAM (1987) Type I (insulin dependent) diabetes: a disease of slow clinical onset. *British Medical Journal*, **294**, 342–345.

Index

ANGLIA LIBRARIES

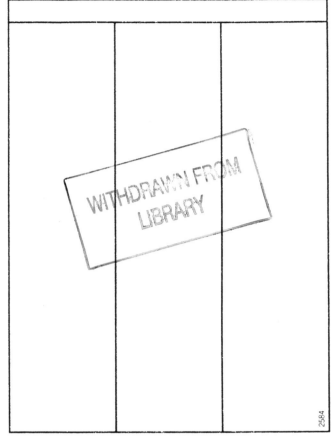

2584